Endocrinological Cancer
Ovarian Function and Disease

Research on Steroids Volume IX

Endocrinological Cancer Ovarian Function and Disease

Proceedings of the IX Meeting of the International Study
Group for Steroid Hormones, Rome, December 5-7, 1979

Editors:

H. Adlercreutz, Finland
R.D. Bulbrook, United Kingdom
H.J. Van der Molen, The Netherlands
A. Vermeulen, Belgium
F. Sciarra, Italy

 1981

EXCERPTA MEDICA, AMSTERDAM–OXFORD–PRINCETON

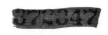

International Congress Series No. 515
ISBN Excerpta Medica 90 219 0444 6
ISBN Elsevier North-Holland 0 444 90149 3

Library of Congress Cataloging in Publication Data

International Study Group for Steroid Hormones.
  Endocrinological cancer — ovarian function and disease.

  Bibliography: p.
  Includes indexes.
  1. Breast — Cancer — Congresses.   2. Prostate gland — Cancer — Congresses.
3. Steroid hormones — Receptors — Congresses.   4. Ovaries — Congresses.
I. Sciarra, F.   II. Title.   [DNLM: 1. Breast neoplasms — Congresses.
2. Endocrinology — Congresses.   3. Prostatic neoplasms — Congresses.
4. Ovary — Physiopathology — Congresses.   WP870 I5835e 1979]
RC280.B8I56   1980   616.99'449   80-20381
ISBN 0-444-90149-3 (U.S.)

Publisher:
Excerpta Medica
305 Keizersgracht
1000 BC Amsterdam
P.O. Box 1126

Sole Distributors for the USA and Canada:
Elsevier North-Holland Inc.
52 Vanderbilt Avenue
New York, N.Y. 10017

Printed in the Netherlands by Casparie, Amsterdam.

Welcoming address

Rome welcomes you with the usual enthusiasm and thanks you for having accepted the invitation to attend the Ninth Symposium of the International Study Group for Steroid Hormones. This shows that our Group, since the first meeting in 1963, almost 17 years ago, is more alive and vital than ever.

The topics to be discussed over the next two days — Endocrinological Cancer, and Ovarian Function and Disease — were both chosen by the International Committee in December 1977, and have not lost their originality and importance even if recently there has been an increasing proliferation of Conferences and Congresses dealing with these topics.

The first of these which is of extreme interest is closely connected to our IV and VII Meetings which concerned 'Steroid protein interactions' and 'Steroid receptor proteins'. From this fascinating subject of molecular biology we hope to broaden our knowledge on the intimate mechanisms regulating cell growth and differentiation and to have ideas for further investigations, especially on the synthesis of compounds capable of modifying the hormone receptor action to dominate the development of hormone dependent neoplasms.

The second topic is equally interesting and concerns all that is new in ovarian physiopathology with special reference to disorders in the menstrual cycle, hyperprolactinaemia syndromes, hirsutism and modern techniques in the detection and treatment of ovarian disorders.

I am confident that the lectures presented and the general exchange of ideas will lead to a better understanding of many, as yet, unsolved problems in this intriguing field of research, and provide a basis for future study programmes.

Rome, December 1979   CARLO CONTI

Acknowledgements

On behalf of the Executive Committee of the International Study Group for Steroid Hormones I express my gratitude to the Chairman, Professor H. Adlercreutz, and members of the Programme Committee, Drs. R.D. Bulbrook, M. Neves e Castro, H.J. van der Molen and A. Vermeulen, for their hard work in the organization of the meeting.

Special thanks go to the members of the Local Organizing Committee Drs. C. Piro, F. Sparano and G. Concolino, but I am especially indebted to Mrs. Marian Shields for all her effort in the preparation of the Meeting and for having taken on the task of revising the English texts for the publication of this volume.

I am taking this opportunity to thank the President of the National Research Council for the use of the Conference Hall.

Support of the Meeting by the following companies is here gratefully acknowledged: Organon International BV, Fidia, Radim, Ravasini, Polifarma, Sigma Tau, Hoechst, Isnardi, Medosan, Industria Chimiche Italiane, Art Market.

CARLO CONTI

Contents

Hormone receptors in prostatic cancer

Diagnostic and prognostic methods

Endocrine treatment of prostatic disease

OVARIAN FUNCTION AND DISEASE

Normal ovarian function

Mechanism of ovulation

Disturbances of the menstrual cycle

Hyperprolactinaemia syndrome

Hirsutism as a clinical problem

Modern diagnostic methods for the detection and management of ovarian disease

BREAST CANCER

Endocrine determinants of risk of breast cancer

R.D. BULBROOK

Imperial Cancer Research Fund, Lincoln's Inn Fields, London, U.K.

Classical studies of the epidemiology of breast cancer have identified several major determinants of risk, most of which are associated with reproductive function. For example, an early age at menarche, a late age at first child or nulliparity, and a late age at menopause are all related to increased risk, while early oophorectomy leads to a marked diminution in incidence (MacMahon et al., 1973). But these studies have not led to a clear understanding of the biological mechanisms involved. In the absence of a unifying hypothesis, refuge has been taken in statements such as 'endocrine features contribute to the aetiology' or 'hormones play an important part', which have very little real meaning.

It might have been expected that the introduction during the last 15 years of reliable analytical methods for the measurement of endocrine function, would have clarified the situation but this has not been the case. Until recently, results obtained from direct measurements of hormones in blood or urine have added further confusion.

In the last few years some interesting leads have appeared. Three endocrine abnormalities* have been tentatively identified which appear to be correlated with an enhanced risk of breast cancer and which fit in with classic aetiological features of the disease. The three determinants of risk involve the ovaries, the adrenal glands and the pituitary.

Ovarian function

Results from work with laboratory animals have shown beyond doubt that the oestrogenic hormones are of cardinal importance in the genesis and maintenance of mammary carcinomas (Noble, 1964). But the oestrogenic status of women with breast cancer is not at all clear. The number of contradictory reports leads to the conclusion that there are certainly no gross abnormalities and that what is being observed is merely a random fluctuation about a normal mean (Wang et al., 1972; Bulbrook et al., 1978).

The role of the second important ovarian hormone, progesterone, has

---

*The word 'abnormality' is not ideal: the term is used here to mean that significant differences between cases (or high-risk groups) and controls have been demonstrated although in almost all instances, the values lie within the normal range.

been much neglected until recently. Grattarola (1964) found that the majority of his patients with breast cancer had endometria which showed a lack of a progestational effect. This, and other evidence, led Sherman and Korenman (1974) to propose that corpus luteum inadequacy, in the face of normal oestrogenic stimulation, might explain the principal epidemiological features of breast cancer. Considerable experimental support for this hypothesis has come from the work of Mauvais-Jarvis et al. (1980) who have shown in a series of incisive investigations that patients with benign breast disease (and hence, at high risk) have subnormal levels of plasma progesterone in the luteal phase of the menstrual cycle. Furthermore, Bulbrook et al. (1978) found a correlation between the calculated risk of developing breast cancer (using the model of Farewell, 1977) and progesterone values: the greater the risk, the lower were the plasma progesterone levels.

Korenman (1980) now seems to have some doubts about the validity of the hypothesis. He cites the findings that young women with a strong family history of the disease have been shown to have normal luteal phase progesterone levels (Henderson et al., 1975) and that normal luteal phases were found in case-control studies (England et al., 1974; Skinner et al., 1975; Sherman, 1979). But the crucial point about such studies is the selection of patients. For example, it appears that none of the women in the England and Skinner studies had anovulatory cycles, which is extraordinary when one considers that the incidence of such cycles in a normal population may be as high as 15% (Doring, 1969). One group of workers studied only women with a normal LH peak (Strax, 1978). Thus, the literature is biased against women with abnormal or anovulatory cycles. A thorough re-investigation of progesteronal status, taking serial cases and random controls would not come amiss.

If it is true that an intermittent corpus luteum dysfunction is an important determinant of risk and that the dysfunction is not all-or-none but quantitative, then what may be required is measurement of oestradiol-progesterone ratios over considerable periods of a woman's reproductive years. In technical terms, such experiments would not be easy to carry out and this may explain why the easy option of studying only those women with 'normal' menstrual cycles has so often been taken.

The attraction of the corpus luteum dysfunction hypothesis is that it would leave the oestrogens as the prime carcinogens (or promoters), in accord with much laboratory evidence. Risk would then be determined by the intensity and duration of oestrogenic stimulation not modified by progesterone secretion. Cycles in adolescents and in women approaching the menopause are characterised by such an abnormality and it would be logical to expect an increased incidence of breast cancer in women with an early menarche or a late menopause. Oophorectomy would diminish both oestrogen and progesterone secretion. The differentiating effect of progesterone might explain the protection afforded by an early first child, given a prolonged exposure to high concentrations.

Adrenal function

The majority of case-control studies show that patients with breast cancer have sub-normal plasma levels of various androgens and also excrete amounts of urinary metabolites at the lower end of the normal range (Wang, 1979). Prospective studies of a large normal population have shown that these abnormalities in adrenal androgen synthesis may precede the clinical appearance of breast cancer by up to a decade (Bulbrook et al., 1971). Similar abnormalities have been found in women with benign breast disease (Wang et al., 1972; Brennan et al., 1973; Thomas et al., 1976), with myasthenia gravis (Papatestas et al., 1977), in kindred of patients with breast cancer (Wang et al., 1975) and in women with a high calculated risk of the disease (Wang et al., 1979).

There has never been a wholly satisfactory physiological explanation for these findings, nor for the curious correlation between androgenic status and response to endocrine ablation (Bulbrook, 1974). A new interpretation will be discussed subsequently.

Pituitary function

The results of most case-control studies have been equivocal. One reason for this is the tardy appreciation of the nycthemeral rhythm of prolactin in which the plasma hormone levels tend to peak at night. When blood samples are obtained in the early hours of the evening, then there is some evidence that higher levels are related to enhanced risk of breast cancer. Early morning samples do not show this relationship (Bulbrook and Wang, 1979).

Relation between endocrine abnormalities

It would be tempting to suggest that the abnormalities in ovarian, adrenal and pituitary function are related. If the primary lesion were an enhanced oestrogenic stimulation due to a defective production of progesterone, then an effect on adrenal androgen production might be expected, since it has been shown that steroidal contraceptives containing small amounts of progestagen, relative to the oestrogenic content, depress plasma dehydroepiandrosterone sulphate levels and that urinary androgen metabolites are sub-normal. These effects are not found when the contraceptives contain large amounts of progestagen (Bulbrook et al., 1973).

Early reports also indicate that women using steroidal contraceptives have increased plasma levels of prolactin, an effect ascribed to the oestrogenic component of the pill (Robyn et al., 1973). But formal evidence that the three endocrine abnormalities occur simultaneously in women with a high risk of breast cancer and are inter-linked is still lacking and new studies will be required to investigate this point.

If this proved to be the case, the next question would be whether administration of progesterone would correct the endocrine imbalance and lead to a diminution in the incidence of breast cancer, as suggested by Mauvais-Jarvis et al. (1980).

References

Brennan, M.J., Bulbrook, R.D., Deshpande, N., Wang, D.Y. and Hayward, J.L. (1973): *Lancet, 1,* 1076.
Bulbrook, R.D. (1974): In: *The Treatment of Breast Cancer,* p.177. Editor: H.J.B. Atkins. Medical and Technical Publishing Co. Ltd., Lancaster, U.K.
Bulbrook, R.D., Hayward, J.L., Herian, M., Swain, M.C., Tong, D. and Wang, D.Y. (1973): *Lancet, 1,* 628.
Bulbrook, R.D., Hayward, J.L. and Spicer, C.C. (1971): *Lancet, 2,* 395.
Bulbrook, R.D., Moore, J.W., Clark, G.M.G., Wang, D.Y., Tong, D. and Hayward, J.L. (1978): *Europ. J. Cancer, 14,* 1369.
Bulbrook, R.D. and Wang, D.Y. (1979): In: *Reviews on Endocrine-Related Cancer.* Editor: B.A. Stoll. In press.
Doring, G. (1969): *J. Reprod. Fertil., 6,* 77.
England, P.C., Skinner, L.G., Cottrell, K.M. and Sellwood, R.A. (1974): *Brit. J. Cancer, 30,* 571.
Farewell, V.T. (1977): *Cancer, 40,* 931.
Grattarola, R. (1964): *Cancer, 17,* 119.
Henderson, B.E., Gerkin, V., Rosario, I., Casagrande, J. and Pike, M.C. (1975): *New Engl. J. Med., 293, 790.*
Korenman, S.G. (1980): In press.
MacMahon, B., Cole, P. and Brown, J.B. (1973): *J. Nat. Cancer Inst., 50,* 21.
Mauvais-Jarvis, P., Sitruk-Ware, R., Kuttenn, F. and Sterkers, N. (1980): In: *Commentaries on Research in Breast Disease.* Editors: R.D. Bulbrook and D. Jane Taylor. Alan Liss, New York. In press.
Noble, R.L. (1964): In: *The Hormones,* p. 559. Editors: V. Thimann and E.B. Astwood. Academic Press, New York.
Papatestas, A.E., Mulvihill, M., Genkins, G., Kornfeld, P., Aufses, A.H., Wang, D.Y. and Bulbrook, R.D. (1977): *J. Nat. Cancer Inst., 59,* 1583.
Robyn, C., Delvaye, P., Nokin, J., Vekemans, M., Badawi, M., Perez-Lopez, F.R. and L'Hermite, M. (1973): In: *Human Prolactin,* p. 167. Editors: J.L. Pasteels and C. Robyn. Excerpta Medica, Amsterdam.
Sherman, B.M. (1979): *Clin. Endocr., 10,* 287.
Sherman, B.M. and Korenman, S.G. (1974): *Cancer, 33,* 1306.
Skinner, L.G., England, P.C., Cottrell, K.M. and Sellwood, R.A. (1975): *Acta endocr. (Kbh.), Suppl. 199,* 128.
Strax, P. (1978): American Cancer Society Estriol Workshop, New York, 1978.
Thomas, B.S., Kirby, P., Symes, E. and Wang, D.Y. (1976): *Europ. J. Cancer, 12,* 405.
Wang, D.Y. (1979): In: *Reviews on Endocrine-Related Cancer,* p. 19. Editor: B.A. Stoll. I.C.I. Pharmaceuticals Ltd., Macclesfield, England.
Wang, D.Y., Bulbrook, R.D. and Hayward, J.L. (1975): *Europ. J. Cancer, 11,* 873.
Wang, D.Y., Moore, J.W., Thomas, B.S., Bulbrook, R.D., Hoare, S.A., Tong, D. and Hayward, J.L. (1979): *Europ. J. Cancer, 15,* 1269.
Wang, D.Y., Swain, M.C., Hayward, J.L. and Bulbrook, R.D. (1972): In: *Recent Results in Cancer Research,* p. 179. Editors: E. Grundmann and H. Tulinius. Springer-Verlag, Berlin.

Effect of diet on estrogen metabolism in women*

H. ADLERCREUTZ[1], B.R. GOLDIN[2], J.T. DWYER[2], J.H. WARRAM[2] and S.L. GORBACH[2]

[1]*Department of Clinical Chemistry, University of Helsinki, Meilahti Hospital, Helsinki, Finland, and*
[2]*Infectious Diseases Service, Department of Medicine, Tufts-New England Medical Center, Boston, MA, U.S.A.*

A number of large epidemiological studies have demonstrated a strong association between the amount of fat and protein in the diet and breast carcinoma mortality (Lea, 1966; Drasar and Irving, 1973; Armstrong and Doll, 1975; Berg, 1975; Carroll, 1975; Miller et al., 1978). Vegetarians have a much lower incidence of breast cancer but the mechanism by which diet lowers the risk of breast cancer is still unknown. Most mammary carcinomas are estrogen dependent. Of all steroid hormones the estrogens have the most extensive enterohepatic metabolism because of the large proportion of estrogens which are excreted with the bile into the intestinal lumen (see review Adlercreutz and Martin, 1980). It is well known that intestinal bacterial enzymatic activity is changed by diet (Finegold et al., 1974; Goldin and Gorbach, 1976, 1977) and that altering the intestinal microflora, particularly by diminishing the number of anaerobic bacteria, e.g. by ampicillin, causes a great increase in the excretion of fecal estrogens (Martin et al., 1975; Adlercreutz et al., 1976). It was therefore decided to investigate whether diet has any influence on estrogen metabolism. The preliminary results obtained indicate that vegetarians excrete much more estrogen in the feces and that this may influence the plasma levels of estrone and estradiol.

Material and methods

Four female subject groups living in the Boston area (U.S.A.) are being investigated: young and old omnivores and young and old vegetarians. This allows a 2 x 2 factorial design of the study. Each group will come to consist of at least 10 subjects, each of whom is investigated 4 times at 4-month intervals. In the young subjects aged 20-30 yrs and with normal menstrual

*This work was supported by contract CB 74104 from the National Cancer Institute through the Breast Cancer Task Force Committee, and by the Ford Foundation, New York.

TABLE 1.

Fecal excretion of estrogens (geometric means; µg/24 hr) in young and postmenopausal omnivorous and vegetarian women*

	Young women Mid-follicular phase			Old women Postmenopausal		
	Estrone	Estradiol	Estriol	Estrone	Estradiol	Estriol
Omnivorous	0.12	0.12	0.11	0.02	0.04	0.04
Vegetarian	0.33	0.29	0.37	0.13	0.13	0.14

*Influence of age and diet is statistically significant for all estrogens.

TABLE 2.

Urinary excretion of estrone, estradiol and estriol (geometric means; µg/24 hr) in young and postmenopausal omnivorous and vegetarian women*

	Young women Mid-follicular phase			Old women Postmenopausal		
	Estrone	Estradiol	Estriol	Estrone	Estradiol	Estriol
Omnivorous	4.5	3.4	7.2	3.6	1.8	3.7
Vegetarian	5.0	3.3	5.1	2.6	1.3	3.5

*Effect of age statistically significant for all estrogens.

cycles, the collection of specimens occurs in the mid-follicular phase. The preliminary data presented here are the results obtained from samples mainly from the 2 first waves of collection periods and at this stage in the work each group consists of 6-8 subjects. Very careful recording of diet was done in order to allow proper selection of vegetarians who limit their animal food intake to not more than 2 types taken regularly.

During the sample collection periods the subjects collect feces and urine over 72 hr and one blood sample is taken on each day of the collection period. During this time the food intake is carefully recorded and a special computer program allows the calculation of 24 nutrients in the food.

Plasma unconjugated estrone and estradiol, urinary conjugated estrone, estradiol and estriol (following hydrolysis) and fecal unconjugated estrone, estradiol and estriol are determined by radioimmunological (RIA) methods involving chromatographic separation of the estrogens on a Sephadex LH-20 column. In addition, plasma testosterone and androstenedione are assayed by RIA and urinary estriol-16α-glucuronide (E3-16G) (Lehtinen and Adlercreutz, 1977) and 'immunoreactive' estriol-3-glucuronide (E3-3G) are determined by direct RIA on diluted urine.

Statistical methods: Linear contrasts of group means have been used as a measure of the main effects and the interaction term. This allows for the unequal number of observations in the four groups. All mean values are geometrical means.

Results

Dietary composition

Total caloric intake is not significantly different for young versus old or omnivore versus vegetarian. Vegetarians consume about 43% as much animal calories as omnivores. Older omnivores consume more protein than young omnivores, while older vegetarians consume less than young vegetarians. The interaction term is significant so this reversal does not appear to be due to chance. It appears that the older vegetarians consume considerably less protein than the older omnivors and both groups of young women are in between. Vegetarians consume about 33% as much animal protein as omnivores regardless of age. Vegetarians consume about 76% as much total fat as omnivores and about 36% as much animal fat.

Thus in terms of these major dietary measures, the groups do not vary greatly in the total amount consumed, but vegetarians do consume substantially less from animal sources although their intake from animal sources is not nil.

Calculation of the intake of micronutrients revealed that vegetarians consume more iron, vitamin A, thiamine and ascorbic acid, whereas calcium, riboflavin and niacin intake was similar in both diet groups.

Hormone analyses

The fecal excretion of estrogens is shown in Table 1. The vegetarian diet results in a much higher excretion both in young and in old women. The change from a western diet to a vegetarian diet results in about 180% and 300% higher fecal excretion values in young and old women, respectively.

The urinary estrogen excretion is not influenced much by diet (Tables 2 and 3). There is only a tendency to lower estriol and estriol conjugate, especially 'immunoreactive' E3-3G, values in vegetarians but this is not statistically significant in this small sample. However, the plasma estrogens are much lower in the vegetarian women as compared to the omnivores and the differences are almost significant (Table 4).

The results for the two androgens measured show a reversal of a diet effect from young to old women which is statistically significant (Table 5). The androgens in young vegetarian women are higher than in young omnivores, but the old vegetarians have lower androgen values than the old omnivores.

TABLE 3.

Urinary excretion of estriol-16α- and of 'immunoreactive' estriol-3-glucuronide (as estriol; geometric means; μg/24 hr) in young and old omnivorous and vegetarian women*

	Young women Mid-follicular phase		Old women Postmenopausal	
	'Immunoreactive' Estriol-3-glucuronide	Estriol-16α-glucuronide	'Immunoreactive' Estriol-3-glucuronide	Estriol-16α-glucuronide
Omnivorous	13.8	3.5	6.4	1.3
Vegetarian	10.2	2.8	4.6	1.1

*Effect of age is statistically significant.

TABLE 4.

Plasma unconjugated estrogens (geometric means, pg/ml) in young and postmenopausal omnivorous and vegetarian women

	Young women Mid-follicular phase		Old women Postmenopausal	
	Estrone	Estradiol	Estrone	Estradiol
Omnivorous	128	125	113	109
Vegetarian	70	91	73	71

Discussion

It has repeatedly been demonstrated that interruption of the enterohepatic circulation of the estrogens caused by various mechanisms results in a decrease of the excretion of E3-3G in urine (Tikkanen et al., 1973; Tikkanen and Adlercreutz, 1973). In vegetarian women the excretion of 'immunoreactive' E3-3G was almost significantly decreased in this small series suggesting that the vegetarian diet may have a similar effect as for example administration of ampicillin. Ampicillin administration causes a huge increase in unconjugated and conjugated estrogens in feces (Martin et al., 1975; Adlercreutz et al., 1976) which is believed to be due, at least partly, to a decrease in bacterial β-glucuronidase activity necessary for the hydrolysis of the biliary estrogen conjugates before the estrogen moiety is absorbed. A vegetarian diet has been shown to result in a decrease in bacterial β-glucuronidase activity in feces (Reddy and Wynder, 1973; Goldin and Gorbach, 1976) hence the high amount of estrogens in feces of vegetarians as compared to omnivores may occur by the same mechanism. In these studies only the unconjugated estrogens in feces were studied, but it has previously been shown that about 98% of the fecal estrogens are unconjugated

TABLE 5.

Androgens in plasma (geometric means; nmol/l) in young and postmenopausal omnivorous and vegetarian women*

	Young women Mid-follicular phase		Old women Postmenopausal	
	Androstenedione	Testosterone	Androstenedione	Testosterone
Omnivorous	3.9	1.2	2.1	0.76
Vegetarian	4.5	1.5	1.2	0.47

*Effect of age is statistically significant. The reversal of diet effect from young to old women is statistically significant.

(Adlercreutz and Martin, 1976). Whether this is also true for vegetarians is not known. The reason for the high excretion of unconjugated estrogens in feces in addition to conjugated estrogens after ampicillin administration may be that unhydrolysed estrogen conjugates are hydrolysed by intestinal bacteria further down in the intestinal tract at a site where absorption is no longer possible.

The reason for the decrease in E3-3G in urine after interruption of the enterohepatic circulation is the fact that it is formed from absorbed estriol in the mucosal cells and immediately excreted in urine without being taken up by the liver. In the human organism E3-3G formation is restricted to the mucosal cells (Dahm and Breuer, 1966).

The antiserum to E3-3G used in the present investigation is not completely specific and the amount of E3-3G found in urine is greater than total E3 measured by a specific method. The compounds cross-reacting are not known but they may at least partly be 2-hydroxylated estrogen metabolites. One of the reasons why statistical significance was not achieved for the difference of E3-3G excretion in urine of vegetarians as compared to omnivores may therefore be that estrogens not influenced by interruption of the enterohepatic circulation are included in the assay. Coupling of the antiserum to a solid phase as used for E3-16G antiserum (Lehtinen and Adlercreutz, 1977) increases specificity of the assay considerably. This technique was used in previous studies also for E3-3G antiserum, but repeated attempts to establish a solid-phase method and utilize the new antiserum used in the present study failed and it was necessary to do the analysis with a technique including separation of free and bound antigen with charcoal suspension (Baker et al., 1979).

The greatly increased fecal excretion of estrogens in vegetarians seems to result in a lowering of the plasma estrogens as compared to omnivores; however, the difference is not statistically significant in this small study. The omnivores have 57% (mean for E1 and E2 in both groups) higher plasma estrogens than the vegetarians.

The postmenopausal women living in Boston have higher estradiol values than expected. Simultaneous repetition of the assay with 3 different antisera and using a number of samples from Finnish postmenopausal women revealed that the values are true and that the Finnish women had considerably lower values. The incidence of mammary cancer is much lower in Finland, but whether this has anything to do with the different plasma estrogen levels remains to be established. The present study is now being extended and the women with the highest plasma estradiol values are being further investigated.*

Thus, all results point to a definite difference in the enterohepatic metabolism of estrogens in vegetarian women as compared to omnivorous women which may ultimately lead to a decrease of the biologically active unconjugated estrogens in plasma. Whether such a decrease may explain the difference in incidence of breast cancer in vegetarians and omnivores remains to be established.

Note added in proof
One of the old postmenopausal omnivorous women was found to have an estrogen-producing tumor and her values slightly increased the mean values of the group.

Acknowledgements

We thank Ms Inga Wiik, Rauni Lehtola and Helena Huhtonen for skillful technical assistance.

References

Adlercreutz, H. and Martin, F. (1976): *Acta Endocr. (Kbh.), 83,* 410.
Adlercreutz, H. and Martin, F. (1980): *J. Steroid Biochem., 13,* 231.
Adlercreutz, H., Martin, F., Pulkkinen, M., Dencker, H., Rimér, U., Sjöberg, N.-O. and Tikkanen, M.J. (1976): *J. Clin. Endocr., 43,* 497.
Armstrong, B. and Doll, R. (1975): *Int. J. Cancer, 15,* 617.
Baker, T., Jennison, K.M. and Kellie, A.E. (1979): *Biochem. J., 177,* 729.
Berg, J.W. (1975): *Cancer Res., 35,* 3345.
Carroll, K.K. (1975): *Cancer Res., 35,* 3374.
Dahm, K. and Breuer, H. (1966): *Z. Klin. Chem. Klin. Biochem., 4,* 153.
Drasar, B.S. and Irving, D. (1973): *Brit. J. Cancer, 27,* 167.
Finegold, S.M., Attebery, H.R. and Sutter, V.L. (1974): *Amer. J. Clin. Nutr., 27,* 1456.
Goldin, B.R. and Gorbach, S.L. (1976): *J. Nat. Cancer Inst., 57,* 371.
Goldin, B.R. and Gorbach, S.L. (1977): *Cancer, 40,* 2421.
Lea, A.J. (1966): *Lancet, 2,* 332.
Lehtinen, T. and Adlercreutz, H. (1977): *J. Steroid Biochem., 8,* 99.
Martin, F., Peltonen, J., Laatikainen, T., Pulkkinen, M. and Adlercreutz, H. (1975): *J. Steroid Biochem., 6,* 1339.
Miller, A.B., Kelly, A., Choi, N.W., Matthews, V., Morgan, R.W., Munan, L., Burch, J.D., Feather, J., Howe, G.R. and Jain, M. (1978): *Amer. J. Epidemiol., 107,* 499.
Reddy, B.S. and Wynder, E.L. (1973): *J. Nat. Cancer Inst., 50,* 1437.
Tikkanen, M.J. and Adlercreutz, H. (1973): *Amer. J. Med., 54,* 600.
Tikkanen, M.J., Pulkkinen, M.O. and Adlercreutz, H. (1973): *J. Steroid Biochem., 4,* 439.

Steroid receptors and breast cancer

W.L. McGUIRE

Department of Medicine/Oncology, University of Texas, Health Science Center at San Antonio, San Antonio, TX, U.S.A.

Considerable progress has been made in the last decade in our approach to patients with breast cancer. Endocrine therapy for advanced disease has now progressed to the point where physicians can confidently select patients who are likely to respond. New information is emerging regarding the use of estrogen receptor (ER) assays to predict which patients will have an early recurrence. It is the purpose of this brief review to present data from my own laboratory on the use of ER and progesterone receptor (PgR) assays in the management of both primary and advanced breast cancer.

Estrogen receptor in the primary breast tumor

It is well appreciated that only about one half of breast cancer patients are cured by surgical and/or radiation therapy of the primary tumor. The majority of these patients have tumors confined to the breast without extension to the axillary lymph nodes (Fisher, 1977). Those patients with regional lymph node involvement will usually present with metastatic disease at some later date. Until the past few years, axillary node positive patients were simply observed following surgery with the hope, albeit slim, of cure. Upon recurrence, palliative endocrine and cytotoxic therapies provided prolongation of life but eventually all patients died of the disease. More recently, the concept of adjuvant therapy with the goal of cure has emerged, particularly in the case of axillary node positive patients. The reasoning is that extension of tumor to regional lymph nodes is operationally equivalent to finding distant microscopic tumor metastases. Rather than waiting until these foci are clinically evident, systemic anti-tumor therapy begun soon after surgery might be very successful since tumor burden is relatively low. There is considerable experimental animal tumor data to support this concept and now many large clinical trials are underway with some preliminary reports showing early success (Bonadonna et al., 1977; Fisher and Wolmark, 1977; Hubay et al., 1980). The question is not whether to use adjuvant therapy but rather which drugs, which patients, and for how long. Since there are considerable arrays of systemic agents available and un-doubtedly many subsets of patients with varying degrees of risk of re-currence and potential response to these agents, a method to select patients

TABLE 1.

Estrogen receptor and recurrence

	Characteristic	Recurrence at 20 months		
		ER−%	vs	ER+%
Age	< 50	32		0
	> 50	36		16
Nodes	Negative	19		6
	Positive	59		26
	1-3	36		25
	> 4	72		27
Primary size	< 2 cm	40		5
	> 2 cm	37		16
Primary location	Outer	31		9
	Inner and central	50		19

(Adapted from Knight et al., 1977)

at risk and the proper adjuvant therapy for particular subsets of these patients is needed.

In San Antonio, we had begun to measure ER in primary breast tumors in the hopes of eventually correlating these data with the response to endocrine therapy at some later date. In many of these patients we had follow up data including time to recurrence and survival, so we decided to look at the natural history of our patient population to see if the ER status was correlated with any particular outcome. To our surprise, we found that regardless of axillary node status, age, size of the primary tumor, or location of the tumor in the breast, those patients with ER− tumors recurred earlier than ER+ patients (Knight et al., 1977). Approximately a year later we re-analyzed our data with the addition of more patients and the elimination of patients who had received any systemic endocrine or cytotoxic therapy. Our earlier conclusions were confirmed and extended to show the ER− patients not only recurred earlier but had worse survival than ER+ patients (Knight et al., 1978). These data are illustrated in Table 1. Subsequently, similar data have been recently reported from other centers around the world which substantiate the results of our pilot study (Rich et al., 1978; Maynard et al., 1978; Allegra et al., 1979; Hahnel et al., 1979). The implications of these findings are considerable. First, we now can identify a subset of axillary node positive patients who have an extremely poor prognosis if left untreated. Second, the ER assay results indicate that the latter group should receive intensive combination chemotherapy and that the ER+ axillary node positive patients should receive an endocrine therapy as part of the adjuvant therapy. In fact, this approach is now being tested. In collaboration with Drs. Hubay, Pearson, and colleagues in Cleveland, we have been assaying ER in primary breast tumors of patients randomized to receive combination chemotherapy with or without antiestrogen therapy. The preliminary data are very encourag-

TABLE 2.

ER and response to endocrine therapy

	Primary biopsy	Metastatic biopsy
ER–	1/6 (17%)	4/47 (8%)
ER+	22/44 (50%)	48/101 (48%)

ing (Hubay et al., 1980). ER+ patients are recurring less frequently if they receive a combination of chemo-endocrine therapy compared to chemotherapy alone. ER– patients recur at the same rate whether or not anti-estrogens are added to the chemotherapy. Independent trials from other centers are needed to confirm these data but the approach is based upon sound physiological principles and the use of ER assays in the primary tumor for prognostic information as well as therapeutic strategy seems assured.

As will be discussed later, the presence or absence of ER in a biopsy of metastatic breast cancer correlates well with the response of that cancer to endocrine therapy. The question remains, however, whether ER assay results at the time of primary surgery are valuable, perhaps years later, if the patient develops metastatic disease. This is of considerable importance since less than 50% of patients presenting with advanced disease have readily accessible lesions for biopsy and assay – whereas practically all patients undergoing primary breast surgery have tissue available for this purpose. The theoretical objection to this approach is that the ER status of a tumor could change between the time of primary surgery and the clinical presentation of advanced disease. This has been examined by various investigators and in the great majority of cases, the ER status is unchanged when comparing primary and metastatic biopsies in the same patient. The most direct test, of course, is to measure ER in the primary tumor and correlate the results with subsequent endocrine therapy for metastatic disease; data from Jensen's laboratory clearly supports such a correlation (Block et al., 1978). Our own data are illustrated in Table 2. We find approximately the same response rate to endocrine therapy of advanced disease in ER+ tumors regardless of whether ER determination was made on the original primary tumor or a subsequent metastatic lesion.

The value of quantitative estrogen receptor assays

In the early days of ER correlations, few laboratories reported quantitative data. It seemed sufficient to merely indicate whether the receptor was present or absent. Our earliest analysis, however, though based on a limited number of patients, indicated that the response rate was the highest in those patients with the highest quantitative tumor ER content (McGuire et al.,

TABLE 3.

Quantitative ER values in primary and metastatic breast cancer

Age	< 50		> 50	
Biopsy	1°	2°	1°	2°
ER value				
< 3	162 (37%)	49 (52%)	279 (23%)	75 (31%)
3-10	90 (20%)	13 (14%)	176 (15%)	39 (16%)
11–100	183 (41%)	28 (29%)	432 (35%)	67 (27%)
100-2000	10 (2%)	5 (5%)	312 (26%)	63 (26%)
Total	445	95	1199	244

TABLE 4.

Quantitative ER and the response to endocrine therapy

	Response	
ER fm/mg	1° Biopsy	2° Biopsy
< 3	1/6 (17%)	4/47 (8%)
3-10	3/7 (42%)	11/24 (45%)
11-100	14/31 (45%)	15/41 (36%)
> 100	5/6 (83%)	22/36 (61%)

1975). As we examine, in Table 3, the actual values in primary vs metastatic biopsies and younger vs older patients, certain features stand out. First, metastatic biopsies are more often ER− than primary biopsies regardless of age. Second, the older patient is much more likely to have a high receptor content than the younger patient regardless of whether the biopsy is from a primary or metastatic lesion. This might be expected since the older patient is more likely to have a favorable response to endocrine therapy. Our actual clinical correlations are shown in Table 4. In almost 200 endocrine trials we find that the response rate is proportional to the absolute receptor content.

Progesterone receptor and response to endocrine therapy

Despite the success of ER assays for prediction, a large number of ER+ patients fail to respond to endocrine therapy. Several years ago we reasoned that since cytoplasmic binding of estrogen to receptor was only the first step in a complex biochemical pathway leading to growth and specific protein synthesis in a breast tumor cell, perhaps certain ER+ tumors failed to respond because of defects distal to the binding step. We hypothesized that progesterone receptor (PgR) might be an ideal marker of estrogen action in

TABLE 5.

Distribution of ER and PgR in 1366 breast cancer patients

	Premenopausal (%)	Postmenopausal (%)
ER–, PgR–	30	19
ER–, PgR+	9	3
ER+, PgR–	12	23
ER+, PgR+	49	55

TABLE 6.

Objective remission of metastatic breast cancer as a function of ER and PgR

	Objective response
ER–, PgR–	3/20 (15%)
ER–, PgR+	—
ER+, PgR–	14/45 (31%)
ER+, PgR+	16/20 (80%)

breast tumor cells as it had been shown to be estrogen dependent in normal reproductive tissue (Horwitz and McGuire, 1975). We developed an assay for PgR which was quite specific and sensitive in breast cancer tissue (Horwitz and McGuire, 1975) and demonstrated that PgR synthesis was strictly controlled by estrogen in both experimental (Horwitz and McGuire, 1977) and human breast cancer cells (Horwitz and McGuire, 1978). The distribution of PgR in a large number of human breast cancer biopsies is shown in Table 5. As anticipated PgR is rarely found in those tumors lacking ER. Conversely, the likelihood of finding PgR in a tumor was proportional to the absolute amount of ER in the tumor. Thus it was likely that PgR would correlate with a favorable response to endocrine therapy. Our own data on clinical response is illustrated in Table 6. As anticipated, those tumors without ER and PgR are unlikely to respond. Tumors containing only PgR are rare and not enough information is available to reach any conclusions. Those patients with both ER and PgR have a remarkably high response rate. The interesting group is that with ER but without PgR. We would have anticipated that few if any of these patients would have responded. Yet the response rate is appreciable even though far below those patients with both receptors. We have considered several possibilities to explain the behavior of this group. First, the assays for PgR are imperfect and it is possible that a few patients in this group are false negative. However, it is doubtful that this could explain the whole result. Second, we must consider the influence of endogenous progesterone in premenopausal women. Saez et al. (1978) have reported that PgR cannot be found in breast tumor cytosols of women with high

TABLE 7.

Quantitative ER vs PgR

		Objective response rate
PgR	+	16/20 (80%)
	−	14/45 (31%)
ER	> 100	17/27 (63%)
	3-100	13/38 (34%)

circulating levels of progesterone during the luteal phase of the menstrual cycle. Presumably all of the cytoplasmic PgR sites have been translocated to nuclei. A nuclear exchange assay might solve this problem. Finally, since PgR synthesis is estrogen dependent, could some postmenopausal women have insufficient circulating estrogen to stimulate PgR in the tumor even when the appropriate biochemical pathways are present? Degenshein and associates (personal communication) have, in fact, biopsied patients before and after a few days of estrogen therapy and found several women who converted to PgR+. So it appears that many of the ER+,PgR− cases who respond to endocrine therapy can be explained.

Quantitative estrogen receptor assays vs progesterone receptor assays

Although the merits of PgR assays are now well documented, one could take the position that since the likelihood of finding PgR in a tumor is correlated with the amount of ER in the tumor and that the likelihood of favorable response is proportional to the amount of ER in the tumor, perhaps PgR is just a signal that a high level of ER is present. If so, PgR measurements would be redundant. Fortunately, the matter can be resolved by direct analysis of the data. We have studied 65 ER+ patients where we have quantitative ER and PgR data as well as objective response to endocrine therapy. The data are illustrated in Table 7. If we use quantitative ER alone to discriminate between low and high response rates in ER+ patients, we find that the best separation obtained is 34% vs 63%. If we use the presence of PgR, the discrimination becomes 31% vs 80%. So we must conclude from our own data that the measurement of ER and PgR is superior to just quantitating ER alone.

The implications for therapy are just emerging. In those patients with both ER and PgR, endocrine therapy is the therapy of choice. The group ER+,PgR− is a little more difficult in that about 30% of these patients will still have a good response. Perhaps many of these responders could be reclassified as ER+,PgR+ if nuclear exchange assays are employed or estrogen stimulation were used. At present, we would not recommend withholding endocrine therapy from this group but would suggest that only those therapies with low morbidity be used (e.g., antiestrogens); this group might be ideal candidates for combined chemo-endocrine therapies.

Acknowledgements

This work was partially supported by the National Cancer Institute (CA 11378, CB 23682) and The American Cancer Society. This review chapter was prepared as a requirement for attending the 1st International Congress on Hormone and Cancer, Rome, October 1979, the Satellite Symposium on Perspectives in Steroid Receptor Studies, Sorrento, October 1979, and the Ninth International Study Group for Steroid Hormones, Rome, December 1979.

References

Allegra, J.C., Lippman, M.E., Simon, R., Thompson, E.G., Barlock, A., Green, L., Huff, K., Do, H.M.T., Aitken, S.C. and Warren, R. (1979): *Cancer Treatm. Rep.,* in press.
Block, G.E., Ellis, R.S., DeSombre, E. and Jensen, E. (1978): *Ann. Surg., 188,* 372.
Bonadonna, G., Rossi, A., Valaqussa, P., Banfi, A. and Veronesi, U. (1977): *Cancer, 39,* 2904.
Fisher, B. (1977): In: *Breast Cancer: Advances in Research and Treatment,* p. 1. Editor: W.L. McGuire. Plenum Press, New York.
Fisher, B. and Wolmark, N. (1977): In: *Breast Cancer: Advances in Research and Treatment,* p. 25. Editor: W.L. McGuire. Plenum Press, New York.
Hahnel, R., Woodings, T. and Vivian, A.B. (1979): *Cancer, 44,* 325.
Horwitz, K.B. and McGuire, W.L. (1975a): *Science, 189,* 726.
Horwitz, K.B. and McGuire, W.L. (1975b): *Steroids, 25,* 497.
Horwitz, K.B. and McGuire, W.L. (1977): *Cancer Res., 37,* 1733.
Horwitz, K.B. and McGuire, W.L. (1978): *J. Biol. Chem., 253,* 2223.
Hubay, C.A. et al. (1980): *Surgery,* submitted for publication
Knight, W.A., Livingston, R.B., Gregory, E.J. and McGuire, W.L. (1977): *Cancer Res., 37,* 3667.
Knight, W.A., Livingston, R.B., Gregory, E.J., Walder, A.I. and McGuire, W.L. (1978): *Proc. Amer. Soc. Clin. Oncol., 19,* 392.
Maynard, P.V., Davies, C.J., Blamey, R.W., Elston, C.W., Johnson, J. and Griffiths, K. (1978): *Brit. J. Cancer, 38,* 745.
McGuire, W.L., Carbone, P.P. and Vollmer, E.P. (Eds.) (1975): *Estrogen Receptors in Human Breast Cancer.* Raven Press, New York.
Rich, M.A., Furmonski, P. and Brooks, S.C. (1978): *Cancer Res., 38,* 4296.
Saez, S., Martin, P. and Chouvet, C. (1978): *Cancer Res., 38,* 3468.

Occupied and unoccupied oestradiol receptors in nuclei and cytosol from human breast tumours

T. THORSEN

Hormone Laboratory, University of Bergen School of Medicine, Bergen, Norway

The amount of occupied receptor in the cytosol is normally low, since the interaction of the steroid receptor complex with the nuclear compartment is a thermodynamically favoured step (Williams and Gorski, 1974). Occupied receptor could be thought to arise in the cytosol in either of two ways: (1) As a result of post-homogenization binding of extracellular oestradiol (Williams and Gorski, 1971) or (2) as a result of a translocation defect (Coffino and Yamamoto, 1976; Thorsen and Støa, 1979). With the methods currently used for receptor assay, failure to detect receptor or serious underestimation may occur, particularly in patients with high concentrations of endogenous oestradiol.

According to a collaborative study under the auspices of The American National Cancer Institute approximately 45% of oestradiol receptor positive tumours gave no objective response to ablative or additive hormone therapy. This would indicate that defects not involving steroid binding to receptor, such as (1) translocation defects, or (2) defects in post-translocation nuclear events, are present in a considerable number of tumours (Shyamala, 1972). We have previously reported that tissue slices from some oestradiol receptor positive mammary tumours are unable to accumulate oestradiol in the nucleus (Thorsen and Støa, 1979). This observation suggests that nuclear oestradiol receptor may be a better indicator of hormone responsiveness than the cytosol receptor alone.

A solid phase hydroxylapatite (HAP) exchange assay (Garola and Mc-Guire, 1977; Thorsen, 1979) has been applied to measure occupied and unoccupied oestradiol receptor in nuclei and cytosols from 110 individual human breast tumours. Results have been compared to DCC assay of oestradiol and progesterone cytosol receptors in the same tumours.

Material and methods

Human breast tumours: Mastectomy specimens were immediately frozen in liquid nitrogen and stored at $-70°C$ for up to 3 weeks.
Radioactive steroids: Oestradiol-17β-(2,4,6,7-^{3}H) and dimethyl-19-nor-

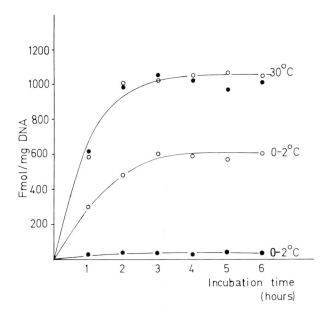

Fig. 1.   Effects of incubation time and temperature on specific binding of oestradiol in nuclear extract. One aliquot (solid circles) was incubated with non-radioactive oestradiol for 4 hr at 4°C to saturate any available binding sites. Excess oestradiol was removed by treatment with dextran/charcoal. The second aliquot (open circles) was treated identically, but without cold ocstradiol. Specific binding was measured in both aliquots by HAP assay. Incubation time was varied between 1 and 6 hr.

pregna-4,9-diene-3,20-dione-17α,21-(17α-methyl-³H) (R 5020) (lot Nos. 1004-063 and 1009-103 were purchased from New England Nuclear, Boston, Mass.).

Methods: DCC assay of oestradiol and progesterone receptors and HAP assay of nuclear and cytosol receptors have been carried out as previously described (Thorsen, 1979). Briefly, the HAP assay entails absorption of receptor to hydroxylapatite, removal of residual cytosol or nuclear extract and incubation of the absorbed receptor with 5 nM ³H-oestradiol at 0-2°C and 30°C for 4 hr. Incubation at both temperatures was carried out in the absence and presence of a 200-fold excess of non-radioactive oestradiol. Nuclear receptor was assayed in a 0.6 M KCl extract of crude nuclear pellets.

Results and discussion

To verify optimal conditions of incubation time and temperature of the HAP assay, the following experiment was carried out: Nuclear extract from pooled tumour tissue was divided into equal parts. One aliquot (solid circles)

TABLE 1.

Measurement of total and unoccupied oestradiol receptor in cytosols before (A) and after (B) complete saturation of binding sites with non-radioactive oestradiol

Tumour	Aliquot A (fmol/mg)		Aliquot B (fmol/mg)	
	Total	Unoccupied	Total	Unoccupied
1	324	286	338	21.3
2	108	56	97	N.S.
3	113	117	118	N.S.
4	264	111	244	18.9
5	58	37	67	N.S.

TABLE 2.

Coefficient of variation, upper confidence interval and sensitivity as calculated from 30 duplicate determinations of non-specific binding at two different incubation temperatures

Incubation temperature (°C)	No. duplicates	Mean non-specific binding (fmol/ml)	Coeff. of variation (%)	Upper confidence limit (%)	Sensitivity (fmol/ml)
30	30	35.5	7.8	123.4	8.3
0-2	30	23.0	7.3	122.0	5.1

TABLE 3.

Interassay precision of the estimates of specific binding calculated from duplicate assays. The coefficients of variation have been calculated as the square root of the sum of variances in the estimates of total and non-specific binding

Range (fmol/ml)	No. duplicates	Mean concentration of specific binding (fmol/ml)		Coefficient of variation (%)	
		30°C	0-2°C	30°C	0-2°C
< 100	15	63	49	13.5	12.2
100-500	18	286	193	7.9	7.7
> 500	8	918	736	7.5	7.4

was incubated at 4°C for 4 hr with 5 nM non-radioactive oestradiol to saturate any unoccupied receptor sites. After charcoal treatment of both aliquots, receptors were measured by the HAP assay at varying incubation times (Fig.

1). Results show that maximal binding is reached after 4 hr at both temperatures. At 30°C there was no difference in binding site concentration between the two aliquots, indicating that complete exchange of occupied receptor had taken place. Similar results were obtained when receptor was assayed in individual cytosols with or without previous saturation of available binding sites (Table 1). Tables 2 and 3 give data on the sensitivity and precision of the method. Precision has been calculated as the square root of the sum of variances in the estimates of total and non-specific binding, and shows that the method works with acceptable reliability.

In Figure 2 representative binding curves and Scatchard plots from nuclear extract (A) and cytosol (B) are given. Association constants were estimated at approximately 1.5×10^9 M^{-1}, which is similar to values given by Garola and McGuire (1977), but significantly lower than those found with the DCC assay (1×10^{10} M^{-1}). This, however, will not influence the estimate of binding site concentration in the single point saturation assay.

A good correlation was observed between unoccupied receptor as measured by HAP assay and the results of DCC assays (Fig. 3). The linear correlation coefficient was 0.95. A survey of the results obtained by HAP assay in a material of 110 individual tumours is given in Figure 4. Values are presented for all tumours containing either occupied or unoccupied receptor or both. The material has been grouped according to age, as a post-menopausal (age above 55 years) and as a pre/paramenopausal group (age 55 years or below). In the cytosol the concentration of unoccupied receptor is significantly higher in the older age group compared to younger women ($p < 0.01$). In the latter group occupied receptor only is found in 40% of tumours. There is no striking difference in occupied receptor in the 2 groups. In the pre/paramenopausal women there is a tendency towards higher incidence and concentration of occupied receptor, which is barely significant by the Wilcoxon two sample test ($p = 0.05$). No significant difference in the concentration of occupied receptor was found in the nuclear compartment. However, both frequency (27 vs 66%) and concentration of unoccupied receptor were significantly lower in the younger group ($p < 0.01$). When total receptor concentrations are compared, cytosol and nuclear, tumours from younger women still have lower values than those in the older age group. This may indicate that the receptor processing induced by oestrogen stimulation in the MCF-7 cell (Horwitz and McGuire, 1978) is operative in solid tumours as well.

Figure 5 presents the relation between unoccupied and occupied cytosol receptors. There is a highly significant negative correlation ($r = -0.76$) between the concentration of unoccupied receptor and the percentage occupied receptor in the cytosol. Premenopausal women (solid circles) have a high ratio of occupied to unoccupied receptor. The mean ratio was 1.5 ± 0.5 (SEM) vs 0.07 ± 0.05 (SEM) in the postmenopausal group.

In Table 4 the material has been grouped according to the tumour content of oestradiol and progesterone receptor as determined by DCC assay. Group

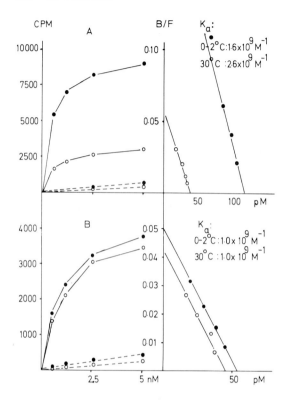

Fig. 2. Representative saturation curves and Scatchard plots from HAP assay of nuclear extract (A) and cytosol (B). Incubation temperature 30°C (solid circles), 0-2°C (open circles). Broken lines: non-specific binding.

I (Oe+, Pg+), group II (Oe+, Pg−), group III (Oe−, Pg+) and group IV (Oe−, Pg−). As could be anticipated a high incidence of occupied nuclear receptor (93%) was found in group I tumours. On the other hand, occupied nuclear receptor was detected in only 8 out of 19 tumours in group II (42%). There was no significant difference in the cytosol receptors in the two groups. This would indicate that defects in translocation or binding to acceptor sites might be present in more than half the tumours in this group. It is of interest to note that McGuire et al. (1977) found that 39% of group II tumours responded to hormone therapy, whereas the response rate in group I tumours was 64%.

It is generally agreed that between 5 and 10% of oestradiol receptor negative tumours will undergo remission after hormone therapy. Occupied nuclear and cytosol receptors have been detected in 9 tumours of group III (82%) and one group IV tumour. All except one of these tumours were from menstruating women, who may have had appreciable amounts of circulating oestradiol. It is suggested that these are 'false negative' tumours.

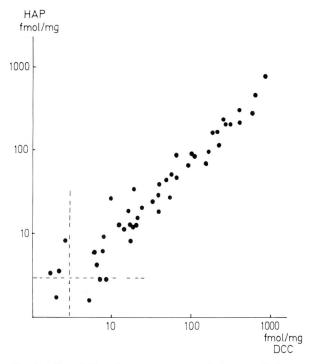

Fig. 3. Correlation between unoccupied oestradiol receptor measured by HAP assay and receptor determined in the same cytosol by DCC assay.

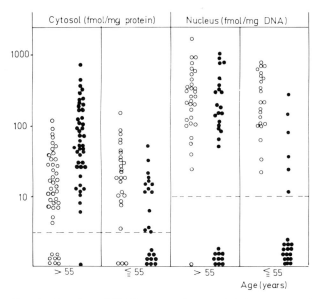

Fig. 4. Results of HAP assay of occupied (open circles) and unoccupied (solid circles) oestradiol receptor in cytosol and nuclear extract from individual human breast tumours.

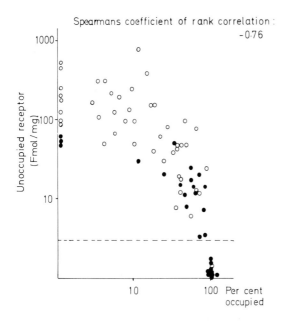

Fig. 5. Relation between unoccupied cytosol receptor and the percentage of occupied receptor. Solid circles: pre/paramenopausal women. Open circles: postmenopausal women.

TABLE 4.

Distribution of nuclear and cytosol receptors as measured by HAP assay in relation to cytosol oestradiol and progesterone receptors measured by DCC assay

Group	Cytosol receptor	% of total	Frequency of nuclear receptors				Frequency of cytosol receptors			
			R_nOe	%	R_n	%	R_cOe	%	R_c	%
I	Oe+ Pg+	36.4	37/40	93	20/40	50	34/40	85	40/40	100
II	Oe+ Pg-	17.3	8/19	42	3/19	16	15/19	79	17/19	90
III	Oe- Pg+	9.7	9/11	82	3/11	27	9/11	82	0/11	0
IV	Oe- Pg-	36.6	1/40	2.5	0/40	0	1/40	2.5	0/40	0

It can therefore be concluded that: (1) Determination of nuclear receptor will probably enhance the predictive value of receptor assays. (2) Total receptor should be measured in the cytosol to ensure the detection of all receptor positive tumours.

References

Coffino, P. and Yamamoto, K.R. (1976): In: *Control Mechanisms in Cancer*, p. 57. Editors: W.E. Criss, T. Ono and J.R. Sabine. Raven Press, New York.

Garola, G. and McGuire, W.L. (1977): *Cancer Res., 37*, 3329.

Horwitz, K.B. and McGuire, W.L. (1978): *J. Biol. Chem., 253*, 2223.

McGuire, W.L., Horwitz, K.B., Pearson, O.H. and Segaloff, A. (1977): *Cancer, 39*, 2934.

Shyamala, G. (1972): *Biochem. Biophys. Res. Commun., 4*, 1623.

Thorsen, T. (1979): *J. Steroid Biochem., 10*, 661.

Thorsen, T. and Støa, K.F. (1979): *J. Steroid Biochem., 10*, 595.

Williams, D. and Gorski, J. (1971): *Biochem. Biophys. Res. Commun., 45*, 258.

Williams, D. and Gorski, J. (1974): *Biochemistry, 13*, 5537.

Relationship of estradiol receptors to tissue and serum α-lactalbumin and serum prolactin in human breast cancer and other human neoplasms

A. MOLTENI[1], R. BAHU[1], E. FORS[1], M. MANGKORNKANOK[1], D. ALBERTSON[1], R.L. WARPEHA[2] and L. BRIZIO-MOLTENI[2]

[1] *Department of Pathology, Northwestern University School of Medicine, Chicago, IL, and* [2] *Department of Surgery, Division of Plastic Surgery, Stritch School of Medicine, Loyola University of Chicago, Maywood, IL, U.S.A.*

Traditionally the identification and classification of breast dysplastic and neoplastic lesions are related to their morphologic description. This approach fails to provide information on their functional status. Various studies have shown that the efficacy of chemotherapy on breast neoplasia is better related to the endocrine and biological classification of the tumors rather than to their histologic description. Breast neoplasias have therefore been studied in relation to their ability to bind hormones such as estrogens (Byar et al., 1979), progesterone (Powell et al., 1979), and glucocorticoids (Allegra et al., 1979). It was also found that protein markers such as α-lactalbumin in tissue and serum are specific for differentiated mammary epithelia (Rolandi et al., 1974; Rose and McGrath, 1975; Schultz and Ebner, 1977). Some breast lesions have been found in association with elevated levels of serum prolactin (Cole et al., 1977; Nagai et al., 1979).

We are reporting the results of our investigation of E_2 binding activity, tissue and serum α-lactalbumin concentration and serum prolactin levels in breast and other human neoplasias in order to better define the biological activity of these neoplasms and hence institute adequate therapy towards a favorable prognosis.

Material and methods

Tissues in this study consisted of 509 primary mammary tumors, 9 non-malignant breast lesions, 48 non-mammary human neoplasias and normal tissues. The specimens for E_2 binding and α-lactalbumin determinations were selected as soon as they were sent to the pathologist for frozen section examination. One gram of tumor, free of other tissue, was frozen in liquid nitrogen and stored at $-80°C$ until the assays could be performed. Normal tissues were obtained from attachments to some excised specimens.

It was not possible to perform all determinations on all specimens, priority being given to the E_2 binding activity study. Serum for prolactin and ∝-lactalbumin was collected in the early morning and approximately 2 hr before surgery.

Estradiol receptor assay

1. Chemical: The cytosol from previously frozen tissue was used to determine the E_2 receptor content using the sucrose density gradient method of Jensen et al. (1971). Although receptors were observed at the 8S and 4S region in the sucrose gradient, in this study receptor content was expressed as the total of the E_2 bound. Protein measurement of the cytosols was performed by the micromethod of Lowry et al. (1951). For breast neoplasias, the values of over 5 fmoles per mg of protein and over 10 fmoles per mg of protein respectively for pre- and postmenopausal women were considered to have positive binding. These values have been suggested by other investigators (Jensen et al., 1971; Jensen and De Sombre, 1977). For all other tumors the dividing line between negative and positive E_2 binding activity was 6 fmoles per mg of protein.
2. Immunofluorescence: Direct immunocytologic staining was performed on 6 μ thick frozen sections according to the method of Lee (1978).

∝-Lactalbumin determination

1. Tissue immunofluorescence: Indirect immunofluorescence with rabbit anti-∝-lactalbumin was performed according to a modification of the method of Coons and Kaplan (1950).
2. Serum radioimmunoassay: A modification of the methods of Kleinberg et al. (1977) and Kleinberg and Todd (1978) and of Schultz and Ebner (1977) was used.

Serum prolactin

Measurement was obtained utilizing the radioimmunoassay kit of Calbiochem, Inc., La Jolla, CA.

Results

Estradiol binding activity

1. Breast neoplasms: 38% of the primary mammary tumors studied have positive E_2 binding activity. In relation to their histologic diagnosis, the highest positive binding was found in infiltrating lobular carcinomas (67%) and the lowest in medullary type of infiltrating ductal carcinoma (Table 1).

TABLE 1.

Relationship of cellular estradiol binding activity to histologic classification in human primary mammary tumors, non-malignant breast conditions and other human neoplasias

		% of positive binding
Breast malignancies		
Infiltrating ductal carcinoma		
Scirrhous		40
Comedo		14
Colloid		40
Medullary		0
Infiltrating lobular carcinoma		67
Tubular carcinoma		40
	Total	38
Non-malignant dysplasias		
Fibrocystic disease of breast		66
Fibroadenoma		20
Gynecomastia		0
	Total	33
Other malignancies		
Kidneys	Renal cell carcinoma	66
	Papillary transitional cell carcinoma	0
	Renal adenoma	0
Adrenals	Cortical hyperplasia	0
	Cortical adenoma	0
Thyroid	Papillary carcinoma	50
	Adenocarcinoma	0
	Colloid adenoma (chronic thyroiditis)	0
Parathyroid	Adenoma	0
	Hyperplasia	0
	Squamous cell carcinoma	0
Lungs	Adenocarcinoma	0
	Squamous cell carcinoma	0
	Large cell carcinoma	0
Colon	Adenocarcinoma	0
Parotid	Squamous cell carcinoma	0
	Pleomorphic adenoma	100
Uterus	Endometrial carcinoma	50
Lymphnodes	Melanoma	0
Testicle	Seminoma	0
	Total	21

Moreover, of 9 non-malignant breast conditions, only 3 (33%) (2 cases of fibrocystic disease and 1 fibroadenoma) were positive.

2. Other neoplasias and normal tissues: E_2 binding activity in normal tissue, primary tumors, and metastatic tumors other than breast is summarized in Table 1. Renal cell and papillary carcinoma of the thyroid were the 2

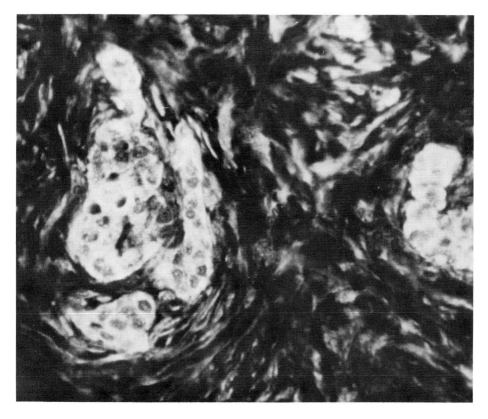

Fig. 1. Infiltrating ductal cell carcinoma exhibiting cytoplasmic fluorescence. N.B. variation in individual cell staining intensity. x 250.

neoplasms with the highest percent of binding (66% and 50%). Positive binding was also found in a pleomorphic adenoma of the parotid and in 50% of the endometrial carcinomas. Although many breast neoplasms showed a positive staining by immunofluorescence (Fig. 1), no direct relationship of the staining intensity to the values of chemical E_2 binding was found.

Tissue and serum α-lactalbumin

α-Lactalbumin measurement in breast neoplasia showed a 63% positive by immunofluorescence of infiltrating ductal adenocarcinoma; 7% of the lobular carcinomas were also positive. Fibrocystic disease and fibroadenomas were both 50% positive. All tumor cells displayed varying degree of intensity of fluorescence but not an uneven distribution of positive and negative cells as cited by Bussolati et al. (1975) (Fig. 2). Of the various types of breast carcinomas, only 4 cases of infiltrating ductal carcinoma (10% of

TABLE 2.

Frequency of α-lactalbumin concentrations in tissue and serum and of prolactin concentration in serum in various breast lesions

Histologic diagnosis	% α-lactalbumin positive tissue immuno-fluorescence	% serum α-lactalbumin positive levels (> 1 ng/ml)	% serum prolactin positive levels (> 30 ng/ml)
Infiltrating ductal adeno-carcinoma	63	10	14
Intraductal carcinoma in situ	0	0	0
Lobular carcinoma	7	0	20
Medullary carcinoma	0	0	0
Fibroadenoma	50	22	22
Fibrocystic disease	50	2	20
Normal breast (non-lactating)	0	0	0

the total) showed elevated serum α-lactalbumin (above 2 ng/ml). Elevated values were also seen in the cases of fibrocystic disease (10%) and 2 of the fibroadenomas (22%) (Table 2).

Serum prolactin

Prolactin was most often elevated in infiltrating ductal carcinomas and fibrocystic disease averaging 20% of the sampling (Table 2). The few gynecomastia and normal breast patients available had serum prolactin values within the normal range (less than 30 μg/ml).

Relationship of E_2 binding activity to α-lactalbumin in mammary neoplasms

Not all tumor samples were of sufficient quantity to have E_2 receptor and immunofluorescence performed, nor was there serum available on each breast lesion patient for α-lactalbumin and prolactin determinations. For the neoplasias where E_2 receptors and α-lactalbumin determinations were performed, no correlation was found between levels of E_2 binding activity and positivity or negativity of α-lactalbumin as seen by immunofluorescence. Neither was it possible to evince a correlation between serum prolactin and serum α-lactalbumin levels (Table 2).

Discussion

Estradiol binding activity is not specific for human breast cancer as it can be measured in other tumors and normal tissues. For breast lesions, our percentage of positives for E_2 binding (38%) is in agreement with Jensen and

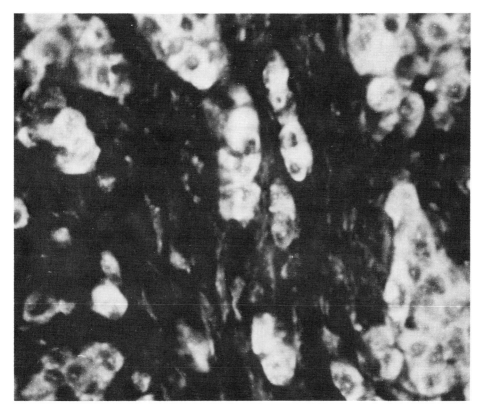

Fig. 2. Infiltrating ductal carcinoma exhibiting cytoplasmic fluorescence with rabbit anti-human α-lactalbumin. x 400.

De Sombre (1977) and MacFarlane and Fazekas (1979), though somewhat lower than McGuire et al. (1978) and Byar et al. (1979). Differences in methodology — sucrose gradient density, as used by Jensen and De Sombre (1977) and ourselves versus charcoal separation, as used by these other investigators, may constitute a possible explanation. Our experience comparing the chemical method for E_2 binding with the immunofluorescence does not seem to show a strict correlation. The results, however, are too limited to allow definite conclusions.

The study of E_2 binding activity in other neoplasias has shown that at least 2 types of tumors (kidney and thyroid) have a higher incidence of positive E_2 binding than breast. For kidney carcinomas, our data are very similar to Concolino et al. (1978). Moreover, human pancreatic tissue also has high E_2 binding activity. This observation coincides with data reported by Sandberg and Rosenthal (1976), and by some of us (Molteni et al., 1979) in normal pancreatic tissue and acinar pancreatic carcinomas. It is worthy of mention that in a tumor of the parotid gland, we have found positive E_2 binding.

α-Lactalbumin is positive in 63% of the infiltrating ductal carcinomas of the breast. These results are similar to those of Schultz and Ebner (1977) who found 65% of human breast tumor extracts were positive for α-lactalbumin. α-Lactalbumin would appear to be very specific when compared to E_2 binding in breast neoplasias since no other tissues than breast are positive. Thus, a positive α-lactalbumin in a metastatic tissue would indicate that the tumor came from the breast, but a negative result would not rule out this possibility since 40% of breast carcinomas are negative by this method. Serum α-lactalbumin does not show any concordance with tissue. This discrepancy between tissue and serum α-lactalbumin could be the result of rapid catabolism or a defective secretory process. The comparison of α-lactalbumin and E_2 receptors in 27 cases of ductal carcinoma failed to reveal a relationship. Nor was there an apparent relationship between serum prolactin and the absence or increased levels of α-lactalbumin. Likewise prolactin levels were independent of the tumor type. The foregoing considerations seem to indicate that in some neoplasms different cell lines coexist, histologically indistinguishable but with different biological activities. These cells may appear morphologically similar but results obtained with the different tests will reveal a varied biochemical profile for each of these neoplasms. Only when a complex profile, including other receptors (e.g., progesterone and androgens) and protein markers such as ACTH and prolactin have been measured may it be possible to institute adequate therapy for each malignancy.

Acknowledgements

The authors wish to thank Mr George Speck for the prolactin determinations and Mrs Rita M. Kaurs for the α-lactalbumin determinations.

References

Allegra, J.M., Lippman, M.E., Thompson, E.B., Simon, R., Barlock, A., Green, L., Huff, K.K., Do, H.M.T., Aitken, S.C. and Warren, R. (1979): *Cancer Res., 39,* 1447.

Bussolati, G., Pich, A. and Alfani, V. (1975): *Virchows Arch. A: Path. Anat. Histol., 365,* 15.

Byar, D.P., Sears, M.E. and McGuire, W.L. (1979): *Europ. J. Cancer, 15,* 299.

Cole, E.N., Sellwood, R.A., England, P.C. and Griffiths, K. (1977): *Europ. J. Cancer, 13,* 597.

Concolino, G., Marocchi, A., Conti, C., Tenaglia, R., Di Silverio, F. and Bracci, U. (1978): *Cancer Res., 38,* 4340.

Coons, A.H. and Kaplan, M.H. (1950): *J. Exp. Med., 91,* 1.

Jensen, E.V., Block, G.E., Smith, S., Kyser, K. and De Sombre, E.R. (1971): *Nat. Cancer Inst. Monogr., 34,* 55.

Jensen, E.V. and De Sombre, E.R. (1977): *Advanc. Clin. Chem., 19,* 57.

Kleinberg, D.L. and Todd, J. (1978): *Cancer Res., 38,* 4318.

Kleinberg, D.L., Todd, J. and Groves, M.L. (1977): *J. Clin. Endocr., 45,* 1238.

Lee, S.H. (1978): *Amer. J. Clin. Path., 70,* 197.

Lowry, O.H., Rosenbough, N.J. and Fair, A.L. (1951): *J. Biol. Chem., 193,* 265.

MacFarlane, J.F. and Fazekas, A.G. (1979): In: *Proceedings of the Society of Surgical Oncology, Atlanta, Georgia, 1979,* Abstract 21.

McGuire, W.L., Horwitz, K.B., Zava, D.T., Garola, R.E. and Chamness, G.C. (1978): *Metabolism, 27,* 478.

Molteni, A., Bahu, R., Battifora, H., Fors, E., Reddy, K., Rao, S. and Scarpelli, D. (1979): *Ann. Clin. Lab. Sci., 9,* 103.

Nagai, R., Kataoka, M., Kobayashi, S., Ishihara, K., Tobioka, N., Nakashima, K., Naruse, M., Saito, K. and Sakuma, S. (1979): *Cancer Res., 39,* 1835.

Powell, B., Garola, R., Chamness, G.C. and McGuire, W.L. (1979): *Cancer Res., 39,* 1678.

Rolandi, B., Barreca, T., Masturzo, P., Poleri, A., Indiveri, F. and Barabino, A. (1974): *Lancet, 2,* 845.

Rose, H.N. and McGrath, C.M. (1975): *Science, 190,* 673.

Sandberg, A.A. and Rosenthal, M.E. (1974): *J. Steroid Biochem., 5,* 969.

Schultz, G.S. and Ebner, K.E. (1977): *Cancer Res., 37,* 4489.

Neutral urinary steroids and estrogen receptors in early breast cancer

D. VANDEKERCKHOVE, E. VANLUCHENE, W. AERTSENS, G. VAN MAELE and J. DE BOEVER

Department of Gynecology, University of Ghent, Ghent, Belgium

Various studies have indicated a possible association between abnormal levels of androgen and corticosteroid metabolites in urine and the predisposition, occurrence and hormone dependency of breast cancer. Bulbrook et al. (1962) reported that patients with early breast cancer excrete lower amounts of androgens but their observation could not be confirmed by other authors (Wade et al., 1969; Cameron et al., 1970; Miller et al., 1975). A lower androgen excretion was found in estrogen receptor negative (ER−) patients than in ER+ patients (Abul Hajj, 1977). In addition, qualitative changes in steroid metabolism were suggested by Pfaffenberger et al. (1977) who found a decrease of the androgen and corticosteroid 5α-reductase activity in breast disease.

In the present study, neutral urinary steroid profiles were determined in early breast cancer (EBC) patients before and after surgery. In the majority, ER content of the tumor was assayed and related to steroid excretion. Control groups consisted of hospitalized patients volunteering for the study.

Material and methods

Urinary steroid excretion was studied in 42 early breast cancer patients, of whom 20 were premenopausal and 22 had been in the postmenopausal condition for at least 2 yrs. A control group consisted of 25 women with no evidence of cancer or endocrinological disease, admitted to the hospital for elective gynecological surgery. Of these subjects 17 were premenopausal and 8 postmenopausal. Patients who had previously undergone castration or had been receiving hormonal treatment during the three months prior to admission were not included in either group. In all hospitalized women a 24-hr urine specimen was collected during admission day 1 (i.e. 2 days before surgery). In 37 patients another sample was obtained on postoperative day 10.

Steroid excretion was determined by glass capillary gas-chromatography (Vanluchene and Sandra, 1979). Estrogen receptors were assayed with a dextran coated charcoal method (De Boever and Vandekerckhove, 1980).

TABLE 1.

Preoperative excretion (mg/24 hr) of some androgen and corticosteroid metabolites in early breast cancer (EBC) patients and in controls

	A	E	DHA	At*	A+E+DHA	5α-THF	THF
Prem.							
EBC							
n	20	20	20	15	20	20	20
Mean	2.16	2.30	0.083	0.29	4.54	1.68	2.22
SD	0.86	0.89	0.13	0.35	1.54	0.97	1.17
Median	2.16	2.31	0	0.17	4.70	1.71	1.90
Controls							
n	17	17	17	9	17	17	17
Mean	1.71	1.96	0.17	0.33	3.84	1.23	1.85
SD	1	0.86	0.23	0.25	1.80	0.71	0.58
Median	1.30	1.83	0.05	0.32	3.29	0.95	1.76
2 α	< .05	NS	NS	NS	NS	< .1	NS
Postm.							
EBC							
n	22	22	22	19	22	22	22
Mean	1	1.42	0.030	0.14	2.45	1.19	2.25
SD	0.50	0.63	0.077	0.13	1.07	0.72	0.67
Median	1.02	1.33	0	0.10	2.33	0.99	2.37
Controls							
n	8	8	8	7	8	8	8
Mean	0.76	1.18	0.086	0.12	2.03	1.04	2.58
SD	0.46	0.66	0.21	0.069	0.99	0.47	1.08
Median	0.65	1.18	0	0.10	1.95	1.07	2.08
2 α	NS	NS	NS	NS	NS	NS	NS
Prem. + Postm.							
EBC							
n	42	42	42	34	42	42	42
Mean	1.55	1.84	0.055	0.21	3.45	1.42	2.24
SD	0.90	0.87	0.11	0.26	1.68	0.88	0.93
Median	1.35	1.82	0	0.14	3.17	1.19	2.17
Controls							
n	25	25	25	16	25	25	25
Mean	1.41	1.71	0.14	0.24	3.26	1.17	2.09
SD	0.96	0.87	0.22	0.21	1.79	0.64	0.83
Median	1.25	1.48	0.040	0.13	2.70	1.06	1.77
2 α	NS	NS	NS	NS	NS	NS	NS

*At = Androstenetriol

Statistical analysis was performed using non-parametric tests. Group differences were calculated with the Mann-Whitney–U test. In the case of two related samples the Wilcoxon test was used. Correlation was expressed by the Spearman rank correlation coefficient (r_s).

TABLE 2.

Excretion (mg/24 hr) of some urinary steroids before and 10 days after simple mammectomy and bilateral salpingo-oophorectomy (premenopausal) and simple mammectomy (postmenopausal), respectively

	A	E	DHA	At*	A+E+DHA	A/E	5 α-THF / THF
Prem. (ovariectomized)							
Preop.							
n	17	17	17	11	17	17	17
Mean	1.87	2.17	0.10	0.26	4.14	0.93	0.70
SD	1.05	1.08	0.15	0.38	1.94	0.40	0.32
Median	1.73	2.14	0	0.11	3.93	0.91	0.74
Postop.							
n	17	17	17	11	17	17	17
Mean	1.38	1.86	0.081	0.33	3.31	0.72	0.51
SD	0.93	1.02	1.16	0.25	1.87	0.26	0.22
Median	1.05	1.49	0	0.25	2.78	0.77	0.50
2α	< .02	NS	NS	NS	< .05	< .01	< .01
Postm. (not ovariectomized)							
Preop.							
n	20	20	20	14	20	20	20
Mean	1.11	1.77	0.029	0.12	2.91	0.67	0.47
SD	0.64	0.84	0.075	0.080	1.23	0.27	0.26
Median	1.08	1.96	0	0.12	2.85	0.74	0.42
Postop.							
n	20	20	20	14	20	20	20
Mean	0.84	1.33	0.061	0.18	2.23	0.62	0.45
SD	0.52	0.67	0.20	0.14	1.23	0.21	0.23
Median	0.74	1.15	0	0.18	1.73	0.65	0.41
2α	< .01	< .01	NS	< .1	< .01	NS	NS

*At = Androstenetriol.

Results

Pre-operative mean excretion of androsterone (A) and etiocholanolone (E) tended to be higher in cancer patients than in controls (Table 1). In the premenopausal subgroup, the difference for A excretion was significant at the $2\alpha < 0.05$ level.

In cancer patients, the levels of A were significantly lower ($2\alpha < 0.01$) on the tenth day after surgery, than before the operation (Table 2). Levels of E were lower in both castrated and non-castrated (postmenopausal) patients, although significance was obtained only in the latter group.

In twenty patients with ER+ tumors the mean excretion of A, E and DHA

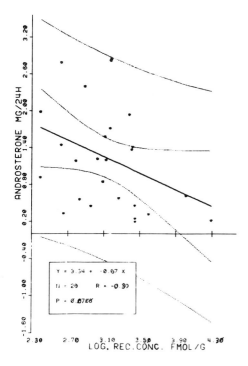

Fig. 1. Regression analysis for androsterone excretion and ER concentration.

was 3.26 mg/24 hr (Table 3). In 20 patients with ER— tumors it amounted to 4.04 mg/24 hr, this difference being not significant.

In ER+ patients, androsterone and 5α-tetrahydrocortisol excretion were both significantly correlated with the ER content (Figs. 1 and 2), Spearman's rank correlation coefficients (r_s) being −0.398 (2α = 0.04) for A and −0.57 (2α = 0.003) for 5α-THF. A similar negative relation (Figs. 3 and 4) was found for the ratios A/E and 5α-THF/THF, r_s being respectively −0.46 (2α = 0.02) and −0.52 (2α = 0.006). The following regression lines were calculated:

$$
\begin{aligned}
A/E &= 2.47 -0.52 \log \text{ER-conc. (fmol/g);} \\
5\alpha\text{-THF/THF} &= 1.57 -0.32 \log \text{ER-conc. (fmol/g);} \\
A &= 3.34 -0.67 \log \text{ER-conc. (fmol/g);} \\
5\alpha\text{-THF} &= 3.14 -0.60 \log \text{ER-conc. (fmol/g).}
\end{aligned}
$$

Discussion

In the present study, both control and EBC patients were hospitalised and urine was obtained under similar preoperative conditions. In contrast to earlier findings, our cancer patients excreted higher 11-deoxy-17-oxosteroids (11-DOKS) than controls. Moreover the increase is more important when dealing with 5α-reduced metabolites. The difference in the time of urine

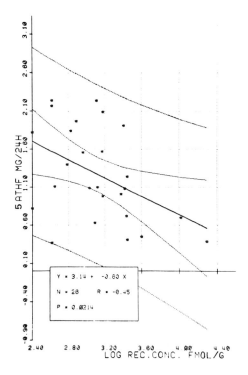

Fig. 2. Regression analysis for 5α-tetrahydrocortisol (5α-THF/THF) and ER concentration.

TABLE 3.

Excretion of some neutral steroids (mg/24 hr) in ER positive and ER negative patients before surgery

	A	E	DHA	A+E+DHA	A/E	5 α-THF / THF
ER positive						
n	20	20	20	20	20	20
Mean	1.37	1.83	0.06	2.26	0.81	0.58
SD	0.84	1.07	0.14	1.67	0.40	0.29
Median	1.30	1.55	0	3.02	0.74	0.52
ER negative						
n	20	20	20	20	20	20
Mean	1.83	2.16	0.05	4.04	0.85	0.66
SD	1.02	0.75	0.08	1.65	0.35	0.32
Median	1.81	2.27	0	4.01	0.77	0.67
2 α	NS	< .1	NS	NS	NS	NS

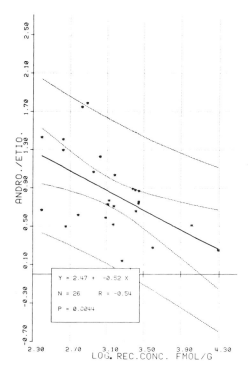

Fig. 3. Regression analysis for androsterone/etiocholanolone ratio and ER concentration.

collection may be important: on day 10 after surgery 11-DOKS in our patients were significantly decreased in comparison with preoperative values.

Higher receptor concentrations appear to be accompanied by lower 5α-reduction of steroids (Figs. 1 to 4). Patients with estrogen receptor negative tumors excrete higher amounts of 11-DOKS. This is in variance with the findings of Abul Hajj (1977) concerning postmenopausal breast cancer patients. It may be of some significance to note that 5α-reduced metabolites are increased both in the EBC patients (compared to controls) and in the ER− patients (compared to ER+ patients) who have a less good prognosis.

The findings of Pfaffenberger et al. (1978), showing an increased ratio of $5\alpha/5\beta$ reduction of steroids in benign breast tumor patients compared to controls, are in part in agreement with our results. These authors used a similar analysis technique based on capillary gaschromatography.

Acknowledgement

The technical assistance of S. Velghe, A. Buyens, E. De Walsche and H. Chrétien is gratefully appreciated.

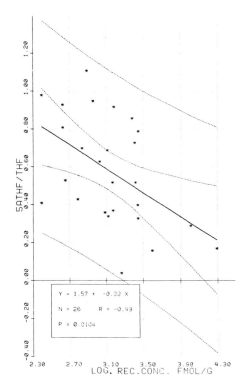

Fig. 4. Regression analysis for 5∝-THF/THF ratio and ER concentration.

References

Abul Hajj, Y.J. (1977): *Europ. J. Cancer, 13,* 749.
Bulbrook, R.D., Hayward, J.L., Spicer, C.C. and Thomas, B.S. (1962): *Lancet, 2,* 1238.
Cameron, E.H.D., Griffiths, K., Gleave, E.N., Stewart, H.J., Forrest, A.P.M. and Campbell, H. (1970): *Brit. Med. J., 4,* 768.
De Boever, J. and Vandekerckhove, D. (1980): *Arch. Int. Physiol. Biochim., 88,* B24.
Miller, W.R., Hamilton, T., Champion, H.R., Walace, I.W.J., Forrest, A.P.M., Prescott, R.J., Cameron, E.H.D. and Griffiths, K. (1975): *Brit. J. Cancer, 32,* 619.
Pfaffenberger, C.D., Malinak, L.R. and Horning, E.C. (1978): *J. Chromatogr., 158,* 313.
Vanluchene, E. and Sandra, P. (1979): In: *Applications of Glass Capillary Gas Chromatography,* Chapter 8. Editor: M. Jennings. M. Dekker Inc., New York (in press).
Wade, A.P., Davis, J.C., Tweedie, M.C.K., Vlarke, C.A. and Haggart, B. (1969): *Lancet, 1,* 853.

Estrogen receptors in breast cancer

J. DE BOEVER[1], K. DE GEEST[1], G. VAN MAELE[2] and D. VANDE-KERCKHOVE[1]

[1] Department of Obstetrics and Gynecology; [2] Medical Information Center, State University of Ghent, Academic Hospital, Ghent, Belgium

The value of estrogen receptor (ER) analysis has been established in the treatment of advanced breast cancer, particularly in identifying those tumors which may respond to endocrine therapy (McGuire et al., 1975). In primary breast cancer, however, the use of ER assays to predict early recurrence and ultimate survival was only recently substantiated (Knight et al., 1977; Bishop et al., 1979). In the present study ER content was determined in breast tumor samples from 180 breast cancer patients.

Material and methods

Tumor samples were collected from 142 patients with early breast cancer and from 38 patients with disseminated disease. Clinical staging was performed according to the international TNM system and histological grading was carried out according to the recommendations of WHO (Scarff and Torloni, 1968). All patients with early i.e. operable (T_{1-3} N_{0-1} M_0) breast cancer underwent a simple mastectomy and axillary dissection by the same group of surgeons of the Department of Gynecology. Postoperative radiotherapy was given to all patients with positive axillary nodes. The early breast cancer patients received no adjuvant therapy. They were followed up for 3 to 36 months (average 18 months) and the recurrence of disease was noted in relation to the presence (ER+) or absence (ER−) of ER. Metastatic disease was detected by physical examination, radiography, bone and liver scans, biochemical procedures and biopsy. Cytoplasmic ER were assayed in the same laboratory using a dextran-coated charcoal assay (De Boever and Vandekerckhove, 1980).

Dissociation constants K_d less than 1×10^{-9} M were considered as specific for ER binding. Protein was determined according to Lowry et al. (1951). Statistical analysis was performed with the Wilcoxon test, the Kurskal-Wallis analysis of variance, the χ^2 test for contingency tables and Spearman correlation coefficient calculations. For the study of prognosis and ER status, graphs were derived from life table analysis of the data at each follow-up time period. Comparisons between 2 curves on each graph were made by the Mantel-Haenzel test.

Results

ER were demonstrated in 58% of all breast cancer specimens, in 56% of the early breast cancer group, and in 66% of the group with advanced breast cancer. Binding capacities ranged from 105 to 77365 fmoles/g wet tissue (3 to 2545 fmoles/mg tissue protein) and K_d values varied between 0.1 and 7×10^{-10} M. Forty-two normal breast tissue samples were examined for ER content and all were found to be ER−. The assay results expressed as fmoles/g wet tissue correlated well ($r_s = 0.94$, p < 0.001) with those presented as fmoles/mg tissue protein (Fig. 1). There was a good correlation ($r_s = 0.82$, p < 0.001) between the binding index, BI (Leung et al., 1973) and the ER concentration calculated from Scatchard plots. An intermediate zone of BI values (BI = 20 to 40) included both ER+ and ER− tumors (Fig. 2).

In the early breast cancer group ER+ tumors were found in 48% of the premenopausal patients and in 62% of the postmenopausal patients (Table 1); these differences are not statistically significant. There were also no statistical differences between pre- and postmenopausal patients with advanced breast cancer for the proportion of ER+ tumors. In both early and advanced breast cancer, the mean ER concentration of the tumor was

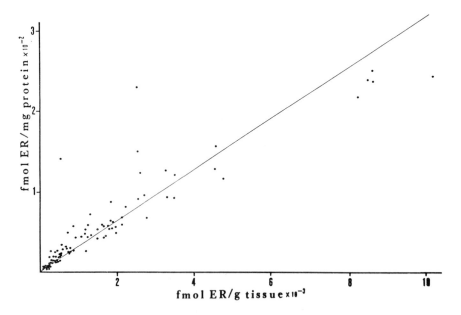

Fig. 1. Relationship between estrogen receptor concentration per g wet tissue and per mg protein in extract of human breast cancers. Estrogen receptors were determined as mentioned in Methods. A correlation ($r_s = 0.94$, p < 0.001) was observed.

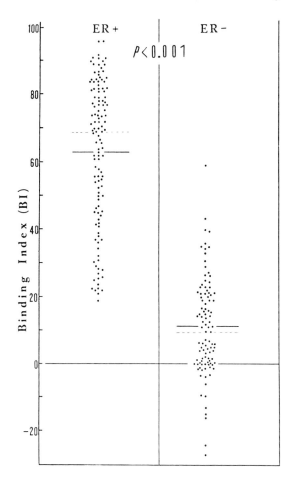

Fig. 2. Distribution of binding index of estrogen receptor positive and negative breast cancer specimen. Binding index is expressed in percentage as BI = (specific estradiol binding/total estradiol binding) x 100, where specific estradiol binding is calculated as difference between total and non-specific estradiol binding respectively in absence and presence of excess of diethylstilbestrol or estradiol. Mean (——) and median (····) values.

significantly higher (p < 0.001) in postmenopausal patients than in premenopausal patients (Table 1 and Fig. 3). There were no statistical differences between ER+ and ER— tumors in patients with early breast cancer in relation to known prognostic factors: axillary nodal status, histological grade, size of tumor, clinical stage, location of tumor; there was also no correlation between these factors and ER levels (Table 1). In the early breast cancer group the rate of recurrence was significantly higher (p < 0.001) in patients with ER— tumors (Fig. 4).

TABLE 1.

Estrogen receptors and prognostic factors in breast cancer

	No. ER+/ No. total	% ER+	ER concentration (fmoles/g wet tissue)	
			Mean	SD
Early breast cancer				
Total No. patients	79/142	56	2991	8546
Menopausal status				
Premenopause	29/61	48	777*	712
Postmenopause	50/81	62	2530	3779
Axillary nodal involvement				
Negative	50/86	58	1634	1289
Positive	33/56	59	2178	3102
Histological grade				
I	36/61	59	1198	1237
II	13/22	59	2377	2812
III	35/59	59	1905	2573
Size of tumor (cm)				
< 2	9/18	50	852	764
2-5	62/107	58	1807	2528
> 5	9/17	53	1594	1473
TNM stage				
I	30/48	63	1563	1647
II	33/53	62	1749	2398
III	22/41	54	2285	2753
Location of tumor				
Inner and central	25/48	52	1782	1596
Outer	52/94	55	2034	3105
Advanced breast cancer				
Total No. patients	25/38	66	4772	13591
Menopausal status				
Premenopause	7/10	70	880*	714
Postmenopause	18/28	64	8987	10448

*Vertical comparison, p < 0.01.
SD = Standard deviation.

When patients with positive axillary nodes (LN+) and patients with negative nodes (LN−) were considered separately, early recurrence was again more frequent in the ER− patients. The LN+ ER− group had a recurrence rate of 50% at 18 months. The LN− ER− patients had the same prognosis as all LN+ patients (Fig. 5).

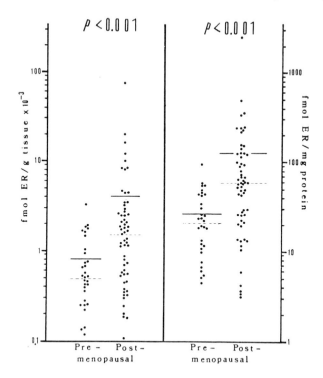

Fig. 3. Estrogen receptor concentrations in premenopausal and postmenopausal women. Estrogen receptor levels in breast cancer tissues from patients with primary or metastatic breast cancer were compared between 31 premenopausal and 60 postmenopausal patients for both ways of expressing estrogen receptor concentrations: fmol/g wet tissue and fmol/mg protein. Mean (——) and median (- - - -) values.

Discussion

The percentage and the binding properties of ER+ tumors in this study group are in agreement with most of the published data. The existence of a correlation between both ways of expressing the ER content, as fmoles/mg protein or as fmoles/g wet tissue, indicates that results are not essentially different if the fresh tumor is cleaned with great care and that consequently protein determinations are not an absolute requirement for reliably classifying a tumor as ER+ or ER−.

The binding index (BI) is less suitable for defining tumors as ER+ or ER−, because there is a range of BI values identical for both tumor types.

The presence or absence of ER did not correlate with various clinical conditions known to be associated with early recurrence; therefore, it appears that ER in primary breast cancer is an independent variable, so its

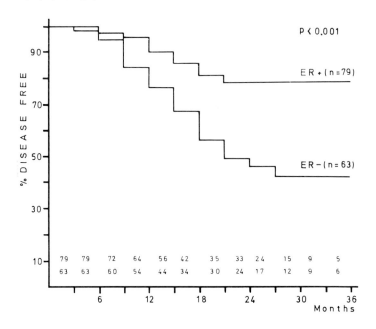

Fig. 4. Recurrence rates in patients with estrogen receptor positive (ER+) and estrogen receptor negative (ER−) tumors. Bottom of figure: numbers of ER+ (upper row) and ER− (lower row) patients who are disease free and under observation at entry and every 3 months thereafter.

presence or absence is a factor worth knowing. Indeed, although ER− tumors were equally distributed among known prognostic factors, the recurrence rate was higher in ER− patients. The observation that LN+ ER− patients constituted a very high risk group with a recurrence rate of almost 50% at 18 months and that the prognosis of LN− ER− patients was similar to that of all LN+ patients, indicates that ER and axillary node status are synergistic in the estimation of recurrence in early breast cancer.

Conceivably, ER determinations in primary tumors may aid in the selection of patients at higher risk of recurrence, and who may benefit from some form of adjuvant therapy.

Acknowledgements

The authors are grateful to the clinical staff of the Department of Gynecology and wish to thank H. Chrétien, T. Dhaeren, D. Leyseele and J. Vekeman for excellent technical assistance and S. Hoste for typing of the manuscript.

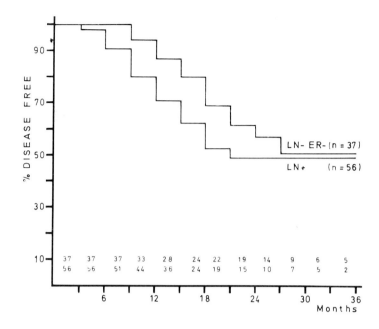

Fig.5. Recurrence rates in patients who had no axillary metastases and with estrogen receptor negative tumors (LN−ER−) and in all patients with axillary metastases (LN+). Bottom of figure: number of LN−ER− (upper row) and LN+ (lower row) patients who are disease free and under observation at entry and every 3 months thereafter.

References

Bishop, H.M., Blamey, R.W., Elston, C.W., Haybittle, J.L., Nicholson, R.I. and Griffiths, K. (1979): *Lancet, 2,* 283.

De Boever, J. and Vandekerckhove, D. (1980): *Arch. Int. Physiol. Biochim., 88,* B24.

Knight, W.A., Livingston, R.B., Gregory, E.J. and McGuire, W.L. (1977): *Cancer Res., 37,* 4669.

Leung, B.S., Manaugh, L.C. and Wood, D.C. (1973): *Clin. Chim. Acta, 46,* 69.

Lowry, O.H., Rosebrough, N.J., Farr, A.L. and Randall, R.J. (1951): *J. Biol. Chem. 193,* 265.

McGuire, W.L., Carbone, P.P. and Vollmer, E.P. (Eds.) (1975): *Estrogen Receptors in Human Breast Cancer.* Raven Press, New York.

Scarff, R.W. and Torloni, H. (1968): *Histological Typing of Breast Tumours.* World Health Organization, Geneva.

Immunofluorescent observation of prolactin receptor in cultured mammary carcinoma cells*

H. TAKIKAWA, R. HORIUCHI and S. TANAKA

Institute of Endocrinology, Gunma University, Maebashi, Japan

The presence of the estrogen receptor in mammary carcinoma cells has been reported by a number of investigators with the use of fluorescent microscopy (Lee, 1978; Pertschuk et al., 1978; Takikawa et al., 1979). It is accepted that prolactin plays an important role in carcinogenesis of mammary tumor as well as estrogens. The presence of prolactin receptors in mammary tumors has been reported by a number of investigators (Franz and Turkington, 1972; Sheth et al., 1974; Holcomb et al., 1976; Yanai and Nagasawa, 1978). The importance of the occurrence of prolactin receptors as an index of the responsiveness of the mammary gland to prolactin has been reviewed by Nagasawa et al. (1979). The localization of prolactin receptors has been studied using an autoradiographic technique (Costlow and McGuire, 1977). As far as we know, only a few reports have appeared on the immunofluorescent detection of prolactin receptor in cultured mammary carcinoma cells. This paper deals with a preliminary experiment using immunofluorescent microscopy for detection of prolactin receptors in cultured cells. Because of their dependence on prolactin DMBA-induced mammary tumors have been used in this study.

Material and methods

Fluorescein isothiocyanate (FITC) was obtained from Sigma Chemical Company, Sephadex G-25 purchased from Pharmacia Fine Chemicals. NIAMDD rat PRL (I-3, 30 IU/mg), NIAMDD rat FSH (I-3, 150 NIH unit/mg), NIAMDD rat LH (I-3, 1 NIH unit/mg), NIAMDD rat GH (I-1, 1.5 IU/mg) and NIAMDD rat TSH (150 NIH unit/mg) were used. Ovine prolactin was obtained from Panlitar-Armour Laboratories, and used for the fluorescent experiment following removal of the other fractions with the use of polyacrylamide gel electrophoresis. Collagenase type II (Worthington Biochemical Corp.), fetal calf serum (Microbiological Associates), Dulbecco's modified Eagle medium (Grand Island Biochemical Co.), kanamycin sulfate (Banyu Pharmaceutical Corp.) and paromycin sulfate (Kyowa Hakko Co.) were used for cell culture experiments. HEPES (N-2-hydroxy-

*This work was supported by a Grant-in-Aid for Cancer Research from the Ministry of Education, Science and Culture, Japan.

ethylpiperazine-N'-2-ethanesulfonic acid) and TES (N-trishydroxymethyl-2-aminoethanesulfonic acid) were obtained from Nakarai Chemicals. Anti-ovine prolactin rabbit serum (anti-prolactin) was kindly prepared by Dr. Wakabayashi, Hormone Assay Center of the Institute.

Preparation of fluorescein isothiocyanate labeled anti-prolactin

Ten mg of anti-prolactin was dissolved in 1 ml of 0.01 M phosphate buffer containing NaCl (PBS), pH 7.8, and 0.1 mg of FITC was dissolved in 0.25 ml of 0.1 M carbonate buffer, pH 9.0. Two hundred and fifty μl of FITC solution was added to 1.0 ml of the anti-prolactin solution, by mixing with a shaking incubator for 4 hr at 5°C. The reaction mixture was applied to a column of Sephadex G-25, which had been equilibrated with PBS. The effluent was monitored at 280 nm for protein and 495 nm for FITC. After removal of the unbound FITC by passing through the column, the effluent was dialyzed against PBS for 24 hr at 5°C, remaining unbound or loosely bound FITC was examined by the Pharmacia gel electrophoresis system.

Cell culture and preparation of microscopic specimen

Mammary tumors were induced in female Sprague-Dawley rats with a single dose of dimethyl benzanthracene (DMBA) in cotton seed oil given by mouth. Tumors were rapidly excised, any necrotic parts of the tumors were removed and the remaining tumor tissue was cut into small pieces. The minced tissue was treated with 0.1% collagenase at 37°C for 1 hr. The cell suspension was filtered through 200 and 400 stainless mesh to remove remaining tissue fragments. The cell suspension was centrifuged at 600 rpm for 5 min and the cell pellets were re-suspended in Dulbecco's modified Eagle medium supplemented with 10% fetal calf serum, antibiotics, 15 mM HEPES and 10 mM TES, inoculated into Falcon plastic dishes and cultured in the medium. After 2 or 3 passages, cloning was done using Nunc microplates. Following treatment with 0.05% trypsin solution containing 0.02% EDTA, the obtained monolayer cells were cultured on non-fluorescent microscopic slide glasses for 2 days, washed with Hanks' solution and extended with refrigerated centrifugation at 1,200 rpm, 4°C for 5 min. The cultured cells were stored at −20°C to be used for microscopic specimens.

Fluorescent microscopic observation

One plate was fixed with alcohol and stained with hematoxylin and eosin for light microscopic observation. The other plates were treated with 0.05% prolactin in carbonate buffer solution in a humid chamber at 20°C for 60 min and washed with PBS 3 times for 5 min. Then the plates were incubated with FITC-labeled anti-prolactin solution at 20°C for 30 min. The plates

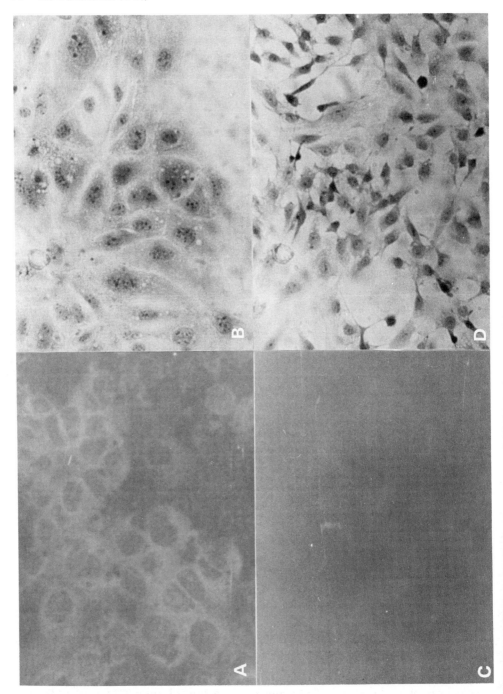

Fig. 1. Epithelial cells of a mammary tumor stained with FITC-labeled anti-prolactin (A), hematoxylin-eosin (B); fibroblastic region stained with FITC-labeled anti-prolactin (C), hematoxylin-eosin (D). (Magnification X300).

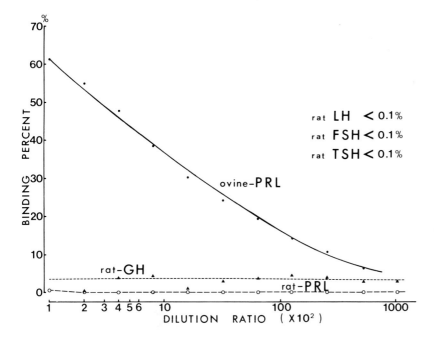

Fig. 2. Binding of anti-ovine prolactin with various pituitary hormones.

were immersed in PBS with three changes of the buffer, dried under cold air and covered with 20% PBS-buffered glycerol. Examination of the prepared specimens was carried out by means of a Nikon fluorescence microscope equipped with a mercury vapor lamp, an exitation filter BG-12 (402 nm) and' a cut filter 0-530 (530 nm) for FITC.

Results and discussion

The periphery of the epithelial cells had a brilliant green fluorescent appearance, while the fibroblastic region of the tumor cells had no fluores-cent appearance. In order to ascertain the specificity of the anti-prolactin, the binding experiments with other pituitary hormones were carried out by radioimmunoassay. As shown in Fig. 2, the antiserum possesses a relatively high specificity for ovine prolactin. The blocking experiment with FITC-unlabeled anti-prolactin succeeded in diminishing specific fluorescence of the cells, and success was also obtained without treatment of prolactin solution (not shown). In the case of estrogen receptors, fluorescence appeared in the cytoplasmic region of the tumor cells (Takikawa et al., 1979), while in this case it appeared in the periphery of the cells. It might be suggested that the estrogen receptor is present in the cytoplasmic area, but that the prolactin receptor is localized or adjacent to the cell membrane. From the results of these experiments it can be seen that this immunofluorescent method may be used to detect cellular localization of the prolactin receptor in mammary tumors.

Acknowledgements

We gratefully acknowledge the kind advice of Dr. K. Wakabayashi and technical assistance of Mrs. A. Nishikawa and Miss K. Tarusawa.

References

Costlow, M.E. and McGuire, W.L. (1977): *J. Endocr., 75,* 221.
Franz, W.L. and Turkington, R.W. (1972): *Endocrinology, 91,* 1545.
Holcomb, H.H., Costlow, M.E., Buschow, R.A. and McGuire, W.L. (1976): *Biochem. Biophys. Acta, (Amst.), 428,* 104.
Lee, S.H. (1978): *Amer. J. Clin. Path., 70,* 197.
Nagasawa, H., Sakai, S. and Banerjee, M.R. (1979): *Life Sci., 24,* 193.
Pertschuk, L.P., Tobin, E.H., Brigati, D.J., Kim, D.S., Bloom, N.D., Gaetjens, E., Berman, P.J., Carter, A.C. and Degenshein, G.A. (1978): *Cancer, 41,* 907.
Sheth, N.A., Ranadive, K.J. and Sheth, A.R. (1974): *Europ. J. Cancer, 10,* 653.
Takikawa, H., Mashio, H. and Adachi, M. (1979): *Cancer Treatm. Rep., 63,* 1146.
Yanai, R. and Nagasawa, H. (1978): *Endocr. Jap., 25,* 511.

Endogenous 17β-oestradiol concentration in breast tumours determined by mass fragmentography and by radioimmuno-assay. Relationship to receptor content

M. EDERY[1], J. GOUSSARD[1], L. DEHENNIN[2], R. SCHOLLER[2], J. REIFFSTECK[2] and M.A. DROSDOWSKY[1]

[1] *Laboratoire de Biochimie C.H.U. Caen and* [2] *Fondation de Recherche en Hormonologie, Fresnes, France*

The value of oestrogen receptor (ER) and progesterone receptor (PR) assays as a guide for breast cancer therapy is now well established (McGuire et al., 1975). The quantitative determination of 'occupied' receptor in addition to 'unoccupied' receptor is of particular importance for premenopausal women having high oestrogen levels and for patients under oestrogen therapy where a substantial portion of the receptors is bound to the endogenous hormone, so that the receptor assay may lead to false negative results (McGuire et al., 1974).

Recent studies suggest that this situation is unlikely, since it has been shown, using exchange assay, that endogenously bound 17β-oestradiol receptor exists in pre- and postmenopausal women (Sakai and Saez, 1976) although the latter have a higher receptor level (Saez et al., 1978). Furthermore, in a selected group of ER positive PR positive postmenopausal women, there was a positive correlation between the levels of 17β-oestradiol receptor and circulating oestrogens (Saez et al., 1979); however, plasma oestrogens may not represent an accurate indicator of tumour status because of the existence of an important plasma-tissue gradient (Cortès-Gallègos et al., 1975).

Several reports have recently appeared demonstrating the presence of 17β-oestradiol in human breast tumours (Millington, 1975; Fishman et al., 1977; Abul Hajj, 1979) in relation to receptor content. Nevertheless, the physiological significance of these results and its relationship to hormone dependence have been differently interpreted. In some studies, radio-immunoassay (RIA) was used and in others gas chromatography-mass spectrometry (GCMS). Although it has been shown that GCMS and RIA give similar results for plasma samples (Wilson et al., 1977), the interpretation of RIA values for tissues remains open to criticism, because the high meta-bolism of the tumour tissue leads to numerous cross reacting substances (Millington, 1977).

In the present work, we compare the values obtained for 17β-oestradiol as measured by RIA and GCMS in a large number of tumour samples. The correlation with the levels of 17β-oestradiol and progesterone receptors is also presented.

Material and methods

Samples of 78 primary breast tumour tissues were obtained fresh from biopsies or mastectomies of patients with cancer of the breast. They were immediately chilled, trimmed free of fat, weighed and directly processed for assays, or stored in liquid nitrogen until used. For the preparation of cytosols, tissues were homogenized under continuous cooling (0-2° C) in 6 volumes of 10 mM Tris-HCl, 12 mM dithiothreitol and 10% glycerol buffer, pH 7.4, using short bursts with an Ultra-Turrax homogenizer. Cytosols were obtained by centrifugation of the homogenates at 100,000 x g for 1 hr in an MSE-65 ultracentrifuge. The total protein content of cytosols was determined by the method of Lowry et al. (1951), using bovine serum albumin as the standard.

ER and PR were determined essentially by identical procedures. The binding reaction was performed at 0-2°C by incubation of aliquots of cytosol (0.1 ml) for 18 hr with 4 nM ^{3}H-R 2858 for ER, 4 nM ^{3}H-R 5020 for PR, either alone or in the presence of competing nonradioactive steroid (2500 nM). In order to minimize interferences with non specific proteins, 100 nM of 5α-DHT was added to the incubation medium for ER and 100 nM of cortisol for PR. After incubation, bound and free steroid fractions were separated by the addition of 0.12 ml of dextran coated charcoal. After continuous shaking for 30 min at 0-2°C, the charcoal was discarded by centrifugation at 800 g for 10 min. Aliquots of supernatant (0.12 ml) were added to 10 ml of scintillation medium and counted for radioactivity in a liquid scintillation spectrometer (Intertechnique SL 4000) with 61% counting efficiency for tritium. Specific binding was calculated from the difference in amount of radioactivity bound in the presence and absence of an excess of unlabelled steroid.

For the assay of endogenous 17β-oestradiol, the tissues were prepared as described by Millington (1975) with further purification on a Sephadex LH 20 column. The yield of extraction as determined by (2,4,6,7-^{3}H)-17β-oestradiol was 80-90%. This yield was independent of the amount of tissue (0.1 to 2 g).

Radioimmunoassay (Thibier and Saumonde, 1975) was performed using an antiserum raised against 17β-oestradiol-6-(O-Carboxymethyl)oxime bovine serum albumin and has been shown to be very specific for 17β-oestradiol (Dray et al., 1971).

Gas chromatography-mass spectrometry: The gas chromatograph was a Girdel instrument (Suresnes, France) fitted with a solid injection system and a high resolution capillary column, (approximately 70,000 theoretical plates), directly coupled to a quadrupole mass spectrometer (Ribermag R

1010B, Rueil-Malmaison, France). The glass open tubular column (25 m x 0.3 mm I.D.) was statically coated with SE-52 stationary phase and operated at 220°C with a helium pressure of 0.8 bar.

Trimethylsilyl ethers (TMS) were used as derivatives and prepared by dissolving the extracts and standard mixtures in 100 μl of N,O-bis(trimethyl-silyl)trifluoroacetamide/pyridine (1 : 1, V.V.) and heating 1 hr at 60°C. After evaporation under a stream of N_2, the residues were dissolved in benzene and an aliquot was deposited on the solid injection needle.

Isotope dilution-mass fragmentography (IDMF) was performed by adding known amounts (400 pg) of deuterium labelled internal standard, $(16,16,17\alpha^2 H_3)$-17β-oestradiol (E_2-d_3), to the tissue extracts before derivatization. The isotopic purity of E_2 is demonstrated by the abundance ratio d_0/d_3 = 0.3%, measured on the molecular ion of 17β-oestradiol-bis(trimethylsilyl ether) at m/e 416 for E_2-d_0 and at m/e 419 for E_2-d_3.

Calculation of the amount of 17β-oestradiol in the tissue extracts was made by using the peak height ratios after correction for d_0 contribution of d_3 (d_0/d_3 = 0.3%) and d_3 contribution of d_0 (4%).

Results

Sensitivity: Since about 10 pg of $^2H_3$-17β-oestradiol-carrier are used per injection, about 2 pg of unlabelled 17β-oestradiol can be reliably determined.
Specificity: The measurement of molecular ion abundance and the high resolution of the capillary column ensure the specificity of the determination. The column causes a minute shift in maxima of deuterated and non labelled 17β-oestradiol (2-3 sec). When the deuterated steroid is omitted, the corresponding peak disappears indicating the absence of interfering endogenous material in the samples.
Accuracy: Samples were fortified with different amounts of hormone and analysed. As shown in Table 1, the results seem quite linear.
Recovery: Since the ^{3}H-17β-oestradiol tracer is added to the sample before

TABLE 1.

Values for 17 β-oestradiol in normal and supplemented samples of tumour tissue

17 β-oestradiol (ng)

Added	Found
—	0.181
1	1.163
2	2.170
5	5.151

56   M. Edery et al.

extraction, subsequent losses during the purification steps are monitored.
Reproducibility: The values obtained following the extraction of 4 samples
of the same biopsy are as follows: 91, 88, 93, 86 pg 17β-oestradiol/g tumour;
mean coefficient variation = 4. This is also an indication of the homogeneity
of the biopsy.

The endogenous concentrations of 17β-oestradiol were measured in 42
human breast cancers using IDMF and RIA methods. The regression analysis
of the data obtained by RIA (x) and by mass fragmentography (y) gives the
equation $y = 0.91x - 65$, the correlation coefficient is $r = 0.88$ ($p < 0.001$
Student's t test).

However, if only the lower values (< 100 pg/g) are used for regression
analysis, no correlation is found between the 2 methods, due to the
dispersion of the RIA values.

17β-Oestradiol was determined using IDMF in 78 human breast cancers;
the 17β-oestradiol and progesterone receptor contents were measured simultaneously. In ER+ tumour (ER > 3 fmol/mg protein), the mean value for
17β-oestradiol is 553 ± 246 pg/g, whereas it is 192 ± 196 pg/g in ER–
tumours (Table 2). In the ER+ group, there is no difference between PR+

TABLE 2.

17 β-oestradiol content in breast tumours (mean ± SD)

Receptor distribution	pg/g tumour	pg/g tumour
ER+, PR+	545.95 ± 246.27 (34)	ER+: 555.33±246.22 (49)
ER+, PR–	576.60 ± 253.60 (15)	
p	NS	
ER–, PR+	278.29 ± 277.96 (7)	ER–: 192.66±196.41 (29)
ER–, PR–	165.41 ± 161.68 (22)	
p	NS	< 0.001

( ) = No. cases.

TABLE 3.

ER level and 17 β-oestradiol content

ER level	17β-oestradiol pg/g tumour
< 3	212.5
3-50	474.1
50-100	642.5
≥ 101	667.0

TABLE 4.

ER level and 17 β-oestradiol content (mean ± SD)

	pg/g tumour	Receptor status (fmol/mg protein)	pg/g tumour
Premenopausal (7)	541 ± 266	ER+: 52.6 (5)	599.7 ± 143.3
		ER− (2)	195.4 ± 200
Postmenopausal (71)	421 ± 292 NS	ER+: 71.2 (44)	550.2 ± 253.3
		ER− (27)	192.4 ± 202.6

( ) = No. cases.

and PR− tumours. Furthermore, a positive correlation is found between the levels of 17β-oestradiol receptor and the 17β-oestradiol contents in the ER+ PR+ group (Table 3).

Although only a small number of tumours of premenopausal women were available there is no evidence that premenopausal women had a higher 17β-oestradiol content than postmenopausal women. Furthermore, in the ER+ group, there is no significant difference in 17β-oestradiol content between pre- and postmenopausal women (Table 4), though the latter have a higher ER content (86 ± 31 fmol/mg protein vs 52 ± 12 fmol/mg protein).

Discussion

Our data reveal that values measured by RIA and IDMF are in good agreement; however, the use of mass fragmentography seems of better validity in providing an accurate methodology to measure steroid concentrations in tumour extracts particularly when low levels of oestrogens are to be assayed.

Using IDMF, we have shown that receptor positive tumours contain a statistically greater 17β-oestradiol concentration than receptor negative tumours, which is consistent with the fact that the hormone controls its own receptor synthesis. Fishman et al. (1977) and Abul Hajj (1979) have presented similar results and concluded that false negative receptor assays due to the presence of endogenous oestrogens are unlikely.

The origin of such endogenous levels of oestrogens remains unclear. It is now established that mammary tumour tissue can synthesize oestrogens in vitro; recent studies indicate either a correlation or an absence of correlation with the 17β-oestradiol receptor content (Varela and Dao, 1978; Abul Hajj et al., 1979a). Abul Hajj et al. (1979a) found that receptor negative tumours synthesize more oestrogens than the positive; they also found a more active 17β-dehydrogenase activity in receptor negative tumours suggesting that oestrogen synthesis in mammary tumours can be attributed to their hormonal independency and their failure to respond to endocrine therapy (Abul Hajj et al., 1979b).

Nevertheless, the aromatase activity of the tumour 'in vitro' may not reflect the real hormonal status of the tumour, since glandular secretion contributes to it in premenopausal women and extraglandular aromatization of androgens (particularly androstenedione) (Hemsell et al., 1974) as well as adrenal secretion of oestrogens (Procope, 1969) are not negligible in postmenopausal women.

Furthermore it is probable that in 40-50% ER+ tumours which are unresponsive to endocrine therapy, additional criteria of selection are necessary for a more precise prediction. A long term programme will establish whether endogenous steroids in conjunction with receptor status provide a better prognostic value for endocrine therapy.

References

Abul Hajj, Y.J. (1979): *Steroids, 34,* 217.

Abul Hajj, Y.J., Iverson, R. and Kiang, D.T. (1979a): *Steroids, 33,* 205.

Abul Hajj, Y.J., Iverson, R. and Kiang, D.T. (1979b): *Steroids, 33,* 477.

Cortes-Gallegos, V., Gallegos, A.J., Sanchez Basurto, C. and Rivadeneyra, J. (1975): *J. Steroid Biochem., 6,* 15.

Dray, F., Terqui, M., Desfosses, B., Chauffournier, J.M., Mowszowicz, I., Kahn, D., Rombauts, P. and Jayle, M.F. (1971): *C.R. Acad. Sci. (Paris), 273,* 2380.

Fishman, J., Nisselbaum, J.S., Menendez-Botet, C.J. and Schwartz, M.K. (1977): *J. Steroid Biochem., 8,* 893.

Hemsell, D.L., Grodin, J.M., Brenner, P.F., Süteri, P.K. and MacDonald, P.C. (1974): *J. Clin. Endocr., 38,* 476.

Lowry, O.H., Rosebrough, N.J., Farr, A.L. and Randall, P.R. (1951): *J. Biol. Chem., 193,* 265.

McGuire, W.L., Carbone, P.P., Sears, M.E. and Escher, G.C. (1975): In: *Estrogen Receptors in Human Breast Cancer,* p. 1. Editors: W.L. McGuire, P.P. Carbone and E.P. Vollmer. Raven Press, New York.

McGuire, W.L., Chamness, G.C., Costlow, M.E. and Shephered, R.E. (1974): *Metabolism, 23,* 15.

Millington, D.S. (1975): *J. Steroid Biochem., 4,* 233.

Millington, D.S. (1977): *J. Reprod. Fert., 51,* 303.

Procope, B.J. (1969): *Acta Endocr. (Kbh.), Suppl., 135,* 1.

Saez, S., Martin, P.H. and Chouvet, C.D. (1978): *Cancer Res., 38,* 3468.

Sakai, F. and Saez, S. (1976): *Steroids, 27,* 99.

Thibier, M. and Saumonde, J. (1975): *J. Steroid Biochem., 6,* 1433.

Varela, R.M. and Dao, T.L. (1978): *Cancer Res., 38,* 2469.

Wilson, D.W., John, B.M., Groom, G.V., Pierrepoint, C.G. and Griffiths, K. (1977): *J. Endocr., 74,* 503.

Receptor studies and survival in human breast cancer

G. CONCOLINO[1], A. MAROCCHI[1], C. D'ATTOMA[1], G. RICCI[1], L. CARDILLO[2] and C. PICARDI[2]

[1] Istituto di Clinica Medica Generale e Terapia Medica V, and [2] Istituto di Clinica Chirurgica Generale e Terapia Chirurgica I, Università di Roma, Rome, Italy.

Many attempts have been made in recent years to identify the molecular mechanism of the hormone dependency of breast cancer. It was thus possible to recognize some common characteristics of normal mammary gland and of hormone-dependent breast neoplasia, and to distinguish hormone-dependent, unresponsive and autonomous breast tumours. Particular attention has been paid to reports that breast cancer patients presenting tumours with both oestradiol (ER) and progesterone (PR) receptors benefit from endocrine therapy (Engelsman et al., 1973; Horwitz et al., 1975; Jensen et al., 1971; McGuire et al., 1975b, 1977; McGuire and Horwitz, 1978). It has also been reported that the response to hormonal treatment may be related to the amount of ER in the tumour cells (Jensen, 1975) and therefore to the presence of PR in these cells, PR synthesis in breast cancer being an oestrogen-dependent phenomenon (Horwitz et al., 1975, 1977). The variable concentration of ER in breast cancer may be due to the heterogeneity of the cell population with ER positive and ER negative tumour cells (Sluyser et al., 1977; Nenci, 1978). The presence of varying proportions of cells, some sensitive, others insensitive to hormonal manipulation, may explain the relapse or ineffectiveness of endocrine therapy in some breast cancer patients. The ER concentration and nodal status at the time of mastectomy have been suggested as prognostic parameters of the neoplastic disease (De Sombre et al., 1978).

To further elucidate the role of ER and PR in breast neoplasia and to evaluate the usefulness of commencing endocrine therapy in receptor positive breast cancer patients, 2 homogeneous groups of mastectomized breast cancer patients, all given radiotherapy, were compared. Receptor studies were performed only in one group. Endocrine therapy was given to some patients in both groups.

Material and methods

The first group of patients refers to 10 pre- and 12 postmenopausal women, aged 33-83 years, examined for the presence of ER, PR and androgen receptor (AR) in the primary tumour. Tumour (T) size ranged between T_1 and T_{3b}; affected nodes (N), assessed on the basis of histologic and not clinical findings, were found in 10 patients, 2 of whom with distant metastases (M), revealed upon X-ray examination.

Receptor studies were performed using tritiated 17β-oestradiol, promegestone (R5020) and dihydrotestosterone (DHT) or metribolone (R1881) as radioligands. Receptor assays were limited to the cytosol fraction preincubated with cold steroids and then submitted to the exchange technique for the measurement of total receptors (free and occupied sites). Dextran-coated charcoal or low temperature agar gel electrophoresis were used to separate bound and free ligands. Some samples were analyzed by means of protamine sulphate precipitation assay.

Eleven patients (all but one with receptor positive tumours) received endocrine treatment: 7 premenopausal patients were ovariectomized and/or treated with tamoxifen (TAM), 20 mg/day; 4 postmenopausal patients (1 with receptor negative tumour) were treated with TAM alone at the same dosage.

The second group of patients comprises 8 pre- and 16 postmenopausal women, aged 38-87 yrs, retrospectively examined for survival, number of recurrences and exitus even in those who received endocrine treatment. Tumour size ranged between T_1 and T_{3b} and affected nodes were found in 9 patients, 1 with distant metastases. Eight patients received endocrine therapy: 5 patients in premenopause or with affected nodes were ovariectomized, and 3 patients in postmenopause were treated with a testosterone derivative (Ectovis), 100 mg/day.

Results

Steroid receptors were found in 17 of the 22 breast cancers. ER and PR were more frequently detected, whilst AR was found only in 2 tumours (9.1%). The distribution (Table 1) of ER and PR in the cytosol fraction was as follows: 68.2% ER positive (ER+) cancers and 54.5% PR positive (PR+), 45.5% ER+PR+ and 22.7% ER−PR−.

TABLE 1.

Distribution of oestradiol (ER) and progesterone (PR) receptors in human breast cancer

	PR+	PR−	Total
ER+	10	5	15
ER−	2	5	7
Total	12	10	22

No correlation was found between the histologic pattern of the tumour and the presence of steroid receptors. Regardless of histologic pattern of the tumour and considering the nodal status at the time of mastectomy, 4 patients with affected nodes (2 of whom with distant metastases) in the first group died 1-3 yrs after mastectomy, irrespective of receptor presence in the primary tumour or of endocrine treatment. Similarly, affected nodes were found in 3 out of the 5 patients in the second group who died 1-3 yrs after mastectomy.

Receptors in primary tumours did not correlate with the number of affected lymph nodes: in the patients with ER+PR+ or ER−PR− breast cancer all the nodes examined were affected by neoplastic disease (Table 2). Fewer affected nodes were found in patients not presenting recurrences 2-5 yrs after mastectomy.

Of the 9 premenopausal patients with ER+ tumours only 1 died 1 yr after mastectomy; of the 6 postmenopausal patients with ER+ tumours, 2 died 1-3 yrs after mastectomy. PR+ tumours were found in 6 pre- and in 6 postmenopausal patients with 1 exitus in each group (Table 3). The relationship between hormonal therapy and overall survival of the 46

TABLE 2.

Correlation between receptors in primary tumours and number of affected lymph nodes

	Affected nodes	
Receptors	A	B
E+ P−	7/10*	1/4*
E+ P−	10/10	10/10
E− P−	8/8	—
E+ P+	15/15	5/7

Breast cancer patients with recurrence and exitus 1-3 yrs (A) and without recurrence 2-5 yrs (B) after mastectomy.
*Nodes affected/nodes examined.

TABLE 3.

Surviving vs dead oestradiol receptor positive and progesterone receptor positive breast cancer patients

Patients	ER+	PR+
Premenopausal	8 vs 1*	5 vs 1*
Postmenopausal	4 vs 2	5 vs 1

*Patients with recurrence and exitus.

TABLE 4.

Correlation between receptors, hormonal treatment and survival in breast cancer patients

	Died	Alive			Total
	Years after mastectomy				
	1-3	1	2-5	> 6	
No. of patients (1st group)	4	5	13		22
No. of receptor positive patients	3	3	11		17
No. of treated patients	3	3	5		11
No. of patients (2nd group)	5	2	10	7	24
No. of treated patients	4	1	2	1	8

patients examined is shown in Table 4. Of the 18 patients in the first group, still alive 1-5 yrs after mastectomy, 8 belong to the 11 patients treated with hormonal therapy on the basis of receptor studies: 4 premenopausal patients with ER+PR+ and 2 with ER+PR– tumours, and 2 postmenopausal patients with ER+PR+ tumours. Of the 19 patients in whom receptor studies were not performed, still alive from 1 to more than 6 yrs after mastectomy, only 4 received endocrine treatment. It is also interesting to speculate on the number of patients in both groups in whom relapse or exitus occurred even under hormonal treatment: 3 out of 4 patients in the first group and 4 out of 5 patients in the second.

Discussion

Steroid receptors play an important role in modulating hormonal action on the genomic expression of the target cells (Jensen et al., 1967; O'Malley et al., 1972; Toft and O'Malley, 1972).

Breast neoplasia possessing ER present some similar characteristics to the normal mammary gland, one of which the hormone dependency (Gardner and Wittliff, 1973; Wittliff et al., 1978). The tumour, however, even in the presence of ER, may be insensitive to hormonal manipulation if defects are present in the ensuing steps of steroid action, e.g. in the translocation, in the transcriptions or posttranscriptional events (Rochefort et al., 1978). Some markers of oestrogen action on the target cells, such as peroxidase activity and synthesis of PR have therefore been considered as parameters of well maintained hormone dependency of the tumour (De Sombre et al., 1975; Horwitz and McGuire, 1975; McGuire et al., 1975a). The possibility of the presence of 2 clones of cells (Sluyser et al., 1977; Nenci, 1978), one with, the other without, receptors, with a difference in growth rates, may explain the lack of response to hormonal treatment (Bruchovsky and Van Doorn, 1977).

The predictability of the response to endocrine therapy based on the presence of ER, PR and AR has, however, been reported by Engelsman et al. (1973), Jensen et al. (1973), Leung et al. (1973), Horwitz et al. (1975), Jensen (1975), McGuire et al. (1975b) who suggest that the treatment of choice could be based on receptor determination.

A combination of endocrine and chemotherapy has been studied, aimed at inhibiting growth of hormone-sensitive and insensitive cells (Wolff and Prahl, 1973; Goldenberg et al., 1975; Tormey et al., 1978; Heuson and Paridaens, 1979).

Although follow-up data was obtained from only a limited number of patients – 22 with and 24 without receptor studies, some of whom received hormonal therapy – attempts were made to demonstrate differences between the 2 groups, in the number of patients with and without recurrence and exitus. From these data it can be concluded that receptor studies help to discriminate hormone-dependent (but not always hormone-responsive) tumours and to select patients to be preferentially treated with endocrine therapy. Hormonal treatment, however, did not influence the survival in patients presenting affected lymph nodes, even in those with ER+PR+ tumours. The survival rate, on the contrary, was higher in patients with less malignant carcinomatous disease. Malignancy was not related to the histologic type but mainly to the stage of the disease. From the large number of patients in both groups still alive 2-5 yrs (or even more) after mastectomy and radiotherapy, it can be concluded that receptor presence in breast cancer is indicative of better prognosis only in patients presenting the less advanced stage. When carcinoma has spread to the lymph nodes or given rise to distant metastases, hormonal therapy alone, even in receptor positive breast cancer patients, can not prolong survival, and therefore a combination of endocrine and chemotherapy should be considered. Bearing in mind that only receptor negative breast cancer patients should not be treated with endocrine therapy, and considering the possibility of the presence of 2 clones of tumour cells, combined endocrine and chemotherapy should be preferred also in the treatment of patients in whom receptor studies have not been performed.

References

Bruchovsky, N. and Van Doorn, E. (1977): In: *Research on Steroids, Vol. VII*, p. 225. Editors: A. Vermeulen, A. Klopper, F. Sciarra, P. Jungblut and L. Lerner. Elsevier/North-Holland Biomedical Press, Amsterdam.

DeSombre, E.R., Anderson, W.A. and Hang, W.H. (1975): *Cancer Res., 35*, 172.

DeSombre, E.R., Greene, G.L. and Jensen, E.V. (1978): In: *Hormones, Receptors, and Breast Cancer, Vol. 10*, p. 1. Editor: W.L. McGuire. Raven Press, New York.

Engelsman, E., Persijn, J.P., Korsten, C.B. and Cleton, F.J. (1973): *Brit. Med. J., 2*, 750.

Gardner, D.J. and Wittliff, J.L. (1973): *Biochim. Biophys. Acta, (Amst.), 320*, 617.

Goldenberg, I.S., Sedransk, N., Volk, H., Segaloff, A., Kelly, R.M. and Haines, C.R. (1975): *Cancer, 36*, 308.

Heuson, J.C. and Paridaens, R. (1979): *The Second Breast Cancer Working Conference, Copenhagen, 1979* (Abstract).

Horwitz, K.B. and McGuire, W.L. (1975): *Steroids, 25,* 497.

Horwitz, K.B. and McGuire, W.L. (1977): In: *Progesterone Receptors in Normal and Neoplastic Tissues,* p. 103. Editors: W.L. McGuire, J.P. Raynaud and E.E. Baulieu. Raven Press, New York.

Horwitz, K.B., McGuire, W.L., Pearson, O.H. and Segaloff, A. (1975): *Science, 189,* 726.

Jensen, E.V. (1975): *Cancer Res., 35,* 3362.

Jensen, E.V., Block, G.E., Smith, S. and DeSombre, E.R. (1973): In: *Breast Cancer: A Challenging Problem,* p. 55. Editors: M.L. Griem, E.V. Jensen, J.E. Ultman and R.W. Wissler. Springer-Verlag, Berlin.

Jensen, E.V., Block, G.E., Smith, S., Kyser, K. and DeSombre, E.R. (1971): *Nat. Cancer Inst. Monogr., 34,* 55.

Jensen, E.V., DeSombre, E.R. and Jungblut, P.W. (1967): In: *Endogenous Factors Influencing Host-Tumor Balance,* p. 15. Editors: R.W. Wissler, T.L. Dao and S. Wood Jr. University of Chicago Press, Chicago.

Leung, B.S., Fletcher, W.S., Lindell, T.D., Wood, D.C. and Krippaehne, W.W. (1973): *Arch. Surg., 106,* 515.

McGuire, W.L., Carbone, P.P., Sears, M.E. and Escher, G.C. (1975b): In: *Estrogen Receptors in Human Breast Cancer,* p. 1. Editors: W.L. McGuire, P.P. Carbone and E.P. Wollmer. Raven Press, New York.

McGuire, W.L., Carbone, P.P. and Wollmer, E.P. (Eds.) (1975a): *Estrogen Receptors in Human Breast Cancer.* Raven Press, New York.

McGuire, W.L. and Horwitz, K.B. (1978): In: *Hormones, Receptors, and Breast Cancer, Vol. 10,* p. 31. Editor: W.L. McGuire. Raven Press, New York.

McGuire, W.L., Raynaud, J.P. and Baulieu, E.E. (Eds.) (1977): *Progesterone Receptors in Normal and Neoplastic Tissues.* Raven Press, New York.

Nenci, I. (1978): *Cancer Res., 38,* 4204.

O'Malley, B.W., Spelsberg, T.C., Schrader, W.T., Chytil, F. and Steggles, A.W. (1972): *Nature (Lond.), 235,* 141.

Rochefort, H., Garcia, M. and Vignon, F. (1978): In: *Hormones Deprivation in Breast Cancer,* p. 276. Editors: M. Mayer, S. Saez and B.A. Stoll. I.C.I. Ltd., Macclesfield, U.K.

Sluyser, M., Evers, S.G. and DeGoeij, C.C.J. (1977): In: *Research on Steroids, Vol. VII,* p. 253. Editors: A. Vermeulen, A. Klopper, F. Sciarra, P. Jungblut and L. Lerner. Elsevier/North-Holland Biomedical Press, Amsterdam.

Toft, D.O. and O'Malley, B.W. (1972): *Endocrinology, 90,* 1041.

Tormey, D.C., Falkson, H., Falkson, G. and Davis, T.E. (1978): *Proc. Amer. Ass. Cancer Res., 19,* 69.

Wittliff, J.L., Lewko, W.M., Park, D.C., Kute, T.E., Baker, D.W.T., Jr. and Kane, L.N. (1978): In: *Hormones, Receptors, and Breast Cancer, Vol. 10,* p. 325. Editor: W.L. McGuire. Raven Press, New York.

Wolff, G. and Prahl, B. (1973): *Arch. Geschwulstforsch., 41,* 363.

Significance of plasma sex hormone binding globulin (SHBG) binding capacity in breast cancer and fibrocystic breast disease

GIAMPIERO GAIDANO, LAURA BERTA, ENRICA ROVERO, PAOLO ANSELMO, PAOLO ROSATTI and CARLA NAVELLO

Cattedra di Patologia Speciale Medica B, Istituto di Medicina Interna dell'Università di Torino, Turin, Italy

Epidemiological data (Feinleib, 1968; De Waard, 1969; Berg, 1975; Lipsett, 1975) and measurement of plasma and urinary sex hormone (Mauvais-Jarvis and Kutten, 1975; Hill et al., 1976a; Hill et al., 1976b; Grattarola, 1978) have demonstrated that hormones are important factors in the aetiology of the benign and malignant diseases of the breast.

Fibrocystic breast disease, characterized by particular hormonal features (hyper-oestrogenism due to absolute or relative luteal deficiency) is very probably a pre-cancerous state (England et al., 1975; Mauvais-Jarvis and Kutten, 1975). In fact, high oestrogen concentrations have been shown 'in vitro' and 'in vivo' to induce neoplastic development in rats (Chan and Cohen, 1974; McCarty and McCarty, 1977). Furthermore, Zumoff et al. (1975) have suggested that the oestrogenic index (oestriol/oestrone + oestradiol) in plasma may discriminate between populations at low or high risk of breast cancer.

The metabolic clearance rate of sex hormone is influenced by specific plasma protein binding, which can modulate the free fraction of the hormones, which are biologically active at the target level (Anderson, 1974). In the present work, the plasma levels of sex hormone binding globulin (SHBG) binding capacity in benign and neoplastic breast diseases were studied in order to clarify whether protein binding can be of clinical significance in these pathological conditions.

Material and methods

The study was carried out in: (1) 14 women with breast cancer, subdivided into 2 groups: 6 premenopausal, aged 28 to 45 yrs, in the follicular phase of the menstrual cycle and 8 postmenopausal women, aged 50 to 75 yrs. The patients had never received any hormonal or cytostatic treatment and did not show hepatic or renal failure. Neoplasia had been recognized and surgically removed 3 months to 2 yrs prior to the present study. (2) 9 women with fibrocystic breast disease, aged 18 to 35 yrs. The control group consisted of 19 premenopausal women, aged 20 to 45 yrs in the follicular

TABLE 1.

Plasma mean values ± 1 SD of SHBG binding capacity (μg DHT bound/100 ml), prolactin (PRL, ng/ml) and 17 β-oestradiol (E_2, pg/ml) in women with breast cancer and fibrocystic breast disease and in normal control women (mean ± 1 SD)

Cases	No.	SHBG (μg DHT bound/100 ml)	E_2 (pg/ml)	PRL (ng/ml)
Normal				
Premenopausal (A)	22	2.56 ± 0.79	110 ± 28	11.3 ± 3.2
Postmenopausal (A')	8	3.10 ± 1.46	75 ± 15	10.2 ± 2.5
Breast cancer				
Premenopausal (B)	8	1.68 ± 0.55	103 ± 32	10.5 ± 2.6
Postmenopausal (B')	9	2.22 ± 1.20	54 ± 10	8.1 ± 2.8
Fibrocystic disease				
Premenopausal only (C)	9	2.39 ± 0.74	122 ± 85	9.3 ± 2.7
	A vs B	$p < 0.05$	N.S.	N.S.
	A' vs B'	N.S.	N.S.	N.S.
	A vs C	N.S.	N.S.	N.S.
	B vs C	$p < 0.05$	N.S.	N.S.

N.S. = $p > 0.05$. Premenopausal subjects were studied in follicular phase of menstrual cycle.

phase of the menstrual cycle, and 8 postmenopausal women, aged 50 to 75 yrs.

All subjects examined were not obese, nor suffering from diabetes mellitus or from any endocrinological disease and had never received any hormonal therapy (including contraceptives).

Blood samples were collected from each subject at 08.00-09.00 hr; plasma was immediately separated by centrifugation and stored at −20°C until assayed.

SHBG binding capacity was measured in an equilibrated Dextran T40/Polyethyleneglycol 6000 system, according to Shanbhag et al. (1973) with some modification (Gaidano et al., 1977). Specific plasma binding was expressed as μg of dihydrotestosterone (DHT) bound/100 ml plasma.

Prolactin (PRL) and 17β-oestradiol (E_2) were measured by radio-immunoassay (RIA) (Sorin-Biomedica, Saluggia, Italy) and expressed as ng/ml and pg/ml, respectively.

Results

The data are given in Table 1. Premenopausal women with breast cancer showed significantly lower mean values of SHBG binding capacity with respect to the corresponding control group. On the contrary, no difference was found between postmenopausal women with breast cancer and the control group.

The women with fibrocystic breast disease did not have different mean values of SHBG binding capacity compared to controls, but their plasma values were significantly higher with respect to those found in premenopausal breast cancer patients.

Plasma prolactin (PRL) and oestrogen mean values were not significantly different in any of the groups studied.

Discussion

Our data are according to the hypothesis that hormonal modulation can play a different role both in the induction and/or in the development of premenopausal or postmenopausal breast cancer, respectively (Stavraky and Emmons, 1974).

The lower levels of SHBG binding capacity observed in premenopausal women can be related to increased adrenal secretion of androgens (Garnham et al., 1969). High levels of plasma androgens have been shown to decrease SHBG synthesis (Anderson, 1974). On the other hand, plasma concentrations of total oestrogen, which were in the normal range in our cases, do not exclude an altered modulation of the 'free fraction'. In fact, an initial decrease of SHBG could be considered, directly related to subsequent neoplasia. The oestrogen free fraction would therefore rise and, consequently, might play a role in the evolution of breast cancer.

In fibrocystic breast disease different plasma hormonal characteristics have been suggested: increased adrenal androgen levels (Grattarola, 1978), relative or absolute progesterone deficiency (Mauvais-Jarvis and Kutten, 1975). The balance of all these factors as well as plasma total oestrogen levels in the normal range, could explain the behaviour of SHBG capacity observed in our cases.

Plasma SHBG binding capacity measurements could assume a significant role both in epidemiological studies of populations at different risk for breast cancer and in monitoring the evolution of fibrocystic breast disease.

References

Anderson, D.C. (1974): *Clin. Endocr., 3,* 69.
Berg, J.W. (1975): *Cancer Res., 35,* 3345.
Chan, P.C. and Cohen, L.A. (1974): *J. Nat. Cancer Inst., 52,* 25.
De Waard, F. (1969): *Int. J. Cancer, 4,* 577.
England, P.C., Skinner, L.G., Cottrell, K.M. and Sellwood, R.A. (1975): *Brit. J. Surg., 62,* 806.
Feinleib, H. (1968): *J. Nat. Cancer Inst., 41,* 315.
Gaidano, G.P., Frairia, R., Berta, L., Boccuzzi, G. and Angeli, A. (1977): *G. Ital. Chim. Clin., 2,* 55.

Garnham, J.R., Bulbrook, R.D. and Wang, D. Y. (1969): *Europ. J. Cancer, 5,* 239.

Grattarola, R. (1978): *Cancer Res., 38,* 3051.

Hill, P., Wynder, E.L., Helman, P., Hickman, R. and Rona, G. (1976a): *Cancer Res., 36,* 1883.

Hill, P., Wynder, E.L., Kumar, H., Helman, P., Rona, G. and Kuno, K. (1976b): *Cancer Res., 34,* 4102.

Lipsett, M.B. (1975): *Cancer Res., 35,* 3359.

Mauvais-Jarvis, P. and Kutten, F. (1975): *Nouv. Presse Méd., 4,* 323.

McCarty, J. and McCarty, O. (1977): *Amer. J. Path., 86,* 705.

Shanbhag, V.P., Sodergard, R., Carstersen, H. and Albertsson, S.A. (1973): *J. Steroid Biochem., 4,* 537.

Stavraky, K. and Emmons, S. (1974): *J. Nat. Cancer Inst., 53,* 647.

Zumoff, B., Fishman, W.L., Bradlow, H.L. and Hellman, L. (1975): *Cancer Res., 35,* 3335.

Endocrine treatment of breast cancer*

O.H. PEARSON, A. MANNI, B. ARAFAH and C. HUBAY

Departments of Medicine and Surgery, Case Western Reserve University School of Medicine, Cleveland, OH, U.S.A.

Hormonal alterations have been shown to induce objective tumor regression in up to 40% of women with advanced (stage IV) breast cancer. A number of different modalities of treatment have been evaluated, and the authors' estimate of the results obtained are summarized in Table 1. Endocrine ablative procedures have provided effective palliation with minimal side effects, although patients undergoing adrenalectomy or hypophysectomy require hormone replacement therapy for life maintenance. Administration of pharmacological doses of steroid hormones can also yield effective palliation in some patients, but there are undesirable side effects particularly with corticosteroids (Cushing's syndrome) and androgens (virilization) although less so with estrogens and progestins. The use of antiestrogen drugs, such as tamoxifen, has produced results comparable to those of surgical hypophysectomy, and this constitutes a major advance in the management of patients with breast cancer, since this drug has minimal side-effects. The use of aminoglutethimide and hydrocortisone to induce a 'medical adrenalectomy' has been shown to induce remissions comparable to those of surgical adrenalectomy. Some patients with breast cancer may obtain more than one remission with sequential use of different modalities of endocrine treatment: thus, premenopausal women who respond to ovariectomy often have a second remission from hypophysectomy, and postmenopausal women who respond to oestrogen treatment may later respond to androgen therapy.

The endocrine factors involved in the growth of hormone responsive human breast cancer have not as yet been completely defined, but studies with antihormone drugs which can presumably affect a single hormone have provided some new insights into the endocrinology of human breast cancer. The physiological basis for endocrine ablative therapy has been the concept that various steroid and peptide hormones play a role in the growth and maintenance of normal breast epithelium, and that the growth of hormone responsive breast cancers may be dependent upon such endocrine stimuli. Thus, ablation of ovaries, adrenal glands and the pituitary gland would lower the circulating titers of these hormones and induce tumor regression in a

*Supported in part by the U.S.P.H.S., grants No. CA-05197, RR-80, and Contract No. NO1-CB-43990, and a grant from the American Cancer Society, Inc., No. PDT-48U.

TABLE 1.

Results of endocrine treatments for stage IV breast cancer

	Response (%)	Duration of response (months)	Menopausal status
Endocrine ablation			
Ovariectomy	40	12	Pre
Adrenalectomy	40	12	Post
Hypophysectomy	40	18	Post
Endocrine addition			
Estrogens	35	12	Post
Progestins	30	8	Post
Androgens	20	6	Post
Corticosteroids	30	3	Post
Antihormones			
Antiestrogen (tamoxifen)	40	18	Pre and Post
Medical adrenalectomy (aminoglutethimide + hydrocortisone)	40	12	Post

manner similar to the atrophy of normal mammary epithelium after such endocrine ablation. The mechanisms by which pharmacological doses of steroid hormones can induce regression of human breast cancer have not been determined. Antiestrogen drugs, such as tamoxifen, appear to act by blocking the entry of estrogens into target organs, and the striking antitumor effects of this drug in women with breast cancer suggest that estrogens play a major role in the growth of these tumors. However, hypophysectomy and androgen therapy have induced remissions in patients after antiestrogen therapy, suggesting that other hormones may play a role in stimulating the growth of some breast cancers.

Estrogen receptor measurements of the tumor have proved to be useful in predicting the response of patients to endocrine therapy. In our experience, two-thirds of the patients with estrogen receptor positive tumors have responded to hypophysectomy or antiestrogen therapy, whereas in patients with receptor negative tumors, the response was nil. This is a useful marker in planning treatment for patients.

In this report, we will review the results of hypophysectomy and antiestrogen therapy in patients with stage IV breast cancer. The effects of antiestrogen therapy after hypophysectomy, and of hypophysectomy and androgen therapy after antiestrogen therapy will be reviewed, as these results appear to provide insight into the endocrinology of human breast cancer. The use of antiestrogen in combination with cytotoxic chemo-

TABLE 2.

Results of hypophysectomy in 199 patients with stage IV breast cancer

| | Patients | | Duration | No. still in | Survival | Patients |
	No.	%	(months)	remission	(months)	still alive
Remissions	84	42	18+ (3-62+)	10	34+*	25
No progression	6	3	13 (12-20)	0	29	0
Failures	109	55	–	–	13+†	6

*p < 0.0001.
† One patient whose survival status is not known is excluded.

(Reproduced from Manni et al., *Cancer*, 1979, *44*, 2330, by permission)

therapy for treatment of women with stage II breast cancer will also be reviewed, and these results indicate that endocrine treatment has an important role to play in this setting.

Hypophysectomy

The results of transsphenoidal microsurgical hypophysectomy in 199 consecutive patients with stage IV breast cancer (Manni et al., 1979a) are presented in Table 2. Forty-two percent of these patients obtained objective remissions of their disease lasting more than 18 months. The majority of these patients were operated upon prior to the use of estrogen receptors for selection of patients. In subsequent studies it was shown that hypophysectomy induced remissions in 65% of women with estrogen receptor positive (ER+) tumors, and that this remission rate was significantly higher than in unselected patients (Manni et al., 1980). We have considered these results to represent an optimal form of endocrine ablative treatment.

Antiestrogen

In an attempt to develop a 'medical hypophysectomy' we first investigated an antiprolactin drug, Lergotrile mesylate (Lilly) for possible antitumor effects (Pearson and Manni, 1978). Despite profound suppression of prolactin secretion by this ergoline derivative, there were only minimal effects on tumor growth in women with stage IV breast cancer.

Following the initial reports of the effects of antiestrogen in women with

TABLE 3.

Results of tamoxifen therapy in 113 patients with stage IV breast cancer

| | Patients | | Duration | No. still in |
	No.	%	(months)	remission
Remissions	56	50	19+	10
			(4-40)	
No progression	8	7	23	0
			(9-45)	
Failures	49	43	–	–

TABLE 4.

Results of tamoxifen therapy in 29 patients post hypophysectomy

| | Patients | | Duration | No. still in |
	No.	%	(months)	remission
Remission	8	25	17+	3
			(4-48.5+)	
No progression	6	21	17+	1
			(11-23)	
Failures	15	52	–	–

breast cancer (Cole et al., 1971; European Breast Cancer Group, 1972), we carried out a clinical trial of tamoxifen in 113 consecutive patients with stage IV breast cancer (Manni et al., 1979b). An update of the results of this study is shown in Table 3. Fifty percent of these patients obtained objective remissions lasting more than 19 months. Forty-nine of these 113 patients were selected because of positive estrogen receptors in their tumors, which probably accounts for the higher incidence of remissions in this series of patients. Nevertheless, it is apparent that the results of antiestrogen treatment are quite comparable to those of hypophysectomy. Since antiestrogens appear to act by blocking the entry of estrogens into the target tissue, the results suggest that estrogens play a major role in maintaining the growth of some human breast cancer.

Antiestrogen following hypophysectomy

We have studied the effects of antiestrogen in patients who had previously obtained remissions from hypophysectomy after which their disease had relapsed (Manni et al., 1979b). An update of these results is shown in Table 4.

TABLE 5.

Response to hypophysectomy after tamoxifen

		No.	Remissions No.	%	Duration (months)	No. still in remission	Failures
(A)	Remissions to tamoxifen	24	15*	62.5	13+	2	9
(B)	Failures to tamoxifen	22	6	27	8.5	0	16
(C)	Arrest of disease on tamoxifen	7	1	14	19+	1	6

*In 3 patients only arrest of disease was documented.

Eight of the 29 patients obtained objective remissions from tamoxifen and an additional 6 patients had arrest of disease lasting more than 17 months. These somewhat surprising results led us to reinvestigate the completeness of hypophysectomy in some of the patients who had obtained remissions from tamoxifen. We found that serum growth hormone and prolactin were undetectable even after provocative stimuli, whereas serum estrone, estradiol and estriol were detectable at low levels by radioimmunoassay. These observations suggest that low levels of circulating estrogens may stimulate the growth of some human breast cancers even in the absence of the pituitary gland.

Hypophysectomy following antiestrogen

We have also studied the effects of hypophysectomy in patients who were initially treated with tamoxifen and failed to respond or who obtained a remission from tamoxifen and then relapsed (Manni et al., 1979b). An update of these results is shown in Table 5. Fifteen of 24 patients who initially responded to tamoxifen obtained further improvement from hypophysectomy lasting more than 13 months. Six of 22 patients who failed to benefit from antiestrogen therapy obtained objective remissions from hypophysectomy lasting 8.5 months. These results suggest that a pituitary factor is involved in the growth of some human breast cancer. Whether lactogenic hormones (growth hormone and prolactin) or some other effect of hypophysectomy are involved remains to be determined.

TABLE 6.

Response to androgens after tamoxifen

	No.	Remissions No.	Remissions %	Duration (months)	No. still in remission	Failures
Remissions to tamoxifen	8	5	62.5	10+	4	3
Failures to tamoxifen	12	4	33	8+	1	8
Arrest of disease on tamoxifen	4	2	50	8+	2	2

Androgen following antiestrogen

The effects of pharmacological doses of androgen (Halotestin, 10 mg bid) have been studied in patients previously treated with antiestrogen or antiestrogen plus hypophysectomy (Manni et al., 1979b). An update of these results is shown in Table 6. It is apparent that androgen therapy was effective in some patients regardless of the previous response to anti-estrogen. It was also effective in some patients after hypophysectomy. Although the mechanism by which pharmacological doses of androgen induces remissions is unknown, these observations suggest that an anti-estrogen effect or an indirect action on the pituitary are not involved under these conditions.

Antiestrogen in stage II breast cancer

Since the 5-year recurrence rate in women undergoing mastectomy for stage II breast cancer is high (50-79%) attempts have been made to use early systemic treatments such as suppression of ovarian and adrenal function and cytotoxic chemotherapy in order to delay or prevent recurrence. Cole (1975) and Nissen-Meyer (1975) have shown that radiation castration can delay recurrence of breast cancer in premenopausal patients with stage I and II disease. Meakin et al. (1977) combined radiation castration with oral prednisone to suppress adrenal function in premenopausal women and found that such treatment not only reduces recurrence rates but also improves survival after 10 years. Fisher et al. (1975) and Bonnadonna et al. (1976) have shown that cytotoxic chemotherapy can delay appearance of re-currence in premenopausal women with stage II breast cancer, but these treatments were ineffective in postmenopausal patients.

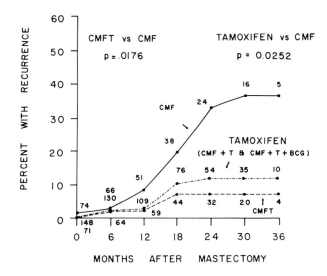

Fig. 1. Life table plot of recurrence rates for ER+ stage II patients divided into treatment groups. Figures over each curve represent number of patients followed for each time period. p values shown compare CMFT vs CMF (p = 0.0176) and all tamoxifen treated patients vs CMF (p = 0.025). (Reproduced by permission from *Surgery*, 1980, *87*, 494).

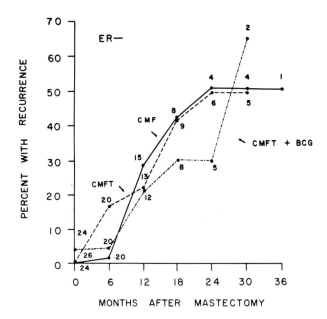

Fig. 2. Life table plot of recurrence rates for ER− stage II patients divided into 3 treatment groups. Figures over each curve represent number of patients followed for each time period. (Reproduced by permission from *Surgery*, 1980, *87*, 494).

We have carried out a prospective, randomized study of cytoxan, methotrexate, 5-fluorouracil (CMF), CMF plus the antiestrogen drug, tamoxifen (CMFT) and CMFT plus immunotherapy as adjuvant treatment in 296 women with stage II breast cancer, and estrogen receptors in the primary tumor were measured. In a preliminary study (Hubay et al., 1980a, 1980b) we found that CMFT was more effective than CMF alone in delaying recurrence after 33 months in women with estrogen receptor positive tumors. These results are shown in Figure 1. An update of these findings at 39 months has shown similar results. The effects of the 3 treatments in women with estrogen receptor negative (ER−) tumors is shown in Figure 2. It is apparent that there was no significant difference in recurrence rate with the 3 treatment regimens. Thus, in women with estrogen receptor positive tumors, antiestrogen treatment induced a delay in recurrence rate over and above any effect of the CMF chemotherapy, and these beneficial effects appear to be occurring in both post- and premenopausal women. A further period of observation is necessary to determine the duration of these effects.

Discussion

Endocrine treatments provide effective palliation for up to 40% of women with advanced breast cancer. Of the variety of endocrine modalities of treatment available, endocrine ablative treatments have in the past provided the optimum results. However, surgical procedures such as adrenalectomy and hypophysectomy are usually performed in medical centers, and such treatment is not available to many patients. The introduction of the antiestrogen drug, tamoxifen, which yields results comparable to those of surgical ablative procedures constitutes a major advance in the endocrine management of patients with stage IV breast cancer. This drug is now widely available and has minimal side effects.

The demonstration that estrogen receptor measurements in the primary or metastatic tumors of patients with stage IV breast cancer are useful in predicting the response to endocrine treatment constitutes another advance in the management of patients with this disease. In our experience, about 30% of women with primary or metastatic breast cancers have undetectable estrogen receptors in the tumors, and the response of these patients to endocrine therapy is virtually nil. Thus, in these patients we use combined cytotoxic chemotherapy as the initial treatment which induces objective remissions in 70% of these patients lasting an average period of one year. In 70% of women with estrogen receptor positive tumors, we find that two-thirds of these patients have objective remissions from hypophysectomy or antiestrogen lasting more than 18 months. In estrogen receptor positive patients who fail to respond to endocrine treatment or who have relapsed after remissions induced by endocrine therapy, 70% respond to subsequent combined cytotoxic chemotherapy with remissions averaging one year. Thus, we find the estrogen receptor measurement in the tumor to be a useful marker for selecting endocrine vs cytotoxic chemotherapy as the initial treatment for patients with stage IV disease.

Studies with the antiestrogen drug, tamoxifen, have yielded insights into the endocrinology of human breast cancer. Since the antitumor effects of tamoxifen appear to be due solely to blocking the entry of estrogens into target tissue, it is apparent that estrogens play a major role in the growth of hormone-responsive human breast cancer. However, the remissions induced by hypophysectomy or pharmacological doses of androgens after anti-estrogen indicate that other endocrine factors are involved in the growth of some human breast cancers. Whether other steroid hormones and/or peptide hormones are involved in stimulating the growth of breast cancer in women remains to be determined.

Our present concept of optimal management of women with stage IV breast cancer is as follows. In women with estrogen receptor positive tumors, we recommend antiestrogen as the initial treatment of choice. Second and third line treatment in these patients is hypophysectomy and androgen therapy. Fourth line treatment is cytotoxic chemotherapy. In women with estrogen receptor negative tumors, cytotoxic chemotherapy is the initial treatment of choice. Second and third line treatments are other forms of cytotoxic chemotherapy and endocrine treatments. When metastatic disease is immediately life-threatening, we use a combination of anti-estrogen and cytotoxic chemotherapy with good results. Whenever tumors involve the central nervous system, radiation therapy is used for these lesions since systemic therapy is usually ineffective in such lesions.

The use of endocrine treatment in earlier stages of the disease (Stages I and II) shows promise of providing better control of breast cancer than when it is reserved to treat the late stages of the disease. The concept behind this approach is that the majority, if not all, women with stage I and II breast cancer have micrometastases at the time of diagnosis, and that it is simply a matter of time before occult metastatic disease appears. If this is the case, can endocrine and chemotherapies presently available and used at this stage delay or prevent recurrences? The results discussed above indicate that endocrine treatments can delay the appearance of recurrence in selected patients, and in one study (Meakin et al., 1977) improved 10-year survival has been demonstrated. Adjuvant, systemic, endocrine and chemotherapy in patients with operable breast cancer is under active study in many centers at the present time, but, as yet, no consensus has developed. However, serious consideration can be given to the use of ovarian suppression and anti-estrogen in premenopausal women and antiestrogen in postmenopausal women with estrogen receptor positive, stage I and II breast cancer, since these modalities of treatment are quite benign.

References

Bonnadonna, G., Brusamolino, E., Valagussa, P. et al. (1976): *New Engl. J. Med., 294,* 405.
Cole, M.P. (1975): In: *Hormones and Breast Cancer, Vol. 55,* p. 143. INSERM, Paris.
Cole, M.P., Jones, C.T.A. and Todd, I.D.H. (1971): In: *Advances in Antimicrobial and Antineoplastic Chemotherapy, Vol. 2,* p. 529. Editors: M. Hejzlar, M. Semonsky and S. Masak. University Park Press, Baltimore.
European Breast Cancer Group (1972): *Europ. J. Cancer, 8,* 387.
Fisher, B., Carbone, P., Economou, S.G. et al. (1975): *New Engl. J. Med., 292,* 117.
Hubay, C.A., Pearson, O.H., Marshall, J.S. et al. (1980a): In: *Breast Cancer – Experimental and Clinical Aspects,* p. 189. Editors: H.T. Mouridsen and T. Palshof. Pergamon Press, Oxford, New York.
Hubay, C.A., Pearson, O.H., Marshall, J.S. et al. (1980b): *Surgery, 87,* 494.
Manni, A., Arafah, B. and Pearson, O.H. (1980): In: *Steroid Receptors in Breast Cancer. Cancer, Suppl.,* in press.
Manni, A., Pearson, O.H., Brodkey, J. and Marshall, J.S. (1979a): *Cancer,* in press.
Manni, A., Trujillo, J.E., Marshall, J.S., Brodkey, J. and Pearson, O.H. (1979b): *Cancer, 43,* 444.
Meakin, J.W., Allt, W.E.C., Beale, F.A. et al. (1977): In: *Adjuvant Therapy of Cancer,* p. 95. Editors: W.E. Salmon and S.E. Jones. Elsevier/North-Holland Biomedical Press, Amsterdam.
Nissen-Meyer, R. (1975): In: *Hormones and Breast Cancer, Vol. 55,* p. 151. INSERM, Paris.
Pearson, O.H. and Manni, A. (1978): In: *Current Topics in Experimental Endocrinology,* p. 75. Editors: L. Martini and V.H.T. James. Academic Press, New York.

Suppression of corpus luteum function in premenopausal women with breast cancer by an FSH/LHRH analogue: D-Leu^6-des-Gly-NH$_2$^{10}

G. TOLIS[1], A. CHAPDELAINE[2], K. ROBERTS[2], N. PAPANDREOU[3]
M. PAPACHARALAMBOUS[3], V. GOLEMATIS[3] and N. FRIEDMANN[4]

[1]*Departments of Medicine, Obstetrics and Gynecology, Royal Victoria Hospital, McGill University, Montreal;* [2]*Maisonneuve Hospital, Université de Montreal, Canada;* [3]*Aghios Panteleimon Hospital and Department of Surgery, University of Athens, Greece; and* [4]*Abbott Laboratories, North Chicago, IL, U.S.A.*

Luteinizing hormone releasing hormone (LHRH) induces follicular maturation and ovulation in women and successful pregnancy can ensue. Similarly, when administered to males with hypogonadotropic hypogonadism, puberty was induced and plasma testosterone levels were elevated with potency and spermatogenesis established. Stimulating effects on pituitary gonadotropins in both male and female patients have been observed after a single administration of LHRH analogues (Mortimer et al., 1974; Zanartu et al., 1974; Nillius and Wide, 1975; Schwarzstein et al., 1975). Chronic administration, to animals and man, gives an initial stimulation and subsequent suppression of gonadal function (Banik and Givner, 1975; Deriks-Tan et al., 1977; Berquist et al., 1979; Casper and Yen, 1979; Lemay et al., 1979). Moreover, chronic administration to rats leads to regression of estrogen dependent mammary tumors (Johnson et al., 1976).

This study was designed to assess the effect of chronic administration of an LHRH nona-peptide analogue (D-Leu^6-des-Gly-NH$_2$^{10}-Pro ethylamide) on ovarian function in premenopausal women with breast cancer.

Material and methods

Three women, aged 27-35 years with resected breast carcinoma with regular (28-30 days) menses of 4 to 6 days duration were studied. Each patient gave informed consent. During the study, patients received no medication which could affect pituitary function.

The study was performed at the Aghios Panteleimon Hospital, where complete physical examinations and routine laboratory evaluations including chemistry, hematology, and urinalysis were performed prior to the initial dosing. These procedures were repeated at the end of the study. All patients

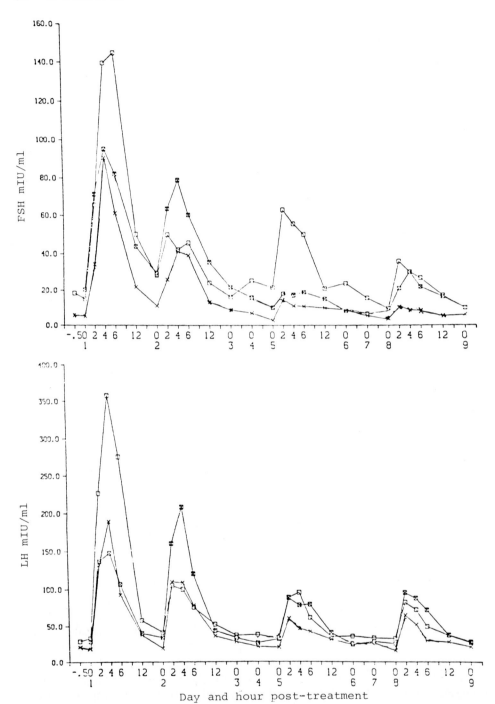

Fig. 1. FSH and LH levels in 3 premenopausal patients receiving daily injections of 10 μg of LHRH analogue for 8 days, first dosing day 7-9 of menstrual cycle.

TABLE 1.

Gonadotropin (FSH, LH), prolactin and sex steroid levels during treatment with the LHRH analogue

Patient No. I

	0	1	2	3	4	5	6	7	8
E_2	207.0	167	92	77	83	92	103	61	124
Pr	1.2	3.1	2.6	2.1	2.6	2.1	5.4	2.6	5.9
FSH									
B	16.5	28.5	16.2	25.5	21.6	24	15.6	9.6	9.9
P	145.2	50.1			63.3			36.0	
LH									
B	31.0	41.1	36.6	37.5	32.1	35.1	32.7	32.1	26.7
P	357.0	105.3			94.8			81.3	
PRL	9.5	7.6	6.1	8.0	9.0	10.3	10.4	8.1	9.5

Patient No. II

	0	1	2	3	4	5	6	7	8
E_2	145	303	335	387	397	365	327	325	340
Pr	0.2	0.3	0.2	0.3	0.3	0.3	0.5	0.5	0.5
FSH									
B	5.7	11.1	8.7	6.9	2.8	9	5.4	3.9	6
P	90.6	41.4			14.7			10.5	
LH									
B	19.5	18.5	27.6	20.7	17.8	23.4	25.8	15.6	21
P	189.0	110.0			60.0			64.0	
PRL	11.2	8.8	12.1	10.5	11.8	17.9	16.3	14	15

Patient No. III

	0	1	2	3	4	5	6	7	8
E_2	58	115	231	394	451	459	324	266	339
Pr	0.2	0.3	0.1	0.2	0.3	0.4	0.7	1.3	1.2
FSH									
B	20.4	29.8	21.7	15.9	10.2	8.2	6.6	8.2	10
P	95.2	79.5			18.9			30.3	
LH									
B	28.2	33.7	32.8	26.2	31.3	11.7	27.9	25	27.7
P	147.3	208.0			87.7			94	
PRL	9.7	6.8	7.2	7.0	10.3		11.5	11.3	8.9

Normal values	Estradiol (E_2) (pg/ml)	Progesterone (Pr) (ng/ml)	FSH (mIU/ml)	LH (mIU/ml)	Prolactin (PRL) (ng/ml)
Follicular phase	20-100	0.2-1.8	5-20	2-30	4-30
Mid-cycle	200-800		12-30	40-200	
Luteal phase	50-300	8-22	5-15	0-20	4-30

B: Basal   P: Peak
0: Pretreatment
1-8: During treatment

were in the 7th to 9th day of the follicular phase of their menstrual cycle at the time of the first administration of the LHRH analogue.

Each patient received subcutaneous injections of 10 μg of the LHRH analogue for 8 consecutive days. Plasma specimens for radioimmunoassay of follicle-stimulating hormone (FSH), luteinizing hormone (LH), prolactin, progesterone, estrone, estradiol, cortisol, and estrone sulfate were collected just prior to each administration of the drug. In addition, on days 1, 2, 5 and 8, plasma specimens were collected 2, 4, 6, 12 and 24 hr after drug administration for determination of these hormones. Samples were stored frozen until analysed (De Villa et al., 1972; Tolis and Franks, 1979).

Results

A sharp increase was observed in FSH and LH levels after each dose of LHRH analogue in all 3 patients. Both hormones showed the highest increase after the first injection in all 3 patients. Each subsequent injection produced a lesser response. A 75% and 62% reduction in the area under the curve for FSH and LH, respectively, was observed between the initial and 8th day gonadotropin responses. However, each patient showed an increase in these hormone levels after the 8th and final dose (Fig. 1).

No consistent patterns of response were detected in levels of prolactin, progesterone, estrone, estradiol, cortisol or estrone sulfate before or after any of the repeated injections of LHRH in these 3 patients. In particular, consistently low levels of progesterone were detected in all specimens from each of these patients (Table 1).

The patients commenced menstruating 4-5 days after the last injection of the LHRH analogue, which represents a shortening of their menstrual cycles by 6-9 days. Subsequent cycles occurred at about 28 days.

The drug was well tolerated with no subjective complaints to the treatment regimen. No changes in the physical examinations, before and after the treatment were observed, there were no significant changes in the clinical laboratory data.

Discussion

This study demonstrates a shortening of the menstrual cycle in premeno-pausal women with breast cancer treated chronically with D-Leu[6]-des-Gly-NH$_2$[10]. The finding of basically unaltered progesterone values in these women indicates a suppression of ovulation with short luteal phase. The fact that serum prolactin levels remained relatively unchanged and within normal range excludes prolactin as a mediator of the suppressed corpus luteum function as it occurs with hyperprolactinemic states (Tolis and Franks, 1979).

The data therefore suggest that the suppression of corpus luteum function is linked with the effects of the analogue upon the pituitary/ovarian axis directly.

The resulting decrease in gonadotropin output is therefore likely to be associated with pituitary 'exhaustion' or 'down regulation' particularly in view of the fact that one would expect the pituitary to be more sensitive to rising estrogen levels at this point in the menstrual cycle (Wang and Yen, 1975).

These results are in agreement with effects of similar analogues on decreasing pituitary responsiveness (Deriks-Tan et al., 1977) and establishment of anovulatory states (Berquist et al., 1979) when the analogue was administered throughout the menstrual cycle. Luteolysis, resulting in premature menstruation, has also been reported in studies with similar analogues administered after mid-cycle (Lemay et al., 1979; Casper and Yen, 1979), implying that LHRH analogues can inhibit progesterone synthesis even without prior interference with the follicular maturationiprocess.

References

Banik, U.K. and Givner, M.L. (1975): *J. Reprod. Fertil.,* 44, 87.

Berquist, C., Nillius, S.J. and Wide, L. (1979): *Lancet,* 2, 215.

Casper, R.F. and Yen, S.S.C. (1979): *Science, 205,* 408.

Deriks-Tan, J.S.E., Hammer, E. and Taubert, H.D. (1977): *J. Clin. Endocr.,* 45, 597.

De Villa, G., Roberts, K., Wiest, W.G., Mikhail, G. and Flickinger, G. (1972): *J. Clin. Endocr., 35,* 458.

Johnson, E.S., Seely, J.H., White, W.F. and De Sombre, E.R. (1976): *Science, 194,* 329.

Lemay, A., Labrie, F., Ferland, L. and Raynaud, J.P. (1979): *Fertil. and Steril., 31,* 29.

Mortimer, C.H., McNeilly, A.S., Fisher, R.A., Murray, M.A.F. and Besser, G.M. (1974): *Brit. Med. J., 4,* 617.

Nillius, S.J. and Wide, L. (1975): *Brit. Med. J., 3,* 405.

Schwarzstein, L., Aparicio, N.J., Turner, D., Calamera, J.C., Mancini, R. and Schally, A.V. (1975): *Fertil. and Steril., 26,* 331.

Tolis, G. and Franks, S. (1979): In: *Clinical Neuroendocrinology, a Pathophysiological Approach,* p. 291. Editors: G. Tolis, F. Labrie, J.B. Martin and F. Naftolin. Raven Press, New York.

Vaitukaitis, J.L. and Ross, G.T. (1973): *Ann. Rev. Med., 24,* 295.

Wang, C.F. and Yen, S.S.C. (1975): *J. Clin. Invest., 55,* 201.

Zanartu, J., Dabancens, A., Kastin, A.J. and Schally, A.V. (1974): *Fertil. and Steril., 25,* 160.

PROSTATE CANCER

Endocrine aspects of aetiology of carcinoma of the prostate

G.D. CHISHOLM and F.K. HABIB

University Department of Surgery/Urology, Western General Hospital, Edinburgh, U.K.

The endocrine dependence of the prostate has been known for centuries. More than 200 years ago, John Hunter recognised and confirmed that the growth of the prostate was dependent upon testicular secretion. Since then, one important fact has remained unchallenged: the development of the prostate gland and the benign enlargement or hypertrophy that occurs in the older male is related to the presence or absence of testes.

The relevance of the study of benign prostatic hypertrophy (BPH) to the development of carcinoma of the prostate (CaP) was first described by Charles Huggins and colleagues whose studies led them to suggest that CaP was an overgrowth of normal prostatic epithelium. To quote Huggins et al. (1941) 'in many instances, a malignant prostate tumor is an overgrowth of adult epithelial cells'. Although carcinoma of the prostate commonly retains the acinar and modified cellular pattern of adult prostatic epithelium, the possibility that these cells maintain the *metabolic* characteristics of normal prostate was not raised until Gutman and Gutman (1938) demonstrated a high acid phosphatase concentration in the malignant cell. The onset of endocrine stimulation in the pubertal male was already known to be associated with a marked increase in the concentration of acid phosphatase in the normal prostatic cell; Huggins suggested that if the malignant cell continued to show this characteristic feature then these cells might also continue to be endocrine responsive. Thus began the era of the control of growth of CaP by endocrine manipulation (Chisholm and O'Donoghue, 1975).

In order to determine whether or not CaP represents a continuum of the endocrine processes that are responsible for BPH, three groups of studies will be reviewed. These studies concern epidemiologic aspects, serum and tissue hormone levels, and morphological aspects.

Epidemiological studies

If the age of presentation alone is considered, then a comparison between BPH and CaP gives no indication of either an age-related incidence or aetiology; both BPH and CaP show parallel increases with age.

Attempts have been made to link the aetiology of CaP with the incidence of BPH but these data must be examined with caution for two reasons: (i) it is difficult to define and to find a male with a normal prostate over the age of 60, and (ii) even the apparently benign prostate may harbour a focus of carcinoma. In most series of BPH 5-15% will have an incidental focus of carcinoma.

Armenian et al. (1974) reported a greater risk of developing CaP in those with BPH compared to the controls. This was a prospective study of 296 cases of BPH and 299 age matched controls who were traced either until death or until the end of the study. The death rate from CaP was found to be 3.7 x greater in the BPH group compared to the controls. Further analysis of the data by matched pairs also showed a significant relative risk of CaP deaths in BPH diagnosed patients compared to the controls. Finally, Armenian et al. (1974) also showed that the death rate from CaP was lower in 77 BPH patients who had had a prostatectomy compared with the non-operated patients with BPH. This led the authors to suggest that a randomised trial of prostatectomy should be carried out in symptom-free patients, with BPH, to see if this affected the incidence of CaP. However, this suggestion was based on the erroneous belief that CaP arises in the posterior aspect of the prostate capsule (see later: morphology).

In the same year, Greenwald et al. (1974) reached a completely different opinion on the relationship between CaP and BPH. These authors followed up 838 patients undergoing prostatectomy and found no increased risk from CaP compared with 802 age-matched surgical controls in the same hospital.

It has been a long-held belief that some abnormality or change in androgen/oestrogen balance was responsible for the change in prostatic growth with age. Various theories have been offered and most have suggested either a decline in androgen levels and/or a relative increase in oestrogens. Epidemiological studies offer some support for the possibility of hyper-oestrogenism. Autopsy studies by Glantz (1964) showed that 500 patients with cirrhosis of the liver had less CaP than the 650 in the control autopsy group. The hyperoestrogenism associated with cirrhosis was thought to have a protective role in CaP. An earlier study by Stumpf and Wilens (1953) had reached a similar conclusion in respect of lower incidence of BPH in 333 cirrhotics.

Other related epidemiological studies looking at weight, height and hair distribution found no differences between the CaP and control groups (Wynder et al., 1971). Likewise, in a study of the anthropometric indices of 286 college men who eventually developed CaP, there were no differences in such variables as somatotype, baldness and gynandromorphy when compared to controls (Greenwald et al., 1974).

Many aspects of sexual behaviour and marital status have been examined in relation to CaP. Some of these studies have used sexual behaviour as an index of maleness and therefore related to the hormone status of the patient; other studies have been directed at the possibility of sexual transmission of an infective agent. Thus it has been shown that the incidence of CaP is strongly associated with the marital status being lower in the never married and higher in the divorced. The incidence of CaP is higher in those with a higher frequency of coitus and higher in those with more children (Owen, 1976). Sexual drive, sexual repression and age of cessation of sexual activity have all been studied as factors influencing the development of CaP – but without detecting any significant trends.

The remarkably high incidence of CaP in the U.S. black population has led to a variety of studies in an attempt to find relevant factors in the aetiology of CaP. Whether or not there is an endocrine factor is unknown since there has been no large scale study of hormone measurements in this group. Nutrition has been offered as an explanation for much of the international variation in rates for many hormone-dependent cancer sites. However, in the U.S. no major nutritional differences between racial groups within a social class have been demonstrated. The high (CaP) incidence in the U.S. black has been compared with the low incidence in the W. African black: apart from the tumour in the W. African black presenting at an earlier age and later stage, no factors have been found to account for the differences in incidence. There was a significant positive association in both groups, with sedentary occupation, sexual activity and venereal disease.

It has been suggested that CaP in the U.S. black is more virulent than in the white; however in a recent study of relative survival rates, there were no differences between the 2 races at 5, 10 and 15 years (Levine and Wilchinsky, 1979).

Serum and tissue hormone levels

Attempts have been made to link the changes in blood levels of hormones with age and therefore with prostatic growth. Data in the past were, in many instances, of limited value because of the methods available for measuring these hormones; with the availability of radioimmunoassay, more precise and consistent data are now available.

The evidence that BPH is under continuing endocrine stimulation is based mainly on the knowledge that the pubertal castrate does not develop benign enlargement, that the hypogonad, such as with Klinefelter's syndrome, can develop benign enlargement and also that castration in the adult leads to a decrease in the size of the gland. In addition oestrogens, androgens, combinations of these, as well as various progestational agents can also affect the size of the gland.

With the knowledge that the active stimulant to prostatic epithelial cell growth is dihydrotestosterone (DHT) rather than testosterone (T) a great deal of interest has focused on blood and tissue levels of T and DHT. Attempts have been made to relate blood hormone levels to the diseased prostate in the hope of determining an endocrine pattern that might distinguish normal from BPH from carcinoma but the results from various centres have not been consistent.

Age: The changes in serum hormones with age include: A decrease of: testosterone metabolites (from age 20-30); free and total T; free and total DHT. An increase of: oestradiol; LH, FSH; SHBG.

Thus, there is the paradox of declining androgen activity with age but the growth of a gland that needs continued androgen support.

BPH: Vermeulen and Sy (1976) found that the mean levels of testosterone in BPH patients aged 60-70 were similar to the control values but in BPH patients aged 70-80 the levels were significantly higher. Ghanadian et al. (1977) found no significant differences in testosterone levels between controls and BPH patients of the same age.

DHT has been shown to be higher in BPH (Vermeulen and Sy, 1976). Ghanadian et al. (1977) found serum values of 81 ± 4 ng/100 ml in BPH compared with 67 ± 3 ng/100 ml in normal age-matched men and although the differences were significant there was a wide variation in both groups. Much of this variation has been explained by the use of the 60+ year old male as a 'normal' control. Habib et al. (1976) assumed all patients over the age of 60 were either BPH or CaP and they found no differences in the circulating androgens of these 2 groups.

In a study of 128 men aged 36-65, Bartsch et al. (1979) classified the prostate size into large, medium and small and found no differences in hormone levels between these 3 groups.

It can be concluded that apart from the elevation in DHT in BPH, which may be a result and not a cause of the enlargement, no consistent changes in blood T or DHT can be related to the aetiology.

Carcinoma: Habib et al. (1976) found no differences in plasma androgen levels between BPH and CaP. However, Ghanadian et al. (1979) found a significantly higher testosterone in CaP but DHT was the same in carcinoma as in controls. In addition, the ratio T/DHT was highly significantly different in those with carcinoma.

These studies have suggested that there is a trend towards higher DHT concentrations in BPH but that this steroid may be depressed towards normal levels in CaP.

Tissue levels: In 1970 Siiteri and Wilson measured the concentration of T and DHT in the epithelial cells of the prostate of men of varying ages, men with BPH and normal prostatic tissue. Surprisingly, the DHT concentration was higher in older men than younger men while BPH tissue had a 5 times greater concentration of DHT than in normal tissue. It was also found that periurethral tissues had a very high concentration of DHT. These studies strongly supported the view that testicular androgen had a direct effect in the aetiology of BPH. It may be that more attention should be paid to androgen metabolism enzymes such as 5α-reductase and 3α-hydroxysteroid-dehydrogenase, in the aetiology of BPH.

Studies of T, DHT and androstanedione in BPH and malignant tissues have shown that there is a higher concentration of androgens compared to BPH (Habib et al., 1976; Hammond, 1978). Since there are no consistent changes in plasma levels it would appear that these differences represent local factors and metabolic changes within the prostate.

Before and after prostatectomy: The implication from some of the studies of serum hormones has been that the prostate 'per se' produces some of the changes. Thus, attention has been directed at the effect of prostatectomy on the levels of T and DHT. Vermeulen and Sy (1976) measured the changes 2-5 months after prostatectomy; they found that the T and DHT levels were significantly higher than before operation and attributed the lower pre-operative values to surgical stress. More recently, studies have shown that there is no significant change in T, DHT or their SHBG binding and that the changes after operation are temporary, returning to normal after 2 months (Ghanadian et al., 1980).

It is also of interest that Mahoudeau et al. (1974) found DHT to be higher in the veins draining the prostate, compared with peripheral venous blood levels.

Other endocrine aspects of prostatic diseases: A wide range of substances has been studied in normal, BPH and malignant tissues (Grayhack and Wendel, 1974). Though certain differences in these substances have been characterised, their relevance in the aetiology of prostatic disease has yet to be clarified. Specific reference will be made to the following:

Prolactin: Prolactin has a synergistic action on androgen-induced weight gain and citric acid secretion by the rat prostate. Other studies have confirmed this interaction and shown, in man, that prolactin does increase prostatic uptake of androgen. Following upon the studies by Jacobi et al. (1978) of bromocriptine and CaP, Farnsworth et al. (1980) have suggested that depleting blood prolactin might reduce the uptake of testicular and adrenal androgens by prostatic tumours and that the effectiveness of this treatment may be related to the density of prolactin receptors.

Steroid receptors: The technical problems of obtaining adequate CaP tissue for steroid receptor measurement as well as the identification of receptors in normal, not hyperplastic, tissues has slowed progress in evaluating receptor proteins in prostatic disease. Recently, Gustafsson et al. (1978) have shown a high correlation between clinical response to human therapy and steroid receptor content. Recently, it has been shown that the concentration of androgen receptors in well differentiated carcinoma is significantly higher than in normal or BPH (Lieskovsky and Bruchovsky, 1979).

Experimental prostatic hyperplasia: Experimental studies in the induction of BPH in dogs have made dramatic progress in identifying endocrine aspects of aetiology of BPH. In 1976, Walsh and Wilson reported that androstanediol induced BPH in the castrate dog (with the epididymis left intact) and that 17β oestradiol had a synergistic effect in this model. It had already been shown, in Wilson's laboratory, that neither T nor DHT alone induced canine prostatic hyperplasia.

Recent studies by De Klerk et al. (1979) have shown surprising differences from these studies. Thus, in the castrate beagle dog, DHT + oestradiol was almost as effective as androstanediol + oestradiol in producing hyperplasia; in the intact beagle dog, DHT + androstanediol without oestradiol induced glandular hyperplasia. These experiments throw no light on any age associated changes but it is evident that some abnormality of testicular secretion, or in the subsequent metabolism of androgens and 5α reduced androgens, may be responsible for the development of canine prostatic hyperplasia. As a corollary to these studies it has also been possible to induce changes in seminal plasma components that are identical to those found in spontaneous canine prostatic hyperplasia.

Morphology

Both Franks (1954) and McNeal (1968) have commented on the greater frequency with which carcinoma of the prostate is located in the periphery of the prostate gland. This peripheral area is often confused with the anatomical posterior lobe but recent studies of prostatic anatomy have indicated that the subdivision of the parenchyma into a central and peripheral zone is more precise in terms of morphology, function and pathology (McNeal, 1968). In consideration of the origins of CaP, McNeal (1969) carried out a detailed histological study of 45 malignant prostates. The origin of carcinoma was limited to a histological area that was neither the posterior 'lobe' nor the subcapsular area. This area was characterised by active rather than atrophic epithelium suggesting an aetiological role of prolonged androgen stimulation. Distinctive premalignant changes were also seen within this active epithelium.

The concept of a mature prostate with 2 morphological zones is not necessarily at variance with other morphological descriptions of the gland; instead, it represents a description based on a more comprehensive description based on the histology. McNeal (1968) described a method of assessing gland activity based on the presence of atrophic changes in the epithelium; significant differences were found between the average activity of the central and peripheral zones of the same gland. Thus various observations (Blacklock, 1976) support the view that the parenchyma of the peripheral zone is more androgen dependent than the central zone. Huggins and Webster (1948) showed that there was a differential effect of oestrogens, degeneration being more marked in the part that is now called the peripheral zone.

Diffuse atrophy of the prostate is a feature of aging processes (focal atrophy is more likely a manifestation of prostatitis). This process of diffuse atrophy appears to commence after about the age of 50 years and is not usually advanced until after 70 years. Again, this change is more marked in the peripheral zone.

Attempts have been made to relate these changes to serum hormone changes, but as we have seen already these changes in serum values in various pathological conditions of the prostate require further evaluation. The endocrine changes are more likely to be intracellular and if changes in the androgen/oestrogen usage by the prostatic epithelial cell could be shown to be the precursor to atrophy, then this would give further support to the concept of differential function by the peripheral and central zones. It might also explain the finding of BPH in the central zone and carcinoma in the peripheral zone. However, even without this evidence we now have an explanation as to how the patient can have both diseases in the same age group in what was once thought to be a gland whose divisions were simply surgical lobes.

References

Armenian, H.K., Lilienfeld, A.M., Diamond, E.L. and Bross, I.D.J. (1974): *Lancet, 2,* 115.

Bartsch, W., Becker, H., Pinkerburg, F.A. and Krieg, M. (1979): *Acta Endocr. (Kbh.), 90,* 727.

Blacklock, N.J. (1976): In: *Scientific Foundation of Urology, Vol. II,* Chapter 16, p. 113. Editors: D.I. Williams and G.D. Chisholm. Heinemann, London.

Chisholm, G.D. and O'Donoghue, E.P.N. (1975): *Vitam. and Horm., 33,* 377.

De Klerk, D.P., Coffey, D.S., Ewing, L.L. et al. (1979): *J. Clin. Invest., 64,* 842.

Farnsworth, W.E., Slaunwhite, W.R., Sharma, M., Oseko, F. and Brown, J.R. (1980): *Urol. Res.,* in press.

Franks, L.M. (1954): *Ann. Roy. Coll. Surg. Engl., 14,* 92.

Ghanadian, R., Lewis, J.G., Chisholm, G.D. and O'Donoghue, E.P.N. (1977): *Brit. J. Urol., 49,* 541.

Ghanadian, R., Puah, C.M. and O'Donoghue, E.P.N. (1979): *Brit. J. Cancer, 39,* 696.

Ghanadian, R., Puah, C.M., Williams, G., Shah, P.J.R. and McWhinney, N. (1980): *Brit. J. Urol., 52,* in press.

Glantz, G.M. (1964): *J. Urol., 91,* 291.

Grayhack, J.T. and Wendel, E.F. (1974): In: *Male Accessory Sex Organs,* Chapter 17, p. 425. Editor: David Brandes. Academic Press, New York.

Greenwald, P., Kirmss, V., Polan, A.K. and Dick, V.S. (1974): *J. Nat. Cancer Inst., 53,* 335.

Gustafsson, J.A., Ekman, P., Snochowski, M. et al. (1978): *Cancer Res., 38,* 4345.

Gutman, A.B. and Gutman, E.B. (1938): *Proc. Soc. Exp. Biol. (N.Y.), 39,* 529.

Habib, F.K., Lee, I.R., Stitch, S.R. and Smith, P.H. (1976): *J. Endocr., 71,* 99.

Hammond, G.L. (1978): *J. Endocr., 78,* 7.

Huggins, C., Stevens, R.E. and Hodges, C.V. (1941): *Arch. Surg., 43,* 209.

Huggins, C. and Webster, W.O. (1948): *J. Urol., 59,* 258.

Jacobi, G.H., Sinterhauf, K., Kurth, K.H. and Altwein, J.E. (1978): *J. Urol., 119,* 240.

Lieskovsky, G. and Bruchovsky, N. (1979): *J. Urol., 121,* 54.

Levine, R.L. and Wilchinsky, M. (1979): *J. Urol., 121,* 761.

Mahoudeau, J.A., Delassalle, A. and Bricaire, H. (1974): *Acta Endocr. (Kbh.), 77,* 401.

McNeal, J.E. (1968): *Amer. J. Clin. Path., 49,* 347.

McNeal, J.E. (1969): *Cancer, 23,* 24.

Owen, W.L. (1976): *J. Chron. Dis., 29,* 89.

Siiteri, P.K. and Wilson, J.D. (1970): *J. Clin. Invest., 49,* 1737.

Stumpf, H.H. and Wilens, F.C. (1953): *A.M.A. Arch. Intern. Med., 91,* 304.

Vermeulen, A. and Sy, W. (1976): *J. Clin. Endocr., 43,* 1250.
Walsh, P.C. and Wilson, J.D. (1976): *J. Clin. Invest., 57,* 1093.
Wynder, E.L., Mabuchi, K. and Whitmore, W.F., Jr. (1971): *Cancer, 28,* 344.

Plasma testosterone, dihydrotestosterone, androstenedione, 3α- and 3β-androstanediols, free testosterone fraction and sex hormone binding globulin capacity in prostatic adenocarcinoma*

F. SCIARRA[1], C. PIRO[1], V. TOSCANO[1], E. PETRANGELI[1], S. CAIOLA[1], F. DI SILVERIO[2], U. BRACCI[2] and C. CONTI[1]

[1]*Istituto di Clinica Medica Generale V, and* [2]*Clinica Urologica, Università di Roma, Rome, Italy*

If approximately 80% of metastatic adenocarcinomas are androgen dependent and initially responsive to endocrine treatment (Franks, 1974; Bracci, 1975; Di Silverio, 1975) the main problems with which we are faced are the choice of management to reduce androgen production and activity, and the parameters to be considered in assessing the effects of therapy. Androgenic support to prostatic cell growth may be reduced by:

1. bilateral orchidectomy which removes about 95% of plasma testosterone (T) (Walsh, 1975);

2. oestrogen administration, which decreases testicular androgen production by lowering pituitary gonadotropin secretion and directly inhibiting gonadal synthesis of sex hormones (Yanihara and Troen, 1972). Additional effects may be the inhibition of DNA polymerase and 5α-reductase activity in prostatic tissue, and the increase in sex hormone binding globulin (Harper et al., 1970; Shimazaki et al., 1971);

3. administration of compounds such as aminoglutethamide which interferes with the synthesis of steroid androgens and cyproterone acetate (CPA), which reduces gonadotropin secretion and competes with the androgens at target tissue level (Breuer and Hoffmann, 1967; Neumann and Steinbeck, 1974; Walsh, 1975).

Plasma T determination has been used to monitor the effects of treatment, but this parameter is insufficient to accurately reflect the androgen situation to which prostatic carcinoma, in particular, is exposed. It has been suggested in fact, that these tumours are sensitive to other circulating androgens and/or to minimum amounts of testosterone (Young and Kent, 1968; Di Silverio et al., 1970; Robinson and Thomas, 1971; Sciarra et al., 1971, 1973; Shearer et al., 1973; Baker et al., 1975; Bracci et al., 1977).

More sophisticated methods are therefore necessary to assess the response of endocrine treatment which is expected to suppress androgen action.

*This work was supported in part by a Grant from the Consiglio Nazionale delle Ricerche, Rome, Italy.

In the present investigation the following indices were taken into consideration: the binding capacity of sex hormone binding globulin (SHBG), which will influence the amount of the free testosterone fraction (FTF), the evaluation of plasma dihydrotestosterone (DHT) representing the levels of active metabolite in the target tissue, of 5α-androstane-3α,17β-diol and 5α-androstane-3β,17β-diol (3α- and 3β-A-diol) as peripheral conversion products of mainly DHT (Di Silverio et al., 1978). In this regard it is worth mentioning that unexpectedly high endogenous concentrations of DHT and 3α-A-diol have been found by various investigators in prostatic carcinoma (Albert et al., 1976; Farnsworth and Brown, 1976; Geller et al., 1979; Krieg et al., 1979).

Material and methods

Thirty-three untreated patients aged between 52 and 65 years, with stage 3-4 prostatic adenocarcinoma (VACURG classification) were studied.

Eight patients underwent bilateral orchidectomy, 8 were treated with cyproterone acetate (200 mg/day), 9 with diethylstilboestrol (3 mg/day) and 8 were submitted to orchidectomy combined with cyproterone acetate (200 mg/day) administration immediately after operation (Table 1).

Blood samples for hormonal assays were collected before and after 2 months of treatment. In 8 cases androgens were assayed for 6-13 consecutive days, starting immediately after the operation or the beginning of treatment.

TABLE 1.

Histological type and treatment in prostate adenocarcinoma cases studied

Cases	Histological type	Treatment
1	Highly differentiated	Bilateral
5	Moderately differentiated	orchidectomy
2	Poorly differentiated	
4	Highly differentiated	Cyproterone acetate
4	Moderately differentiated	(200 mg/day)
2	Highly differentiated	Diethylstilboestrol
5	Moderately differentiated	(3 mg/day)
2	Poorly differentiated	
1	Highly differentiated	Bilateral
4	Moderately differentiated	orchidectomy
3	Poorly differentiated	+
		Cyproterone acetate
		(200 mg/day)

Plasma T, $\triangle^4$-androstenedione (A), DHT, 3α- and 3β-A-diols were evaluated using a RIA technique after chromatographic separation of the compounds on celite microcolumns (535) using isoctane/benzene at different ratios. The antisera employed for steroid assays were: anti T-3-oxime-BSA for T, anti DHT-3-oxime-BSA for DHT, 3α- and 3β-A-diols, anti A-11-oxime-BSA for 4-androstenedione (Toscano et al., 1980).

The equilibrium dialysis method described by Vermeulen et al. (1971) was used for the determination of FTF and SHBG.

Results reported are the mean of 2 determinations in plasma samples obtained between 8 and 9 a.m.

Results and discussion

Plasma androgen levels in prostatic adenocarcinoma stage 3-4 before treatment

Mean values of T in these patients were 412 ± 84 SD ng/dl, i.e. lower than those found in normal males (Table 2).

In stage 2 prostatic carcinoma, however, T was higher (493 ± 95 SD ng/dl) than in stage 3-4 (412 ± 84 SD ng/dl) and comparable to that of normal elderly men (Young and Kent, 1968; Robinson and Thomas, 1971; Shearer et al., 1973) (Table 2).

In stage 3-4 T values appear to be comparable to those found in other neoplastic diseases (385 ± 121 SD ng/dl); this finding may reflect the state of debilitation of these patients, as also observed by Young and Kent (1968).

In prostatic carcinoma stage 3-4, moreover, SHBG is more elevated (5.9 ± 0.18 x 10^{-8} M) than in young controls and comparable to that of normal subjects after 50 years (Table 2) in agreement with the findings of Vermeulen et al. (1974) and Klosterhalfen et al. (1975). Consequently the percent of free T (1.90 ± 0.2) the active fraction of total T, is decreased (Table 2) and less DHT (35 ± 9.6 SD ng/dl) is found in the peripheral

TABLE 2.

Hormonal pattern and SHBG capacity in stage 3-4 prostatic adenocarcinoma before treatment (Mean ± S.D.)

	Controls (n 12) (18-25 yrs)	Controls (n 10) (50-70 yrs)	Prostatic carcinoma (n 33) (stage 3-4)
T (ng/dl)	765 ± 186	498 ± 145	412 ± 84
SHBG (x10^{-8} M)	3.5 ± 0.7	5.1 ± 0.18	5.9 ± 0.18
FTF (% total T)	2.53 ± 0.51	2.18 ± 0.2	1.9 ± 0.2
DHT (ng/dl)	45.6 ± 13.5	—	35 ± 9.6
3α-A-diol (ng/dl)	28.7 ± 8.6	17.5 ± 8.3	15.4 ± 6.7
3β-A-diol (ng/dl)	54.9 ± 29	30.6 ± 9.5	6.2 ± 2.2
$\triangle^4$-androstenedione (ng/dl)	116 ± 28	131 ± 38	128 ± 32

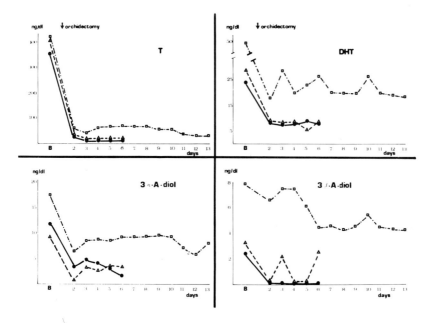

Fig. 1. Effects of orchidectomy on plasma androgens and SHBG during immediate postoperative period.

circulation. Similarly the 3α- and the 3β-A-diols show a reduction (15.4 ± 6.7 SD and 6.2 ± 2.2 SD ng/dl, respectively) following the DHT pattern (Table 2).

In conclusion the values of these parameters in patients with advanced prostatic adenocarcinoma are almost comparable to those of normal elderly male subjects and are of no prognostic significance or aid in the diagnosis of this neoplasia.

Effects of orchidectomy

With bilateral orchidectomy the principal source of androgens is removed and a dramatic fall has been observed in their blood concentration (Young and Kent, 1968; Di Silverio et al., 1970; Robinson and Thomas, 1971; Vermeulen et al., 1971; Sciarra et al., 1973; Shearer et al., 1973; Bracci, 1975; Bracci et al., 1977; Di Silverio et al., 1978).

In general T, DHT, 3α- and 3β-A-diols values were very low or even undetectable in the immediate post-orchidectomy days. In 1 case, however, levels remained higher than those in the other 2 cases, suggesting that the adrenal cortex may be responsible for the production of compounds, transformed peripherally into active metabolites (Fig. 1).

Measurements repeated 2 months later, confirmed the marked reduction

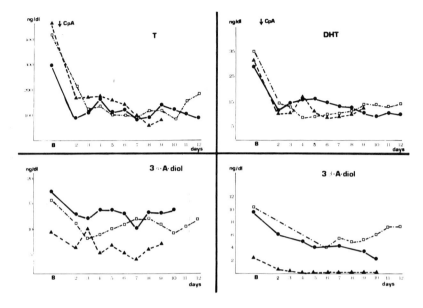

Fig. 2. Effects of cyproterone acetate (CPA) administration on plasma androgens and SHBG during days immediately after beginning of treatment.

of T, DHT and A-diols, which had reached very low values even in the patient presenting a minor reduction immediately post-castration (Table 3).

SHBG was markedly increased and FTF concomitantly decreased. A, on the contrary, showed a less marked reduction, as it was consistently produced by the adrenal cortex.

It can therefore be concluded that bilateral orchidectomy removes most of the circulating androgens, especially those with strong biological activity. Weak androgens continue to be secreted, however, by the adrenal cortex, providing substrates for the peripheral formation of active compounds such as DHT.

Effects of cyproterone acetate

Administration of 200 mg/day of CPA to non-orchidectomized patients, causes a significant decrease in plasma T (Sciarra et al., 1971; Bracci et al., (1977), DHT and 3α-,3β-A-diol (Di Silverio et al., 1978) values which however were still higher, during the days immediately after the beginning of the treatment, than those observed after orchidectomy (Fig. 2).

Two months later these androgens were still present in appreciable amounts in the peripheral circulation, especially A, which was only slightly decreased during CPA treatment. SHBG, on the other hand, increased moderately, values being lower than those found after orchidectomy.

TABLE 3.

Hormonal pattern and SHBG capacity in stage 3-4 prostatic adenocarcinoma 2 months after orchidectomy (Mean ± S.D.)

	Prostatic carcinoma (n 8)	
	pre-treatment	2 months after orchidectomy
T (ng/dl)	412 ± 84	16 ± 1.6
SHBG ($\times 10^{-8}$ M)	5.9 ± 0.18	8.8 ± 1.4
FTF (% total T)	1.9 ± 0.2	0.8 ± 0.06
DHT (ng/dl)	30 ± 12	5.4 ± 0.8
3α-A-diol (ng/dl)	14.6 ± 6.9	4.7 ± 1.7
3β-A-diol (ng/dl)	5.5 ± 3.5	1.26 ± 0.6
Δ^4-androstenedione (ng/dl)	128 ± 32	87 ± 10

TABLE 4.

Hormonal pattern and SHBG capacity in stage 3-4 prostatic adenocarcinoma after 2 months cyproterone acetate (CPA) administration (200 mg/day) (Mean ± S.D.)

	Prostatic carcinoma (n 8)	
	pre-treatment	2 months CPA
T (ng/dl)	447 ± 110	148 ± 73
SHBG ($\times 10^{-8}$ M)	5.6 ± 0.2	7.3 ± 0.9
FTF (% total T)	1.8 ± 0.25	1.5 ± 0.2
DHT (ng/dl)	34 ± 5.6	17.6 ± 6
3α-A-diol (ng/dl)	15.7 ± 7.5	7.7 ± 2.8
3β-A-diol (ng/dl)	12.8 ± 5.5	5.2 ± 4.3
Δ^4-androstenedione (ng/dl)	125 ± 25	106 ± 7

Consequently, FTF and DHT were higher than in castrated patients and the 3α- and 3β-A-diols showed a slight reduction (Table 4).

CPA is not therefore effective as gestagen in terms of its capacity to suppress androgen levels, but may still inhibit the activity, at prostatic cell level, of the metabolites still present in the peripheral circulation.

Effects of diethylstilboestrol

The response to diethylstilboestrol treatment (3 mg/day) was characterized by a significant decrease in T and DHT values, which were lower than those observed after CPA therapy, but higher than those post-orchidectomy

TABLE 5.

Hormonal pattern and SHBG capacity in stage 3-4 prostatic adenocarcinoma after 2 months diethylstilboestrol administration (3 mg/day) (Mean ± S.D.)

	Prostatic carcinoma (n 9)	
	pre-treatment	2 months diethylstilboestrol
T (ng/dl)	430 ± 98	99 ± 28
SHBG (×10^{-8} M)	5.5 ± 0.22	22 ± 2.5
FTF (% total T)	2.1 ± 0.3	0.62 ± 0.3
DHT (ng/dl)	38.5 ± 9.5	11 ± 3.5

TABLE 6.

Hormonal pattern and SHBG capacity in stage 3-4 prostatic adenocarcinoma 2 months after orchidectomy associated with cyproterone acetate (CPA) administration (200 mg/ day) (Mean ± S.D.)

	Prostatic carcinoma (n 8)	
	pre-treatment	2 months after orchidectomy + CPA
T (ng/dl)	443 ± 95	18.8 ± 8
SHBG (×10^{-8} M)	6.0 ± 0.17	9.1 ± 1
FTF (% total T)	1.82 ± 0.18	0.8 ± 0.06
DHT (ng/dl)	40 ± 11	7.9 ± 3
3α-A-diol (ng/dl)	15.9 ± 5.9	1.6 ± 1.02

(Sciarra et al., 1971). SHBG, however, showed the maximal elevation so that FTF fell to values below those observed following the other forms of treatment and is therefore available only in minor amounts for trans-formation into DHT, which was likewise decreased (Vermeulen et al., 1969; Klosterhalfen et al., 1975) (Table 5).

This form of treatment, therefore, inducing a consistent reduction of androgenic activity without the mutilation of orchidectomy, could be the treatment of choice. A serious limitation which cannot, however, be overlooked is the frequent occurrence of cardiovascular side effects, which has been the cause of death in many patients (Baker et al., 1975; Bracci, 1975).

Effects of orchidectomy associated with cyproterone acetate

According to Bracci and Di Silverio (Bracci, 1975; Di Silverio, 1975; Bracci

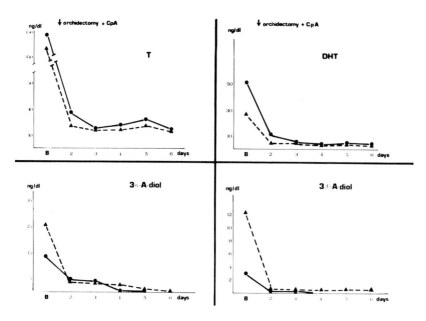

Fig. 3. Effects of orchidectomy associated with cyproterone acetate administration (CPA) on plasma androgens and SHBG during immediate postoperative period.

et al., 1977) the best management for advanced prostatic adenocarcinoma is orchidectomy, in combination with administration of CPA. This treatment results in a maximal decrease in androgen production and an inhibition of the action, at target tissue level, of the small amounts of active androgens derived from the peripheral transformation of adrenal metabolites.

Furthermore, CPA does not present those complications observed during oestrogen treatment.

T, DHT, 3α- and 3β-A-diol levels in our patients thus treated showed a dramatic fall during the immediate postoperative period (Fig. 3) and were still low 2 months later (Table 6).

SHBG was markedly increased and consequently FTF decreased associated with a marked reduction in DHT. The values of these parameters were almost comparable to those found after castration alone.

Conclusions

It is not possible, on account of the small number of patients studied and the short period of observation, to draw definite conclusions from the present investigation.

Nevertheless, it is worthwhile stressing that the hormone pattern before treatment in patients with stage 3-4 prostatic adenocarcinoma shows no correlation with the histologic type of the tumour, and is very similar to that of elderly normal males.

Evaluations of these parameters after the various forms of endocrine treatment, provide sufficient information to assess the residual androgenic situation.

On the basis of these data, bilateral orchidectomy appears to be the most valuable treatment in advanced prostatic adenocarcinoma, in terms of reducing androgen production. CPA might then be administered in order to inhibit the effects of androgens of adrenal origin.

At present, 1 year after orchidectomy, or orchidectomy plus CPA treatment, only 2 patients show a deterioration in local and general conditions, although plasma androgens remained very low or undetectable. The histological type of the 2 carcinomas, however, was poorly differentiated. The remaining patients are all in satisfactory clinical conditions, even those treated for almost 6 months with CPA alone.

Only longitudinal follow-up will indicate the practical usefulness to monitor the effects of endocrine treatment of metastatic prostate adenocarcinoma by determining circulating androgens, such as DHT and androstanediols, which represent the products of the general and not the local metabolism at prostatic level.

More information can possibly be obtained by measuring simultaneously DHT and 3α- and 3β-androstenediols in the peripheral circulation and tumour tissue as suggested by Geller et al. (1979).

References

Albert, J., Geller, J., Geller, S. and Lopez, D. (1976): *J. Steroid Biochem., 7*, 301.

Baker, H.W.G., Burger, H.G., De Kretser, D.M., Hudson, B., Rennie, G.C. and Straffon, W.G. (1975): *J. Urol., 113*, 824.

Bracci, U. (1975): In: *Hormonal Therapy of Prostatic Cancer*, p. 177. Editors: U. Bracci and F. Di Silverio. Cofese, Palermo, Italy.

Bracci, U., Di Silverio, F., Sciarra, F., Sorcini, G., Piro, C. and Santoro, F. (1977): *Brit. J. Urol., 49*, 161.

Breuer, H. and Hoffmann, W. (1967): *Naturwissenschaften, 54*, 616.

Di Silverio, F. (1975): In: *Hormonal Therapy of Prostatic Cancer*, p. 47. Editors: U. Bracci and F. Di Silverio. Cofese, Palermo, Italy.

Di Silverio, F., Gagliardi, V., Sorcini, G. and Sciarra, F. (1970): *Boll. Soc. Centro-Merid. Isole, 7*, 196.

Di Silverio, F., Sciarra, F., Piro, C., Toscano, V., Amicarelli, A. and Bracci, U. (1978): In: *Proceedings Italian Society of Urology.* p. 1. Editor: C. Corbi.

Farnsworth, W.E. and Brown, J.R. (1976): *Endocr. Res. Commun., 3*, 105.

Franks, L.M. (1974): In: *Treatment of Prostatic Hypertrophy and Neoplasia*, p. 1. MTP Medical and Technical Publ., Lancaster, U.K.

Geller, J., Albert, J. and Loza, D. (1979): *J. Steroid Biochem., 11, 1B*, 631.

Harper, M.E., Fahmy, A.R. and Pierrepoint, C.G. (1970): *Steroids, 15*, 89.

Klosterhalfen, H., Becker, H. and Burchardt, P. (1975): In: *Hormonal Therapy of*

Prostatic Cancer, p. 193. Editors: U. Bracci and F. Di Silverio. Cofese, Palermo, Italy.
Krieg, M., Bartsch, W., Janssen, W. and Voigt, K.D. (1979): *J. Steroid Biochem., 11, 1B,* 615.
Neumann, F. and Steinbeck, H. (1974): In: *Handbook of Experimental Pharmacology,* p. 235. Editors: O. Eichler, A. Farah, H. Herken and A.D. Welch. Springer, Berlin-Heidelberg-New York.
Robinson, M.R.G. and Thomas, B.S. (1971): *Brit. Med. J., 4,* 391.
Sciarra, F., Sorcini, G., Di Silverio, F. and Gagliardi, V. (1971): *J. Steroid Biochem., 2,* 313.
Sciarra, F., Sorcini, G., Di Silverio, F. and Gagliardi, V. (1973): *Clin. Endocr., 2,* 110.
Shearer, R.J., Hendry, W.F., Sommerville, I.F. and Fergusson, J.D. (1973): *Brit. J. Urol., 45,* 668.
Shimazaki, J., Horaguchi, T. and Ohki, Y. (1971): *Endocr. Jap., 18,* 179.
Toscano, V., Petrangeli, E., Adamo, M.V., Foli, S. and Caiola, S. (1980): *J. Endocrinol. Invest., 3, Suppl. 1,* 112.
Vermeulen, A., Rubens, R. and Verdonck, L. (1974): *J. Clin. Endocr., 34,* 730.
Vermeulen, A., Stoica, T. and Verdonck, L. (1971): *J. Clin. Endocr., 33,* 759.
Vermeulen, A., Verdonck, L., Van der Straeten, M. and Orie, N. (1969): *J. Clin. Endocr., 29,* 1470.
Walsh, P.C. (1975): *Urol. Clin. N. Amer., 2,* 125.
Yanihara, T. and Troen, P. (1972): *J. Clin. Endocr., 34,* 968.
Young, H.H. and Kent, J.R. (1968): *J. Urol., 99,* 788.

Characterization of a transplantable androgen-dependent human prostatic carcinoma (PC 82)

J.C. ROMIJN, G.J. VAN STEENBRUGGE, K. OISHI, J. BOLT-DE VRIES, W. HÖHN* and F.H. SCHRÖDER

Department of Urology, Erasmus University, Rotterdam, The Netherlands

At present, our knowledge of the biological behavior of prostatic cancer is still incomplete. The experimental approach to this problem has been hindered by a lack of suitable model systems. In the last few years, however, experimental model systems of animal origin have been developed (Pollard and Luckert, 1975; Noble, 1977; Smolev et al., 1977). In this paper the establishment and characterization of a model system of human origin will be described.

Establishment of the PC 82 tumor line

The tumor line, PC 82, was established in July 1977 from a prostatic tumor that was removed by total perineal prostatectomy. Small pieces of tumor tissue were transplanted subcutaneously on nude mice. After about 8 weeks slowly growing tumor nodules became apparent in the male recipients. Since then, the tumor line has been maintained by serial transplantation. In 70-80% of the male mice tumor nodules appear within 2 months after transplantation of small pieces (about 50 mg) of tumor tissue. The nodules consist of soft masses that are well supplied by blood from the host. Metastases into regional lymphnodes or into other organs have never been observed.

Histological observations

The original tumor was classified as a moderately differentiated adeno-carcinoma of the prostate (Fig. 1). The histology of the PC 82 tumor (Fig. 2) shows a cribriform pattern with relatively little stroma between the acini; the appearance is still similar to that of the original tumor. The histology of tumor tissue from subsequent mouse passages did not reveal any change until now.

*Present address: Urologische Klinik, Universität Erlangen, D8520 Erlangen, F.R.G.

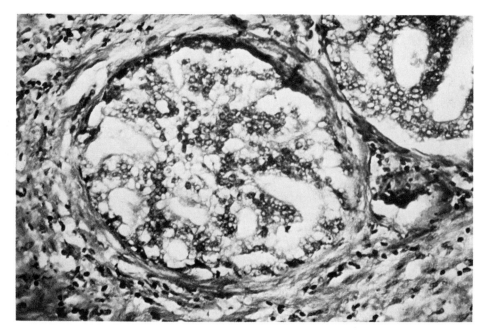

Fig. 1. Original histology of the prostatic carcinoma PC 82.

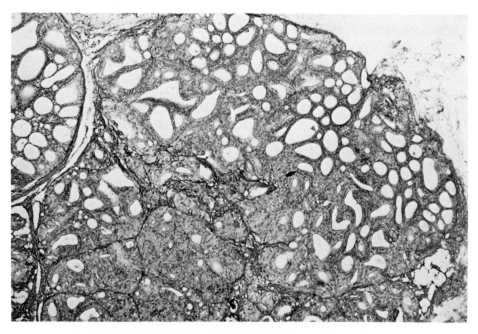

Fig. 2. Histology of a PC 82 tumor of the seventh mouse passage.

TABLE 1.

Take rate in male and female nude mice

	No.of takes	%
Females	0/24	0
Males	30/46	65

Tumor tissue of the 7th mouse passage was used. All mice received two transplants, on the right and the left shoulder. Only mice that survived more than 8 weeks after transplantation were scored.

Hormone dependence

The original tumor tissue was transplanted onto 4 male and 2 female nude mice. In the females the xenografts were resorbed completely within a few weeks. In the males however, slowly growing nodules appeared after 8 weeks. In the seventh mouse passage a group of female mice was included once more. As shown in Table 1, none out of 24 transplants (12 mice, bilaterally) in females grew, whereas the success rate for transplants from the ṣame tumor tissue in males showed the usual percentage of takes (65%).

In another experiment, male mice carrying a tumor have been castrated. In this case the tumor immediately stopped growing and a considerable reduction of tumor size was observed after some time (90% reduction after 2-3 weeks).

Preliminary experiments have shown that androgen receptors, measured by an exchange assay using ^{3}H-labeled dihydrotestosterone with a nuclear preparation, are present in PC 82 tumor tissue. The amount of receptor was estimated to be at least 1500 molecules per nucleus.

Growth rate

Human prostatic carcinoma is a relatively slow growing tumor. The growth rate of the PC 82 tumor has been studied by caliper measurements of the tumor dimensions. A parameter for the tumor volume was calculated from:

$$I_v = (d_1 \times d_2)^{3/2},$$

where d_1 and d_2 represent the smallest and largest diameter respectively. It is shown in Figure 3 that, after an exponential phase the growth rate gradually slows down with increasing tumor size. Eventually the growth may stop completely. In such big tumors some fluid is present in the center of the tumor which contains necrotic elements and secretory products. It will be clear that (comparative) growth rate measurements in terms of doubling times can be performed only during the exponential phase, i.e. in tumors with an average diameter of less than 1 cm (I_v = 1000). Figure 4 shows a representative growth curve. The doubling time calculated from such curves is 18 ± 5 days (mean ± Ṡ.D.; n = 20).

Biochemical properties

By an immunohistochemical technique it has been shown that human prostate-specific acid phosphatase is present in large amounts in the original tumor as well as in PC 82 tumor tissue (Höhn, Jöbsis and Schröder, to be published). Acid phosphatase in mouse serum has been estimated by a (standard) biochemical assay (Table 2). In tumor-bearing mice the serum level of acid phosphatase was elevated, especially in the mice with very large tumors (mouse numbers 7 and 8). The fluid recovered from the center of very large tumors did contain extremely high levels of acid phosphatase (Table 2). Most of the elevated enzyme activity was inhibited by tartrate.

The activity of lactate dehydrogenase (LDH) was slightly, but not significantly, increased in serum from tumor-bearing mice. Analysis of the isoenzyme composition was carried out by means of gel electrophoresis. Because of the different electrophoretic mobility of the mouse and the human isoenzymes (especially those containing the A-subunit), some human isoenzymes (LDH-4 and LDH-5) can be separated from the other isoenzymes

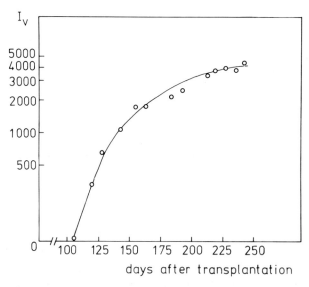

Fig. 3.   Growth curve of PC 82 tumor in a male nude mouse (5th mouse passage). I_v is a parameter for the tumor volume: I_v = 1000 corresponds to a tumor with an average diameter of 1 cm.

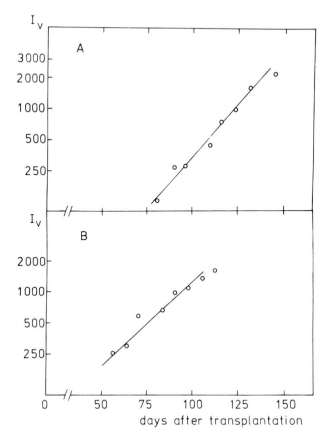

Fig. 4. Representative growth curves of PC 82 in male nude mice.
(a) 5th mouse passage (calculated doubling time 15 days);
(b) 7th mouse passage (calculated doubling time 19 days).

as well as from the corresponding mouse isoenzymes. By this method the presence of human LDH-5 in the serum from a PC 82 tumor-bearing mouse could be clearly demonstrated. In PC 82 tumor extracts human LDH-5 was the predominant isoenzyme.

Conclusion

The results described indicate that the PC 82 tumor line has retained several important properties of the human prostatic carcinoma. This includes the histological characteristics and a relatively slow growth rate. Androgen dependence of the PC 82 tumor line is demonstrated by the lack of growth in female subjects and the regression after castration. To our knowledge,

TABLE 2.

Acid phosphatase levels in mouse serum and in tumor fluid

Sample	Total acid phosphatase	Tartrate-inhibited acid phosphatase
	(IU/l)	(IU/l)
Control (n = 10)	0.9 ± 0.6	0.2 ± 0.2
1	1.6	0.2
2	1.4	0.7
3	2.9	1.6
4	3.9	3.1
5	7.4	3.9
6	12.2	10.6
7	29.1	17.1
8	31.5	27.2
TF 1	17600	15500
TF 2	124000	108000
TF 3	46000	40000

Enzyme levels were measured in sera from nude mice without tumors (control) and nude mice with PC 82 tumor (Nos. 1-8). Left column: levels inhibited by 0.1 M tartrate. The tartrate-labile fraction might be indicative for prostate specific acid phosphatase. TF 1-3: tumor fluid.

only one other prostatic tumor line with more or less similar properties has been described until now (Reid and Shin, 1978). The results from the biochemical studies indicate the functional activity and prove the human origin of the PC 82 tumor line. Therefore we conclude that this tumor line is an appropriate model system for further studies on prostatic carcinoma, e.g. on the response to hormonal manipulations and chemotherapeutic treatment.

References

Noble, R. (1977): *Cancer Res., 37,* 1929.
Pollard, M. and Luckert, P.H. (1975): *J. Nat. Cancer Inst., 54,* 643.
Reid, L.C.M. and Shin, S. (1978): In: *The Nude Mouse in Experimental and Clinical Research,* Chapter 15, p. 313. Editors: J. Fogh and B.C. Giovanella. Academic Press, New York.
Smolev, J.K., Heston, W.D.W., Scott, W.W. and Coffey, D.S. (1977): *Cancer Treatm. Rep., 61,* 273.

In vitro metabolism of androgens by rat prostate*

J.-C. PLASSE[1], A. REVOL[1] and B.P. LISBOA[2]

[1] *Hospices Civils de Lyon, Hôpital Jules Courmont-Sainte Eugénie, Saint Genis Laval, France;* [2] *Universitäts-Frauenklinik Eppendorf, Hamburg, F.R.G.*

Since the early experiments showing the important role of 5α-dihydro-testosterone in the metabolism of testosterone by prostate, numerous metabolites of testosterone have been characterized in vivo or in vitro in this organ. The aim of the present study was to investigate the interconversion of some physiological androgenic steroids by rat prostate.

Material and methods

Incubation

Ventral rat prostates were obtained from 200-300 g Sprague-Dawley rats. A 10% (w/v) homogenate was prepared in Krebs-Ringer-Tris-HCl buffer (pH 7.4). Twenty five μCi corresponding to 200 μg of testosterone, androstenedione, 5α-androstanedione, 5α-androstane-3α,17β-diol, 5α-androstane-3β,17β-diol, androsterone and epiandrosterone were separately incubated with a portion of the prostate homogenate corresponding to 1 g fresh tissue, in a medium supplemented with 0.2 μmol manganese, 0.2 mmol magnesium, 2 mmol nicotinamide and a NADPH regenerating system (0.2 mmol isocitrate, 28 I.U. isocitrate dehydrogenase, 8 μmol NADP). Incubations were run for 1.5 hr at 38°C under air.

Extraction

Extraction of incubated steroids and metabolites was provided by means of XAD 2 column chromatography. Separation of steroids was obtained through liquid chromatography on Sephadex LH 20 developed with a heptane-chloroform-methanol (85:11:4, v:v) solvent mixture, and monitored by the elution of radioactive standards.

Identification

Identifications and evaluations were done after preparing TMSi derivatives of

*This work was supported by the DFG (SFB-34 Endokrinologie).

TABLE 1.

Results of metabolic transformations obtained after incubations of rat prostate homogenate with selected steroids (Results expressed as nmol of substrate transformed per min and g of fresh tissue)

Incubated steroids	Metabolites								
	T	A_4-dione	dHT	A-dione	A	epiA	A-3α,17β	A-3β,17β	Polar compounds
T (testosterone)		0.60	0.71				0.18	0.08	0.5
A_4-dione (androstenedione)	0.14		0.02	1.30	0.30	0.04	0.02	0.01	0.03
dHT (5α-dihydrotestosterone)				0.08	0.02		2.16	0.25	0.41
A-dione (5α-androstanedione)			0.04		3.07	0.09	0.09	0.01	0.25
A (androsterone)			0.06	3.29		0.09	0.08	0.01	0.10
epiA (epiandrosterone)								0.06	
A-3α,17β (5α-androstane-3α,17β-diol)			2.95	0.07	0.04			0.03	0.32
A-3β,17β (5α-androstane-3β,17β-diol)			0.08				0.01		0.32

the steroids by radiogaschromatography on 2 columns coated with SE 30 or QF 1.

Results and discussion

Results of biochemical transformations expressed in nanomoles of substrate transformed per min and per g of fresh tissue are included in Table 1.

5α-Reductase activity

5α-Reductase can transform both testosterone and androstenedione into 5α-reduced metabolites. Under our experimental conditions this enzyme appears more active with androstenedione than testosterone (0.97 nmol of testosterone 5α-metabolites and 1.65 nmol of androstenedione 5α-metabolites) as substrates.

17β-Hydroxysteroid dehydrogenase

Unsaturated steroids e.g. testosterone and androstenedione are transformed to a larger extent. Oxidation of testosterone at C-17 in rat prostate seems quantitatively more important than the 17β-hydroxy-reduction of androstenedione (0.6 nmol of androstenedione from testosterone and 0.14 nmol of testosterone from androstenedione). When comparing oxidative and reductive pathways of testosterone it should be pointed out that the rates of reductive and oxidative pathways are similar; the latter may play a role in the regulation of testosterone metabolism in prostate. In contrast, 17β-hydroxysteroid dehydrogenase exhibits a very weak affinity towards 5α-reduced metabolites of both testosterone and androstenedione. However, relationships between the formation of 17-oxo and 17β-hydroxysteroids exist for 3α- and/or 3β-hydroxymetabolites. Enzymic reactions tend to result in the formation of the 'active' derivatives of androgens: 17β-hydroxy metabolites.

3α-Hydroxysteroid dehydrogenase

5α-Reduced metabolites are good substrates for 3α-hydroxysteroid dehydrogenase. In the 17-oxo pathway there is complete equilibrium between androsterone and 5α-androstanedione, both compounds showing poor androgenic activity. In the 17β-hydroxy pathway the rates of oxidation and reduction for the interconversion between 5α-dihydrotestosterone and 5α-androstane-3α,17β-diol are different. Equilibrium between the 3-oxo and 3α-hydroxy forms tends to favour the formation of 5α-dihydrotestosterone. Our results confirm those of Malathi and Gurpide (1977) who considered

TABLE 2.

'In vitro' metabolic pathway of testosterone in rat prostate

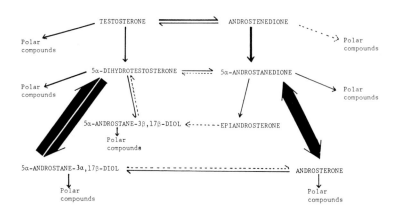

5α-androstane-3α,17β-diol in human prostate as a terminal metabolite in direct enzymic equilibrium with 5α-dihydrotestosterone. As a consequence of the rapid conversion of 5α-androstane-3α,17β-diol into 5α-dihydro-testosterone, the former compound could act as a source of substrate for the latter.

3β-Hydroxysteroid dehydrogenase

In both pathways, 17-oxo or 17β-hydroxy, 3β-hydroxysteroid dehydro-genase causes the formation of 3β-hydroxy metabolites. The very weak re-verse conversion of 5α-androstane-3β,17β-diol into 5α-dihydrotestosterone de-monstrates the importance of 3β-androstanediol which is probably one of the active forms of testosterone in the prostate. Recently, further metabolism of 5α-androstane-3β,17β-diol in the prostate has been shown in man: 7α-hydroxy derivatives have been characterized (Morfin et al., 1979). The possible importance of these 7α-hydroxy derivatives in the prostate remains uncertain.

Hydroxylase activities

Earlier experiments demonstrated the presence of 6β- and 6α-hydroxylase activities in rat prostate (Plasse et al., 1971; Plasse and Lisboa, 1974). Most of the hydroxylated derivatives of testosterone and androstenedione are well known and can be characterized by radiogaschromatography. On the other hand, it is more difficult by the same method, to identify the numerous hydroxylated metabolites of 5α-reduced compounds. Hydroxylated compounds were found in all incubations. The conversion ratio of the incubated steroid is higher in the 17β-hydroxy pathway than in the 17-oxo pathway. The results are given in Table 1. We were able to quantify 6β-hydroxylase only in the testosterone incubation: 0.34 nmol of testosterone can be converted per min and g of tissue. In vitro and quantitatively, this transformation represents a major pathway besides the oxidative and reductive pathways of testosterone.

On the basis of these results pathways of testosterone metabolism in rat prostate in in vitro experiments are summarized in Table 2.

In conclusion, the metabolism of testosterone results in the biosynthesis of at least 2 active compounds (5∝-dihydrotestosterone and 5∝-androstane-3β,17β-diol) both of the 17β-hydroxy pathway. 17-Oxo derivatives with weak physiological activity probably play a regulatory role in the biosynthesis of active forms. In vitro studies of enzymic equilibria can provide useful information concerning the potential pathways for in vivo biosynthesis or metabolism of steroids.

References

Malathi, K. and Gurpide, E. (1977): *J. Steroid Biochem.*, *8*, 141.
Morfin, R.F., Charles, J.-F. and Floch, H.H. (1979): *J. Steroid Biochem.*, *11*, 599.
Plasse, J.-C., Gustafsson, J.-Å. and Lisboa, B.P. (1971): *Steroidologia, 2*, 193.
Plasse, J.-C. and Lisboa, B.P. (1974): *Acta Endocr. (Kbh.), Suppl., 184*, 153.

Role of mesenchyme in the early cytodifferentiation of human prostate

P. KELLOKUMPU-LEHTINEN, R. SANTTI and L.J. PELLINIEMI

Department of Anatomy and Laboratory of Electron Microscopy, University of Turku, Turku, Finland

Light microscopic studies have shown that human prostate develops as a derivative of the urogenital sinus close to the openings of the mesonephric ducts (Lowsley, 1912). The glands constituting the prostate appear as epithelial buds growing from the sinus wall into the surrounding mesenchyme. The buds grow into solid, branching cords, which start to develop a lumen and are thus transformed into tubules and alveoli. The lack of the male accessory sex organs in patients with androgen insensitivity implies an essential role of androgens in the prostatic development of man.

The development of the prostate in rodents involves precisely timed epithelio-mesenchymal interactions. Findings on sex reversed mice heterozygous for testicular feminization (Ohno, 1977) and the cultures of epithelio-mesenchymal recombinations (Cunha and Lung, 1979) have revealed that androgens act on mesenchyme, and that the mesenchyme may be the main determinant in the embryonic development of the prostate. In agreement with these experimental findings, a defect in stromal-epithelial interaction has been postulated to be responsible for prostatic maldevelopment in the prune belly syndrome (DeKlerk and Scott, 1978) and the lack of growth capacity of adult human prostate epithelium mechanically separated from its stroma (Franks, 1970). The occurrence of an active 5α-reductase in human prostatic stroma might also be taken as evidence that this tissue has the capacity to respond to androgens (Cowan et al., 1977).

The aim of the present study was to examine the ultrastructure of the developing prostate in man with special attention to morphological signs of epithelio-mesenchymal interactions. The changes in the epithelium and adjacent mesenchyme of the urogenital sinus were examined and correlated with the cytodifferentiation of testicular Leydig cells in the same individuals.

Material and methods

Male embryos, aged 6 to 15 weeks, were obtained from legal abortions. The ages were determined from foot-length or crown-rump length according to Streeter (1920). The fixative contained 0.24 mol/1 glutaraldehyde and 4.1

mmol/l CaCl₂ in 0.1 mol/l sodium cacodylate-HCl buffer, pH 7.4. Tissue samples were postfixed in 39 mmol/l osmium tetroxide in 0.2 mol/l s-collidine-HCl buffer, pH 7.4. Sections were stained with uranyl acetate and lead citrate.

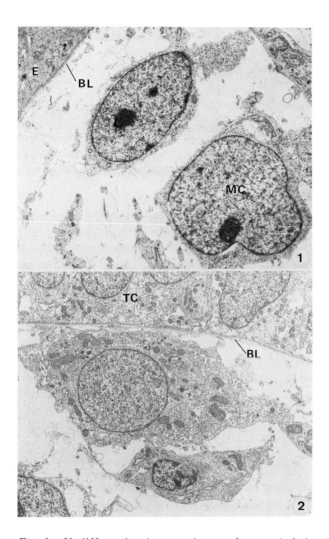

Fig. 1. Undifferentiated mesenchyme of urogenital sinus wall (6-week-old embryo). E, epithelium; BL, basal lamina; MC, mesenchymal cell. x 4000 (Reproduced from Kellokumpu-Lehtinen et al., 1979, by courtesy of the Editors of the *Anatomical Record.*)

Fig. 2. Primitive Leydig cell (6-week-old embryo) lying close to basal lamina (BL) of testicular cord (TC). Note agranular endoplasmic reticulum in cytoplasm. x 3400 (From Kellokumpu-Lehtinen et al., 1979).

Results and discussion

The mesenchyme adjacent to the epithelium of the urogenital sinus is loose and composed of roundish primitive cells in the region into which the mesonephric and paramesonephric ducts open in the 6- and 7-week-old male embryos (Fig. 1). Primitive, round to ovoid Leydig cells are seen in the developing testes at this age (Fig. 2). In the 9th week the cellular density of the mesenchyme increases, and the cells develop into elongated fibroblastic cells with markedly increased granular èndoplasmic reticulum (Fig. 3). These changes indicate increased synthetic activity of the cells which is confirmed by the accumulation of collagen fibers in the intercellular space. In several places the mesenchymal cells have cytoplasmic processes in close contact with the continuous basal lamina. The mesenchymal changes implying incipient prostatic development correlate with the Leydig cell differentiation. Leydig cells grow large and their number increases. Their cytoplasm is closely packed with agranular endoplasmic reticulum (Fig. 4). Ultrastructurally they have the characteristics of the steroid-secreting cells. The temporal relationship between the cytodifferentiation of Leydig cells and mesenchymal cells of the urogenital sinus is consistent with the hypothesis that fetal androgens induce the prostatic development also in man. The epithelial cells of the urogenital sinus have a primitive appearance and do not achieve morphological characteristics of secretory prostatic cells at this developmental stage. The differentiation of the mesenchyme before the epithelial outgrowth suggests that the mesenchyme has an important role in the cell proliferation accounting for the glandular morphogenesis.

Light microscopic development of the prostatic glands begins in the tenth developmental week by formation of several outgrowths of the epithelium into the surrounding condensed mesenchyme. By the end of the 11th week a lumen appears in the terminal portion of some solid cellular cords completing the acinar structure for the first time. The epithelium of these primitive glands consists of 3 to 5 cell layers. Most of the epithelial cells are round and apolar. Between the 11th and 16th weeks a few luminal cells become structurally polarized and columnar with a round nucleus in the middle of the cell, and a supranuclear Golgi complex (Fig. 5). The appearance of apical cytoplasmic granules with electron dense or flocculent content and similar material in the lumen implies incipient secretory activity (Fig. 6). Even though some of the epithelial cells have signs of secretory activity, most of them are less differentiated and resemble the basal cells in normal adult prostate and prostatic carcinoma cells. In a few glands the basal lamina is discontinuous, and there epithelial cells grow into the mesenchyme and contact the underlying mesenchymal cells (Fig. 7). Junctional specializations of the cell membrane to maintain close cell to cell contact on the respective cell boundaries are not seen. The direct epithelio-mesenchymal contacts seen in association with the polarization of the epithelial cells and the appearance of secretory activity suggest that the mesenchyme could regulate epithelial differentiation into secretory cells. Similar findings have been made by Cutler (1977) in the developing salivary gland, where the epithelio-mesenchymal contacts appear after the establishment of the morphogenetic branching patterns, but prior to the functional differentiation. Close cellular contacts between the epithelium and mesenchyme are also necessary for the

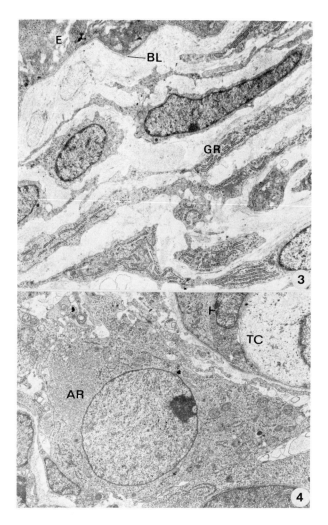

Fig. 3. Elongated mesenchymal cells (9-week-old fetus) with abundant granular endoplasmic reticulum (GR). E, epithelium; BL, basal lamina. x 3900 (From Kellokumpu-Lehtinen et al., 1979).

Fig. 4. Ultrastructure of Leydig cell (9-week-old fetus). Amount of agranular endoplasmic reticulum (AR) markedly increased. TC, testicular cord. x 3500 (From Kellokumpu-Lehtinen et al., 1979).

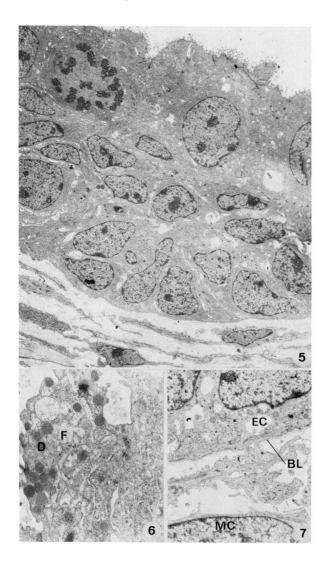

Fig. 5. Electron micrograph of acinar epithelium with apical columnar cells and basal triangular cells and mesenchyme of developing prostate gland (15-week-old fetus). x 3700 (From Kellokumpu-Lehtinen et al., 1980).

Fig. 6. Secretory granules with electron dense (D) or flocculent (F) content in apical portion of epithelial cell (13-week-old fetus). x 8100 (From Kellokumpu-Lehtinen et al., 1980).

Fig. 7. Basal lamina (BL) with gap through which epithelial cells (EC) are growing to make close contact with mesenchymal cell (MC) (15-week-old fetus). x 5200 (From Kellokumpu-Lehtinen et al., 1980).

tubulo-morphogenesis of the kidney (Wartiovaara et al., 1974). These findings lead us to hypothesize that stromal influences on the proliferation and differentiation of the epithelial cells continue throughout life and play an important role both in normal and pathological prostatic growth.

References

Cowan, R.A., Cowan, S.K., Grant, J.K. and Elder, H.Y. (1977): *J. Endocr., 74*, 111.
Cunha, G.R. and Lung, B. (1979): *In Vitro, 15*, 50.
Cutler, L.S. (1977): *J. Embryol. Exp. Morphol., 39*, 71.
DeKlerk, D.P. and Scott, W.W. (1978): *J. Urol., 120*, 341.
Franks, L.M., Riddle, P.N., Carbobell, A.W. and Gey, G.O. (1970): *J. Path., 100*, 113.
Kellokumpu-Lehtinen, P., Santti, R. and Pelliniemi, L.J. (1979): *Anat. Rec., 194*, 429.
Kellokumpu-Lehtinen, P., Santti, R. and Pelliniemi, L.J. (1980): *Anat. Rec.,* in press.
Lowsley, O.S. (1912): *Amer. J. Anat., 13*, 299.
Ohno, S. (1977): In: *Morphogenesis and Malformation of the Genital System*, p. 99. Editors: R.J. Blandau and D. Bergsma. Alan R. Liss Inc., New York.
Streeter, G.L. (1920): In: *Carnegie Inst. Wash. Publ. 55, Contrib. to Embryol. Vol., 11*, p. 143.
Wartiovaara, J., Nordling, S., Lehtonen, E. and Saxén, L. (1974): *J. Embryol. Exp. Morphol., 31*, 667.

120

Hormone receptors in prostatic tissue*

P.S. RENNIE and N. BRUCHOVSKY

Department of Cancer Endocrinology, Cancer Control Agency of British Columbia, Vancouver, British Columbia, Canada

The marked dependence of the prostate on gonadal steroids is assumed to be a specific biological property conditional upon the presence of intracellular receptors for steroidal hormones. Although efforts to identify receptor molecules in prostatic tissue have met with considerable success, the issue as to whether a positive or negative receptor test is a relevant consideration in the treatment of prostatic carcinoma has not been resolved.

Androgen receptors

Androgen receptors have been demonstrated in normal prostate by Wagner et al. (1975), Mobbs et al. (1978), Ekman et al. (1979a), Griffiths et al. (1979), Lieskovsky and Bruchovsky (1979) and Shain et al. (1980); however a careful study by Krieg et al. (1979) using the techniques of agar-gel electrophoresis failed to reveal the presence of receptors. As well, there have been numerous confirmations of the presence of androgen receptors in benign prostatic hyperplasia (Wagner et al., 1975; De Voogt and Dingjan, 1978; Ghanadian et al., 1978a; Menon et al., 1978; Mobbs et al., 1978; Shain et al., 1978; Sirett and Grant, 1978; Ekman et al., 1979a; Griffiths et al., 1979; Krieg et al., 1979; Lieskovsky and Bruchovsky, 1979; Pertschuk et al., 1979; Shain et al., 1980). Carcinoma of the prostate, both primary (Wagner et al., 1975; De Voogt and Dingjan, 1978; Ghanadian et al., 1978b; Mobbs et al., 1978; Griffiths et al., 1979; Krieg et al., 1979; Lieskovsky and Bruchovsky, 1979; Pertschuk et al., 1979; Sidh et al., 1979; Shain et al., 1980) and metastatic (Ekman et al., 1979b; Shain et al., 1980) is characterized by a broad range of receptor concentrations. On theoretical grounds, the high concentration of dihydrotestosterone both in carcinomatous and hyperplastic tissue would favor a large shift of androgen receptors into the nuclear compartment (Menon et al., 1978; Lieskovsky and Bruchovsky, 1979); however the most recent experimental data suggest that the greater proportion remains lodged in the cytoplasm (Griffiths et al., 1979; Shain et al., 1979).

*Our projects are supported by grants from the Medical Research Council of Canada and the National Cancer Institute of Canada.

Estrogen receptors

The occurrence of estrogen receptors in normal prostate has been reported by Wagner et al. (1975), and Ekman et al. (1979a), but questioned by Griffiths et al. (1979) who could not confirm this observation. Similarly, estrogen receptors have been detected in benign prostatic hyperplasia by some investigators (Hawkins et al., 1975; Wagner et al., 1975; Bashirelahi et al., 1976; Hawkins et al., 1976; De Voogt and Dingjan, 1978; Pertschuk et al., 1979) but not by others (Shain et al., 1978; Ekman et al., 1979a; Griffiths et al., 1979). Estrogen receptors have been found in primary carcinoma of the prostate with regularity (Wagner et al., 1975; Bashirelahi and Young, 1976; De Voogt and Dingjan, 1978; Pertschuk et al., 1979; Sidh et al., 1979) except in the experiments of Griffiths et al. (1979). Metastatic carcinoma is apparently devoid of estrogen receptors (Ekman et al., 1979b).

Progestin receptors

Evidence documenting the distribution of progesterone receptors in normal (Mobbs et al., 1978; Ekman et al., 1979a), hyperplastic (Asselin et al., 1976; Dubé et al., 1976; Cowan et al., 1977; Gustafsson et al., 1978; Menon et al., 1978; Ekman et al., 1979a), and carcinomatous (Gustafsson et al., 1978; Ekman et al., 1979b) prostates has been remarkably consistent. According to Cowan et al. (1977), the progesterone receptor-like binding sites are a feature of the prostatic stroma rather than the epithelium.

Glucocorticoid and prolactin receptors

Information on the content of glucocorticoid receptors in prostate is scant; in reports by Ekman and his colleagues, the absence of glucocorticoid receptors in normal and hyperplastic tissue (Ekman et al., 1979a) is contrasted with their presence in metastatic carcinoma (Ekman et al., 1979b). As reviewed by Griffiths et al. (1979), prolactin receptors have been described in the rat prostate but no studies of a similar nature have been conducted on human prostate.

Clinical application of receptor tests

The success of the estrogen receptor test in predicting the hormonal status of breast cancer has fostered mounting interest in the potential use of steroid receptor determinations in the medical and surgical management of prostatic cancer. In breast cancer, patient selection with the estrogen receptor test increases response rates from 15-35% to 60% or slightly higher. Since the response rate in unselected patients with prostatic cancer is already 60-80%, the impact of any specific receptor test on this predetermined high rate is unlikely to be very important. Nevertheless, it remains possible that the receptor test might be useful in identifying the small percentage of nonresponders in the group of patients with untreated metastatic disease, and, furthermore, it might be applied to the selection of the minority of patients who will benefit from endocrine therapy of reactivated disease.

Preliminary correlations with response to treatment reported by Mobbs et al. (1978, 1979) suggest that in patients with low endogenous androgens, hormonal sensitivity of prostatic carcinoma is not directly related to the concentration of androgen receptors. Partial responses to hormonal manipulation were observed only when the androgen binding capacity of cytosol protein was between 0.4-1.0 fmol/mg tissue. Tumors which failed to respond to therapy were characterized by values above and below this range.

In a similar study, Ekman et al. (1979c) detected significant quantities of androgen receptors (0.3-2.0 fmol/mg tissue) in 20 of 25 specimens of primary prostatic carcinoma. The response rate in 18 clinically evaluable patients with receptor-positive tumors was 80%; in 5 patients with receptor negative tumors, it was only 20%.

Such observations contrast with the experience of De Voogt and Dingjan (1978) who were unsuccessful in demonstrating any consistent relationship between the quantity of androgen receptors in extracts of carcinomatous tissue and the clinical course of a number of previously treated and untreated patients. On the other hand, since 3 of 4 patients who benefited from therapy had tumors with a high content of estrogen receptors, these investigators suggested that the presence of estrogen receptors might have prognostic significance.

This impression has gained support from the investigations of Sidh et al. (1979); they observed subjective and objective regression of endocrine treated disease in 9 of 15 patients with tumors characterized by an estrogen-binding capacity that was large in comparison to the number of androgen-binding sites. On the other hand, specimens of prostatic carcinoma from 17 of 18 patients with progressive disease, and 6 of 7 patients with stable disease, were characterized by a greater capacity to bind androgens than estrogens. The authors inferred that patients with tumors deficient in estrogen receptors but containing a full measure of androgen receptors are less likely to respond to endocrine manipulations.

Alternative approaches

The usefulness of measuring the whole tissue concentration of dihydrotestosterone for predicting clinical responsiveness of prostatic carcinoma has been studied by Geller and co-workers (1979a, b). In 11 patients with advanced untreated disease, androgen content appeared to correlate better with ultimate response to antiandrogen than histologic grading. Significant amounts of dihydrotestosterone were found in prostatic tissue of two patients who clinically relapsed after prior treatment with estrogen and castration or castration alone. In three non-castrated patients treated with hormonal agents, the prostatic concentration of dihydrotestosterone was well above normal. These results raise the interesting possibility that recurrent prostatic carcinoma is not necessarily hormone resistant; it is likely that in some patients therapy has been inadequate and simply failed to eliminate dihydrotestosterone from the carcinomatous cell.

Nuclear androgen receptors and significance

In an earlier report, we reviewed the technical problems that hinder the accurate measurement of the concentration of androgen receptors in the cytoplasm of the human prostate (Lieskovsky and Bruchovsky, 1979). From a conceptual standpoint, one of the more serious of these is the strong possibility that most of the physiologically active receptor is localized in the nucleus owing to the elevated concentration of dihydrotestosterone especially in hyperplastic and carcinomatous tissue. We were persuaded by this line of reasoning to measure the quantity of receptor in highly purified nuclei. The following results, expressed in terms of molecules per nucleus, were obtained: normal prostate 900 ± 180 (mean ± S.E.M.); hyperplastic prostate, 1600 ± 260; well-differentiated carcinoma, 1800 ± 160 (Bruchovsky et al., 1980a). The two-fold increase in the amount of receptor in carcinomatous nuclei appeared to be explained by the chance finding that such nuclei contained twice as much DNA as nuclei from normal tissue. We implied, therefore, that the concentration of receptor in carcinomatous tissue is elevated in proportion to the DNA content of the nucleus.

In an extension of this work, the nuclear concentration of dihydrotestosterone was measured by radioimmunoassay and compared to the amount of receptor. The number of molecules per nucleus of dihydrotestosterone was 11,000 ± 3000 (mean ± S.E.M.), 50,000 ± 6000, and 36,000 ± 7000, respectively in normal, hyperplastic and carcinomatous prostates (Bruchovsky et al., 1980a, b). Thus, irrespective of the normal or abnormal condition of the prostate, the nucleus of the prostatic cell is characterized by an apparent capacity to accumulate dihydrotestosterone in excess of the quantity of receptor. This feature is most pronounced in hyperplastic prostate.

In view of the direct relationship between the amounts of nuclear receptor and DNA, we investigated the binding reaction between the two molecules in more detail (Rennie, 1979; Bruchovsky et al., 1980a). Extracts of nuclei from rat ventral prostate were digested with micrococcal nuclease to yield receptor-chromatin complexes of varying sizes; the complexes were separated in linear 7.6 − 76% (v/v) glycerol density gradients. With extensive digestion of DNA, receptor labeled with radioactive dihydrotestosterone was released from the chromatin. After 5% digestion of DNA to acid soluble products, only a trace amount of labeled receptor was detected in the unbound form. In the latter instance, most of the receptor was recovered from the gradients in association with five A_{260} peaks representing oligo-meric and monomeric nucleosomes with a repeat length of 182 ± 3 (mean $\pm$ S.E.M.) base pairs. The concentration of receptor was highest in the A_{260} peaks which contained large oligomers of nucleosomes and lowest in fractions containing monomers. Similar experiments were performed with chromatin from nuclei of normal and hyperplastic human prostates; free receptor was recovered only after the chromatin was digested with micro-coccal nuclease. We concluded from these observations that the androgen receptor is bound to linker DNA in both rat and human prostate.

To determine whether the nuclear receptor is essential for the expression of hormonal sensitivity, we compared the amount of nuclear androgen-binding and the activities of acid phosphatase and plasminogen activator in the transplantable prostatic adenocarcinoma of Nb rats. Androgen-stimulated tumors were found to have more nuclear receptor and less acid phosphatase activity than autonomous tumors (Rennie et al., 1980a). Also, the plasminogen activator activity was seven-fold lower in the androgen-stimulated tumors than in the latter (Rennie et al., 1980b). These observations are consistent with the view that a diminished concentration of nuclear androgen receptor in prostatic carcinoma is associated with an increasing grade of malignancy.

Acknowledgement

We thank Kathy Barrett for typing this manuscript.

References

Asselin, J., Labrie, F., Gourdeau, Y., Bonne, C. and Raynaud, J.-P. (1976): *Steroids, 28,* 449.
Bashirelahi, N., O'Toole, J.H. and Young, J.D. (1976): *Biochem. Med., 15,* 254.
Bashirelahi, N. and Young, J.D. (1976): *Urology, 8,* 553.
Bruchovsky, N., Rennie, P.S. and Shnitka, T.K. (1980b): In: *Proceedings of the First International Congress on Hormones and Cancer.* Editors: S. Iacobelli, R.J.B. King, H.R. Lindner and M. Lippman. Raven Press, New York. In press.
Bruchovsky, N., Rennie, P.S. and Wilkin, R.P. (1980a): In: *Steroid Receptors, Meta-bolism and Prostatic Cancer,* p.57. Editors: F.H. Schröder and H.J. De Voogt. Excerpta Medica, Amsterdam.
Cowan, R.A., Cowan, S.K. and Grant, J.K. (1977): *J. Endocrin., 74,* 281.
De Voogt, H.J. and Dingjan, P. (1978): *Urol. Res., 6,* 151.
Dubé, J.Y., Chapdelaine, P., Tremblay, R.R., Bonne, C. and Raynaud, J.-P. (1976): *Hormone Res., 7,* 341.
Ekman, P., Snochowski, M., Dahlberg, E., Bression, P., Högberg, B. and Gustafsson, J.-A. (1979a): *J. Clin. Endocr., 49,* 205.
Ekman, P., Snochowski, M., Dahlberg, E. and Gustafsson, J.-A. (1979b): *Europ. J. Cancer, 15,* 257.
Ekman, P., Snochowski, M., Zetterberg, A., Högberg, B. and Gustafsson, J.-A. (1979c): *Cancer, 44,* 1173.
Geller, J. (1979a): In: *Steroid Receptors and the Management of Cancer, Vol. I,* Chapter

8, p. 113. Editors: E.B. Thompson and M.E. Lippman. CRC Press, Inc., Boca Raton.

Geller, J., Albert, J. and Loza, D. (1979b): *J. Steroid Biochem., 11,* 631.

Ghanadian, R., Auf, G., Chaloner, P.J. and Chisholm, G.D. (1978a): *J. Steroid Biochem., 9,* 325.

Ghanadian, R., Auf, G., Chisholm, G.D. and O'Donoghue, E.P.N. (1978b): *Brit. J. Urol., 50,* 567.

Griffiths, K., Davies, P., Harper, M.E., Peeling, W.B. and Pierrepoint, C.G. (1979): In: *Endocrinology of Cancer, Vol II,* Chapter 1, p. 1. Editor: D.P. Rose. CRC Press, Inc., Boca Raton.

Gustafsson, J.-A., Ekman, P., Pousette, A., Snochowski, M. and Högberg, B. (1978): *Invest. Urol., 15,* 361.

Hawkins, E.F., Nijs, M. and Brassinne, C. (1976): *Biochem. Biophys. Res. Comm., 70,* 854.

Hawkins, E.F., Nijs, M., Brassinne, C. and Tagnon, H.J. (1975): *Steroids, 26,* 458.

Krieg, M., Bartsch, W., Janssen, W. and Voigt, K.D. (1979): *J. Steroid Biochem., 11,* 615.

Lieskovsky, G. and Bruchovsky, N. (1979): *J. Urol., 121,* 54.

Menon, M., Tananis, C., Hicks, L.L., Hawkins, E.F., McLoughlin, M.G. and Walsh, P.C. (1978): *J. Clin. Invest., 61,* 150.

Mobbs, B.G., Johnson, I.E. and Connolly, J.G. (1979): In: *Prostate Cancer and Hormone Receptors,* p. 13. Editors: G.P. Murphy and A.A. Sandberg. Alan R. Liss, Inc., New York.

Mobbs, B.G., Johnson, I.E., Connolly, J.G. and Clark, A.F. (1978): *J. Steroid Biochem., 9,* 289.

Pertschuk, L.P., Zava, D.T., Gaetjens, E., Macchia, R.J., Wise, G.J., Kim, D.S. and Brigati, D.J. (1979): *Ann. Clin. Lab. Sci., 9,* 225.

Rennie, P.S. (1979): *J. Biol. Chem., 254,* 3947.

Rennie, P.S., Bruchovsky, N., Noble, R.L. and Mo, S. (1980a): *Biochim. Biophys. Acta,* in press.

Rennie, P.S., Bruchovsky, N., Noble, R.L. and Mo, S. (1980b): *Biochim. Biophys. Acta,* in press.

Shain, S.A., Boesel, R.W., Lamm, D.L. and Radwin, H.M. (1978): *Steroids, 31,* 541.

Shain, S.A., Boesel, R.W., Lamm, D.L. and Radwin, H.M. (1980): *J. Clin. Endocr., 50,* 704.

Shain, S.A., Boesel, R.W., Radwin, H.M. and Lamm, D.L. (1979): In: *Prostate Cancer and Hormone Receptors.* p. 33. Editors: G.P. Murphy and A.A. Sandberg. Alan R. Liss, Inc., New York.

Sidh, S.M., Young, J.D., Karmi, S.A., Powder, J.R. and Bashirelahi, N. (1979): *Urology, 13,* 597.

Sirett, D.A.N. and Grant, J.K. (1978): *J. Endocr., 77,* 101.

Wagner, R.K., Schulze, K.H. and Jungblut, P.W. (1975): *Acta Endocrinol. (Kbh.), Suppl., 193,* 52.

The Dunning tumor as a model for human prostatic carcinoma*

E. DAHLBERG, M. SNOCHOWSKI and J.-Å. GUSTAFSSON

Departments of Chemistry and Medical Nutrition, Karolinska Institutet, Stockholm, Sweden

Prostatic carcinoma, which comprises 17% of male tumors, is the second most common malignancy in American men, and although it often occurs without clinical symptoms, it accounts for over one third of cancer deaths in men over 55 years of age. More than 95% of the prostatic malignancies are adenocarcinomas. These tumors usually arise in the peripheral zones of the gland and most often multifocally or are extensively distributed within the gland. A significant correlation exists between tumor grade and prognosis, irrespective of tumor stage. Contrary to the common belief that skeletal metastases appear at an early stage as a contrast to lymph node metastases, it has recently been found that prostatic carcinoma may metastasize to lymph nodes early in the course of the disease. These and other clinically relevant studies have recently been reviewed (Mainwaring, 1976; Catalona and Scott, 1978; Klein, 1979; Mawhinney and Neubauer, 1979).

The observation that the testes are necessary for the maintenance of the prostate in animals was made by William Harvey over 300 years ago (Whitteridge, 1964), and castration or estrogen administration was introduced by Huggins and Hodges (1941) as important alternatives in the therapy of prostatic cancer. The role of androgens as regulatory factors involved in the physiology and pathology of the prostate has been considerably elucidated during recent years by numerous studies initiated by the findings of Bruchovsky and Wilson (1968) that testosterone is reduced to 5α-dihydrotestosterone in the prostate, and that this metabolite is taken up by the cell nuclei. The nuclear uptake occurs following binding of the steroid to a cytoplasmic receptor protein, as was initially shown for the uptake of estradiol-17β into the cell nuclei of the rat uterus by Jensen et al. (1968). Several recent reviews cover this subject (King and Mainwaring, 1974; Liao, 1976; Higgins and Gehring, 1978; Shain and Boesel, 1978; Voigt and Castro, 1978). The need for model systems for prostatic carcinoma is based upon both ethical and practical considerations, and valuable information could be expected from suitable model systems concerning tumor etiology,

*This study was supported by grants from the Swedish Cancer Society and from Leo Research Foundation.

mechanisms of carcinogenesis and tumor progression, the metastasizing process, hormonal actions, tumor genetics and immunity, and therapeutical effects. Several general limitations of tumor model systems have been discussed by Handelsman (1977) and Merchant (1977). The particular drawbacks of induced tumors and in vitro models have been discussed by Higuchi (1977) and by Merchant (1976), respectively, and of in vivo models by Mathe (1976). The specific problems related to extrapolation of results from model systems to the situation in man have been discussed by Lasagna (1958).

Spontaneous transplantable prostatic adenocarcinomas are potentially useful models for human prostatic malignancy. Spontaneous prostatic adenocarcinoma is frequent only in man, but does occur in aged animals of other species, particularly in rats. Transplantable tumors have been developed from such material, the most extensively studied of which are those developed by Dunning (1963), and by Pollard (1973). Recently Shain et al. (1977) reported that the aged AXC rat has a high frequency of spontaneous adenocarcinoma of the prostate, but this model system has not yet been as extensively studied as the Dunning tumor. The AXC rat tumor was reported to have an altered androgen metabolism and diminished amounts of cytosolic androgen receptors (Shain et al., 1977). The tumor described by Pollard may be cultured and propagated in vitro (Chang and Pollard, 1977), and the effects of various treatments have been reported (Pollard et al., 1977; Müntzing et al., 1979). The model described by Dunning (1963) has been thoroughly investigated and several tumor lines have been developed. The interest has been focused particularly on 2 lines, one dependent and the other one independent of androgens for growth. Apart from different growth properties, these lines have different testosterone-metabolizing capacity. Furthermore, the androgen-dependent but not the androgen-independent line has been reported to possess a 5α-dihydrotestosterone-binding protein sedimenting at about 3.5 S on sucrose density gradients (Voigt and Dunning, 1974; Voigt et al., 1975). The R-3327 tumor has been reported to respond to estrogens and antiandrogens (Smolev et al., 1977a, b) and the effects of cytostatic drugs on the tumor have been described (Block et al., 1977; Müntzing et al., 1977). Also, the effect of surgery, immunotherapy and chemotherapy have been investigated using cell kinetic techniques (Weissman et al., 1977). The Dunning tumor has been used for studies on immunological tumor-host-interactions (Claflin et al., 1977; Lopez and Voigt, 1977; Rao et al., 1978), and its ultrastructure has been described (Seman et al., 1978). Isaacs et al. (1979), using enzymatic methods, were able to distinguish the androgen sensitivity from the differentiation in R-3327 sublines. The Dunning tumor was recently reported to contain binding sites for prolactin (Witorsch, 1979). Apart from the paper by Voigt et al. (1975), studies on steroid receptors in the R-3327 adenocarcinoma have not appeared until recently (Markland et al., 1978; Dahlberg et al., 1980; Heston et al., 1979; Markland and Lee, 1979; Wilson and

French, 1979). Since the data so far obtained from the numerous studies on this tumor model suggest that it is the best single model available for prostatic cancer in man, we considered it of interest to compare its contents of steroid hormone receptors to those obtained from human tissues with the same techniques. The human data stem from our papers on steroid receptors in metastases from cancer of the prostate (Ekman et al., 1979a, 1980) and benign prostatic hyperplasia and 'normal' prostate (Ekman et al., 1979b).

Material and methods

Tumors were transplanted from intact male donors to intact male recipients subcutaneously, and pieces of tumor were frozen at $-80°C$ for analyses. Cytosol was prepared as the 105 000 x g supernatant from a 1:3 (w:v) homogenate. Cytosolic protein and DNA in the pellets were estimated using modified methods of Lowry et al. (1951) and Burton (1956), respectively, at 3 dilutions to check parallelism to the standard curves. Receptor quantifications were carried out by incubating cytosol with ^{3}H-ligand at 6 doses in the absence or presence of a 100-fold excess of unlabeled ligand at 0-4°C for 16-20 hr, and following separation of free and protein-bound radioactivity by treatment with dextran-coated charcoal, Scatchard plots were used to calculate binding parameters from data corrected for non-specific binding according to Chamness and McGuire (1975). For the determination of androgen and progestin receptors, ^{3}H-methyltrienolone and ^{3}H-R 5020 were used, respectively. Glucocorticoid and estrogen receptors were determined with ^{3}H-dexamethasone and ^{3}H-R 2858, respectively. Our criteria for interpretation of the Scatchard plot data, details of methodology and original references have been given elsewhere (Snochowski et al., 1977; Dahlberg et al., 1980; Ekman et al., 1979a, b).

Results and discussion

As can be seen in Table 1, most of the Dunning R-3327 tumors contained androgen and estrogen receptors (8/9 and 5/6, respectively). However, the tumors lacked detectable amounts of progestin and glucocorticoid receptors in all cases analyzed (7 and 4, respectively). The apparent equilibrium dissociation constant (K_d) for the binding of ^{3}H-methyltrienolone was higher than in metastases from human prostatic carcinoma, and more similar to that recorded for the binding to human benign prostatic hyperplasia (BPH). The apparent equilibrium B_{max} values (maximum number of binding sites) for methyltrienolone in the Dunning tumor, on the other hand, were more similar to those obtained in human metastatic cancer of the prostate than in BPH. The finding that the rat model contains estrogen receptors in the majority of cases contrasts to the situation in both

TABLE 1.

Comparison between steroid receptor contents in the Dunning R-3327 rat prostatic adenocarcinoma and human benign prostatic hyperplasia and human prostatic cancer metastases

	Dunning tumor	Human benign prostatic hyperplasia	Human metastatic prostatic carcinoma
Ratio protein to DNA (95% confidence interval)	16-32	17-20	4-16
Androgen receptor			
Receptor presence	8 of 9	40 of 40	4 of 5
K_d range (nM)	0.7-4.3	0.2-1.9	0.1-0.5
B_{max} range (fmol/g tissue)	1490-25100	166-3460	110-28500
Estrogen receptor			
Receptor presence	5 of 6	0 of 26	0 of 5
K_d range (nM)	0.6-1.8		
B_{max} range (fmol/g tissue)	638-5810		
Progestin receptor			
Receptor presence	0 of 7	29 of 39	2 of 5
K_d range (nM)		0.1-1.3	0.7-0.9
B_{max} range (fmol/g tissue)		277-3820	424-1410
Glucocorticoid receptor			
Receptor presence	0 of 4	0 of 7	3 of 5
K_d range (nM)			1.7-6.2
B_{max} range (fmol/g tissue)			4730-13600
Reference	Dahlberg et al. (1980)	Ekman et al. (1979b)	Ekman et al. (1979a)

human cancer metastases and BPH, where estrogen receptors seem to be absent. However, we have detected receptors for estrogens in some 'normal' human prostates (Ekman et al., 1979b). Progestin receptors seem to be present in the majority of BPH specimens as well as in some metastases, but were not detectable in the Dunning tumors analyzed. Some 'normal' human prostates contained progestin receptors, but none contained glucocorticoid receptors. Glucocorticoid receptors were not detected in BPH, nor in the Dunning tumor, but were present in some metastases.

Another parameter that is different in the human metastatic cancer of the prostate and in the Dunning tumor is the ratio of protein to DNA. This ratio was higher in the Dunning tumor than in the metastases, and more similar to the ratio found in human BPH. Since the DNA content but not the protein content parallels the degree of anaplasia in a tumor, this finding may reflect some biological difference between the Dunning tumor and metastatic carcinoma of the human prostate.

In view of these differences between the investigated rat tumor model and its human counterpart, it seems essential to interpret data obtained from studies on the Dunning tumor with due caution when attempting to extrapolate these data to the human situation. On the other hand, at least the human prostatic carcinoma is a histologically heterogeneous tumor (Tannenbaum, 1977), and we still know little about the steroid hormone receptor activities of truly normal human prostates due to the difficulties in obtaining and in defining the normality of a prostate (Ekman et al., 1980). Hence, in conclusion, the Dunning tumor does not seem to be an optimal model for human prostatic carcinoma. Partly this may be explained by the heterogeneity of the human prostatic cancer metastases (Ekman et al., 1979a, 1980). Although it is possible that some understanding of human cancer of the prostate may be gained from studies on e.g. the Dunning tumor, the validity of such results should be judged after taking differences in hormone responsiveness into account.

References

Block, N.L., Camuzzi, F., Denefrio, J., Troner, M., Claflin, A., Stover, B. and Politano, V.A. (1977): *Oncology, 34,* 110.
Bruchovsky, N. and Wilson, J.D. (1968): *J. Biol. Chem., 243,* 2012.
Burton, K. (1956): *Biochem. J., 62,* 315.
Catalona, W.J. and Scott, W.W. (1978): *J. Urol., 119,* 1.
Chamness, G.C. and McGuire, W.L. (1975): *Steroids, 26,* 538.
Chang, C.F. and Pollard, M. (1977): *Invest. Urol., 14,* 331.
Claflin, A.J., McKinney, E.C. and Fletcher, M.A. (1977): *Oncology, 34,* 105.
Dahlberg, E., Snochowski, M. and Gustafsson, J.-Å. (1980): *The Prostate, 1,* in press.
Dunning, W.F. (1963): *Nat. Cancer Inst. Monogr., 12,* 351.
Ekman, P., Dahlberg, E., Gustafsson, J.-Å., Högberg, B., Pousette, Å. and Snochowski, M. (1980): In: *Hormones and Cancer,* p. 361. Editors: S. Iacobelli et al. Raven Press, New York.
Ekman, P., Snochowski, M., Dahlberg, E., Bression, D., Högberg, B. and Gustafsson, J.-Å. (1979b): *J. Clin. Endocr., 49,* 205.
Ekman, P., Snochowski, M., Dahlberg, E. and Gustafsson, J.-Å. (1979a): *Europ. J. Cancer, 15,* 257.
Handelsman, H. (1977): *Oncology, 34,* 96.
Heston, W.D.W., Menon, M., Tananis, C. and Walsh, P.C. (1979): *Cancer Lett., 6,* 45.
Higgins, S.J. and Gehring, U. (1978): *Advanc. Cancer Res., 28,* 313.
Higuchi, M. (1977): In: *Tumors of the Male Genital System,* p. 27. Editors: E. Grundmann and W. Vahlensieck. Springer-Verlag, Berlin.
Huggins, C. and Hodges, C.V. (1941): *Cancer Res., 1,* 293.
Isaacs, J.T., Isaacs, W.B. and Coffey, D.S. (1979): *Cancer Res., 39,* 2652.
Jensen, E.V., Suzuki, T., Kawashima, T., Stumpf, W.E., Jungblut, P.W. and De Sombre, E.R. (1968): *Proc. Nat. Acad. Sci. (Wash.), 59,* 632.
King, R.J.B. and Mainwaring, W.I.P. (1974): *Steroid-Cell Interactions.* Butterworths & Co. Ltd., London.
Klein, L.A. (1979): *New Engl. J. Med., 300,* 824.
Lasagna, L. (1958): *Ann. N.Y. Acad. Sci., 76,* 939.

Liao, S. (1976): In: *Receptors and Mechanism of Action of Steroid Hormones, Vol. 1,* Chapter 5, p. 159. Editor: J.R. Pasqualini. Marcel Dekker, New York.

Lopez, D.M. and Voigt, W. (1977): *Cancer Res., 37,* 2057.

Lowry, O.H., Rosebrough, N.J., Farr, A.L. and Randall, R.J. (1951): *J. Biol. Chem., 193,* 265.

Mainwaring, W.I.P. (1976): In: *Steroid Hormone Action and Cancer,* p. 152. Editors: K.M.J. Menon and J.R. Reel. Plenum Press, New York.

Markland, F.S., Chopp, R.T., Cosgrove, M.D. and Howard, E.B. (1978): *Cancer Res., 38,* 2818.

Markland, F.S. Jr and Lee, L. (1979): *J. Steroid Biochem., 10,* 13.

Mathe, G. (1976): *Biomedicine, 24,* 225.

Mawhinney, M.G. and Neubauer, B.L. (1979): *Invest. Urol., 16,* 409.

Merchant, D.J. (1976): *Semin. Oncol., 3,* 131.

Merchant, D.J. (1977): *Oncology, 34,* 100.

Müntzing, J., Kirdani, R.Y., Murphy, G.P. and Sandberg, A.A. (1979): *Invest. Urol., 17,* 37.

Müntzing, J., Kirdani, R.Y., Saroff, J., Murphy, G.P. and Sandberg, A.A. (1977): *Urology 10,* 439.

Pollard, M. (1973): *J. Nat. Cancer Inst., 51,* 1235.

Pollard, M., Chang, C.F. and Luckert, P.H. (1977): *Oncology, 34,* 129.

Rao, B.R., Nakeff, A., Eaton, C. and Heston, W.D.W. (1978): *Cancer Res., 38,* 4431.

Seman, G., Myers, B., Bowen, J.M. and Dmochowski, L. (1978): *Invest. Urol., 16,* 231.

Shain, S.A. and Boesel, R.W. (1978): *Invest. Urol., 16,* 169.

Shain, S.A., McCullough, B., Nitchuk, M. and Boesel, R.W. (1977): *Oncology, 34,* 114.

Smolev, J.K., Coffey, D.S. and Scott, W.W. (1977b): *J. Urol. (Baltimore), 118,* 216.

Smolev, J.K., Heston, W.D.W., Scott, W.W. and Coffey, D.S. (1977a): *Cancer Treatm. Rep., 61,* 273.

Snochowski, M., Pousette, Å., Ekman, P., Bression, D., Andersson, L., Högberg, B. and Gustafsson, J.-Å. (1977): *J. Clin. Endocr., 45,* 920.

Tannenbaum, M. (1977): In: *Urological Pathology,* p. 303. Editor: M. Tannenbaum. Lea and Febiger, Philadelphia.

Weissman, R.M., Coffey, D.S. and Scott, W.W. (1977): *Oncology, 34,* 133.

Whitteridge, G. (1964): *The Anatomical Lectures of William Harvey.* Livingstone with the Royal College of Physicians, Edinburgh and London.

Wilson, E.M. and French, F.S. (1979): *J. Biol. Chem., 254,* 6310.

Witorsch, R.J. (1979): *Hormone Res., 10,* 268.

Voigt, W. and Castro, A. (1978): In: *Endocrine Control in Neoplasia,* p. 291. Editors: R.K. Sharma and W.E. Criss. Raven Press, New York.

Voigt, W. and Dunning, W.F. (1974): *Cancer Res., 34,* 1447.

Voigt, W., Feldman, M. and Dunning, W.F. (1975): *Cancer Res., 35,* 1840.

Distribution of dihydrotestosterone and of nuclear androgen receptors between stroma and epithelium of human benign hyperplastic prostatic tissue*

D.A.N. SIRETT, S.K. COWAN, A.E. JANECZKO and J.K. GRANT

University Department of Steroid Biochemistry, Royal Infirmary, Glasgow, U.K.

The development of benign hyperplasia of the human prostate (BPH) is apparently initiated by a local proliferation of the stromal component of the tissue (Mostofi, 1970; Pradhan and Chandra, 1975). The resulting fibro-muscular nodules incorporate glandular elements to a variable extent as the hyperplasia progresses. The investigation of any putative interaction between stroma and epithelium in the hyperplastic tissue has been facilitated by the development in our laboratory of a procedure for the separation of the two components (Cowan et al., 1976). The essential role of androgens in the development and maintenance of the diseased prostate suggested that we examine their mechanism of action in the separated fractions. Early work on this theme demonstrated that BPH stroma contains much larger amounts of testosterone 5α-reductase activity than the epithelial component (Cowan et al., 1977). Reduction of testosterone is an essential preliminary to androgen action in most target tissues; the distribution of 5α-reductase activity suggested that the stroma may be androgen-responsive as well as the epithelium. In continuation of this study, we now present measurements of endogenous dihydrotestosterone (DHT) and of nuclear androgen receptors in the separate BPH tissue components.

Material and methods

The preparation of stromal and epithelial fractions from fresh BPH tissue has been described (Cowan et al., 1976). Androgen receptors in nuclear extracts from the separated fractions were determined by the procedure previously applied to whole tissue samples (Sirett and Grant, 1978). Briefly, extracts were prepared from crude nuclei using buffered potassium chloride (0.5 mol/l), and subjected to an exchange assay by incubation with [^{3}H] DHT (0.1-20 nmol/l) at $15°$C for 18-20 hr. Separation of protein-bound and free steroid was achieved by chromatography on columns of Sephadex LH20.

*This work was supported by grant no. SP1230 of the Cancer Research Campaign.

TABLE 1.

DHT content in BPH tissue components

	DHT	
	pg/mg protein	ng/mg DNA
Whole tissue	97 ± 16*	4.7 ± 0.7
Stroma	93 ± 15	5.0 ± 1.2
Epithelium	468 ± 98	6.2 ± 2.6

*Mean ± S.E.M. for 6 patients.

Endogenous androgens were extracted with ether from homogenates of whole tissue, stroma and epithelium. DHT was separated by column chromatography on Lipidex-5000, and measured by radioimmunoassay. Further details will be given elsewhere (Sirett et al., 1980).

Arginase activity was determined in homogenates of whole tissue, stroma and epithelium by the assay of urea released from arginine added as substrate, as described in the Worthington Enzyme Manual (1972).

Protein was determined by the method of Lowry et al. (1951), and DNA by that of Burton (1956).

Results

The concentrations of DHT measured in whole tissue, epithelium and stroma from 6 specimens of BPH tissue are shown in Table 1. The whole tissue values are consistent with those reported by other workers (Siiteri and Wilson, 1970; Hammond, 1978). The results are presented in terms of the protein content or the DNA content of the homogenates. On a protein basis the DHT is considerably enriched in epithelium, compared to stroma or whole tissue. Examination of the data in terms of DNA content indicates a more even distribution of the androgen between epithelium and stroma.

Nuclear androgen receptor measurements for components from 8 tissue specimens are summarized in Table 2, and typical results are plotted according to Scatchard (1949) in Figure 1. Both the equilibrium dissociation constant and the concentration of receptor sites are similar in the 2 fractions. In a further series of tissue samples, nuclear androgen receptors were measured in whole tissue, stroma and epithelium. Arginase activity was determined in aliquots removed from the homogenates prior to isolation of the nuclei. Table 3 summarizes the results as the ratio of receptor content (fmol) to arginase activity (μmol/hr). For both measurements the results are

TABLE 2.

Androgen receptor in nuclear extracts from BPH tissue components: [³H]DHT binding

	K_d (nmol/l)	Concentration (fmol/mg DNA)
Stroma	2.14 ± 0.29*	556 ± 76
Epithelium	1.75 ± 0.29	697 ± 182

*Mean ± S.E.M. for 8 patients.

TABLE 3.

Ratio of nuclear androgen receptor content (fmol/g wet tissue) to arginase activity (μmol/hr/g wet tissue) in BPH components (x 10^9)

	Receptor/arginase
Whole tissue	3.85 ± 0.43 (4)*
Stroma	9.92 ± 1.75 (5)
Epithelium	2.70 ± 0.56 (5)

*Mean ± S.E.M. for (n) patients.

calculated in terms of the wet weight of the tissue used to prepare the fractions.

Discussion

The dihydrotestosterone content of BPH epithelium is considerably greater than that of stroma when the results are expressed in terms of protein content (Table 1). However, a proportion of the stromal protein is likely to be associated with extracellular fibrous and connective elements which are absent from the epithelial component. In terms of DNA content, similar levels of DHT are observed in both components, suggesting that on a 'per cell' basis there is an even distribution of the steroid between epithelium and stroma.

Nuclear extracts prepared from both the epithelial and stromal fractions contain androgen receptors (Fig. 1). The binding affinities are similar, as are the concentrations of receptor sites measured (Table 2). In fact, the distribution of nuclear androgen receptors seems to correspond to that of

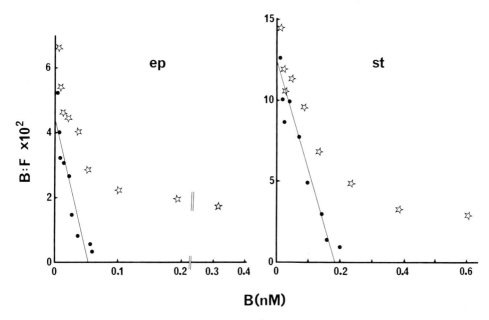

Fig. 1. Scatchard plots of the binding of [³H]DHT to nuclear extracts from BPH epithelium (ep) and stroma (st). Points shown are mean values from incubations (20 hr, 15°C) in duplicate. ☆, experimental points; ●, points corrected for non-saturable binding.

the homogenate DHT, although, considering the low number of tissue samples in each series, the result may be fortuitous. The amount of DHT present is much greater than the amount of receptor detected.

Scrutiny of the original account of our separation procedure suggests that the 'stromal' fraction retains a proportion of the epithelium (Cowan et al., 1976). The possibility arises that the receptor detected in nuclear extracts from the stromal fraction derives from such residual epithelium. For a few tissue samples we have measured both receptor content and arginase activity, so that the latter can be used as a marker for epithelial elements (Cowan et al., 1977). Our results suggest that in these cases the distribution of arginase activity does not parallel that of the nuclear receptor (Table 3). The ratio of receptor to arginase activity is consistently higher for the 'stromal' fraction than for the epithelial fraction, with whole tissue samples giving intermediate values. A constant ratio might be expected if both receptor and arginase were limited to epithelial cells, independent of the efficiency of the separation procedure. We have to assume, of course, that receptor is not selectively degraded in some way in the epithelial component.

In conclusion, the results reported here indicate that endogenous dihydro-testosterone, when related to DNA content, is distributed evenly between epithelial and stromal components of BPH tissue. This does not correspond to the observed distribution of testosterone 5α-reductase activity. Furthermore, the presence of considerable concentrations of androgen receptor in nuclear extracts, detected by exchange assay, suggests that both components are sensitive to androgens, at least to the extent that they possess receptors capable of translocation to cell nuclei. Confirmation of this result will require the preparation of a stromal fraction which is demonstrably free from epithelial contamination.

References

Burton, K. (1956): *Biochem. J. 62,* 315.
Cowan, R.A., Cowan, S.K., Giles, C.A. and Grant, J.K. (1976): *J. Endocr., 71,* 121.
Cowan, R.A., Cowan, S.K., Grant, J.K. and Elder, H.Y. (1977): *J. Endocr., 74,* 111.
Hammond, G.L. (1978): *J. Endocr., 78,* 7.
Lowry, O.H., Rosebrough, N.J., Farr, A.L. and Randall, R.J. (1951): *J. Biol. Chem., 193,* 265.
Mostofi, F.K. (1970): In: *Urology, Vol. 2,* p. 1065. Editors: M.F. Campbell and J.H. Harrison. W.B. Saunders Co., Philadelphia.
Pradhan, B.K. and Chandra, K. (1975): *J. Urol., 113,* 210.
Scatchard, G. (1949): *Ann. N.Y. Acad. Sci., 51,* 660.
Siiteri, P.K. and Wilson, J.D. (1970): *J. Clin. Invest., 49,* 1737.
Sirett, D.A.N., Cowan, S.K., Janeczko, A.E., Grant, J.K. and Glen, E.S. (1980): *J. Steroid Biochem., 13,* 723.
Sirett, D.A.N. and Grant, J.K. (1978): *J. Endocr., 77,* 101.
Worthington Enzyme Manual (1972): p. 149. Worthington Biochemical Corporation, Freehold, New Jersey.

Characterization of androgen receptors in a rat prostate adenocarcinoma*

O.A. LEA and F.S. FRENCH

Department of Pediatrics, School of Medicine, University of North Carolina, Chapel Hill, NC, U.S.A.

The R 3327 adenocarcinoma discovered by W. Dunning in 1961 (Dunning, 1963) developed spontaneously in the prostate of Copenhagen rats. Since then the tumor has been successfully transplanted to genetically compatible hosts. This tumor, which is slow growing, well differentiated and androgen responsive, appears to be a good model for the human disease. A detailed knowledge of the mode of androgen action in tumor cells will be instrumental for the understanding of how tumor growth is regulated. One of the earliest steps in the mechanism of androgen action is the binding of hormone to a specific soluble receptor.

The present investigation was aimed at characterization of tumor cytosol receptor and comparison with receptors found in normal tissues.

Material and Methods

Tumor-bearing Copenhagen-Fisher rats were obtained from the Papanicolaou Cancer Research Center, Miami, USA, and were used for studies on tumor and dorsal prostate receptors. Other organs studied were obtained from Sprague-Dawley rats. All rats were castrated 20 hr prior to tissue removal. Cytosols were labeled in vitro by incubating overnight at 0°C with 15 nM tritiated 5α-dihydrotestosterone, DHT, or testosterone. For a detailed description of experimental procedures see Lea et al. (1979a).

Results

'Prostatein' was not detected in cytosols prepared from tumor or dorsal prostate using a specific immunoassay (Lea et al., 1979b).

When tumor cytosol was studied by sucrose gradient centrifugation at a low salt concentration (0.05 M), the labeled receptor sedimented as an 8 S

*This work was supported by U.S. Public Health Service Grant HD 04466.

CYTOSOL

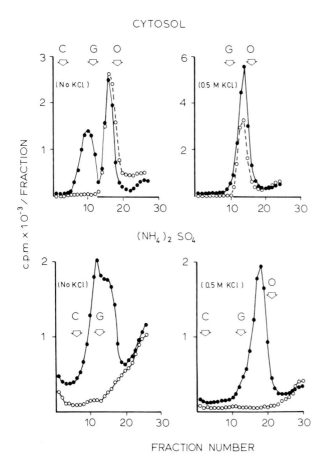

Fig. 1. Sucrose density gradient centrifugation of tumor cytosol (upper panels) and of cytosol proteins precipitated by 33% saturated ammonium sulfate (lower panels). Samples were incubated overnight at $0°C$ with 15 nM ^{3}H-DHT (●——●) or with 15 nM ^{3}H-DHT and 1.5 μM cold DHT (○–––○). Excess free steroid was removed by incubation with 0.1% Dextran-coated charcoal for 15 min prior to application on 5-20% sucrose gradients. Gradients shown in left panels were prepared in 50 mM tris-HCl buffer, pH 7.4, containing 10 mM β-mercaptoethanol and 10% (v/v) glycerol. Samples and gradients shown in right panels were adjusted to 0.5 M with respect to KCl. Gradient tubes were fractionated and numbered from the bottom. Arrows: sedimentation of the following internal reference markers: C, catalase (11.2 S); G, Bovine γ-globulin (6.9 S) and O, ovalbumin (3.6 S).

species. A second DHT-binding component with a lower sedimentation rate was not saturated by adding a 100-fold excess of cold steroid and represents nonspecific binding to protein(s) of low affinity (Fig. 1). High ionic strength shifted the receptor peak to the 4-5 S region where it overlapped with the nonspecific binding protein (Fig. 1). Receptor could be separated from

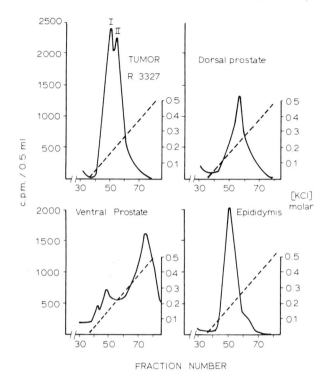

Fig. 2. Chromatography of cytosol receptors on phosphocellulose (Whatman p-11) columns. Cytosols (5 ml) were incubated overnight at $0°C$ with saturating amounts ^{3}H-DHT (15 nM) and loaded on 0.9 x 7 cm columns. Following washing with tris-HCl buffer (50 mN, pH 7.4 containing 10 mM β-mercaptoethanol) adsorbed proteins were eluted with a linear 0-0.7 M KCl gradient in 125 ml buffer. Broken line: KCl concentration as measured with an ion-specific electrode. Temperature was kept at $4°C$. Each fraction equals 1.3 ml.

nonspecific binding proteins by precipitation with 33% saturated ammonium sulfate. Receptor was recovered from the precipitate only partly in the 8 S form (Fig. 1). If the precipitate was dissolved in buffers of high ionic strength (0.5 M) the receptor sedimented as a single peak of sedimentation coefficient 5.0 S (Fig. 1).

Tumor cytosol receptors were retained on phosphocellulose column and were eluted with 0.15-0.25 M KCl (Fig. 2). Two DHT-binding components were observed. The first peak eluted (peak I, Fig. 2), which constituted more than 80% of recovered receptor, was shown to have a sedimentation coefficient of 5.1 S when analyzed on salt-containing sucrose gradients. Gel filtration on Sephadex G-200 in the presence of 0.5 M KCl, revealed a Stokes radius of 53 Å. From these data a molecular weight of 118,000 Daltons was calculated (Siegel and Monty, 1966). Another receptor form (form II, Fig. 2)

TABLE 1.
Molecular forms of androgen receptor

	Tumor R 3327	Dorsal prostate	Ventral prostate	Epididymis Testis Seminal vesicles
Sedimentation coefficient				
Low salt	7.9 ± 0.4	N.D.	3-9*	5-8*
High salt (0.5 M KCl)	I: 5.1 ± 0.2 II: 3.5 ± 0.2	I: N.D. II: 3.5 ± 0.3	A: 3.6 ± 0.1 B: 3.0 ± 0.2	I: 5.0 ± 0.3 II: 3.5 ± 0.2
Gel filtration (Stokes) radius (Å) (in 0.5 M KCl)	I: 53 ± 1 II: 37 ± 1	I: 53 ± 2 II: 38 ± 2	A: 35 ± 1 B: 22 ± 1	I: 53 ± 1 II: 36 ± 2
Molecular weight (Daltons)	I: 118,000 ± 7,000 II: 56,000 ± 5,000	I: N.D. II: 58,000 ± 6,000	A: 55,000 ± 5,000 B: 29,000 ± 2,000	I: 115,000 ± 6,000 II: 55,000 ± 5,000
Frictional ratio (f/f_0)	I: 1.64 ± 0.03 II: 1.47 ± 0.07	I: N.D. II: 1.49 ± 0.1	A: 1.40 ± 0.05 B: 1.05 ± 0.05	I: 1.66 ± 0.04 II: 1.43 ± 0.08
I KCl I at elution from phosphocellulose (M)	I: 0.17 ± 0.02 II: 0.23 ± 0.02	I: ~0.2 II: 0.24 ± 0.02	A: 0.40 ± 0.05 B: 0.28 ± 0.08	I: 0.18 ± 0.04 II: ~0.25, 0.40**
Dissociation half life of DHT-receptor complex at 0°C	~200 hr	N.D.	38 hr*	40 hr*
Thermal stability (heating at 20-37°C for 10-30 min)	I: Stable II: Unstable	I: Unstable II: Unstable	Unstable. A is converted to B	Unstable

N.D.: Not determined;
*Wilson et al. (1978);
**In seminal vesicles only.

which was eluted at slightly higher ionic strength, showed a sedimentation coefficient of 3.5 S and a gel filtration radius of 37 Å (Table 1).

In general, tumor cytosol receptors showed a high degree of homology with receptors from epididymis (Fig. 2) and testis (Table 1), both with respect to physico-chemical properties and relative abundance of the two receptor forms. Both receptors were also present in the dorsal prostate (Fig. 2), but here the 3.5 S from was predominant. In ventral prostate a receptor of size and symmetry similar to the small form (form II) was observed. The ventral prostate receptor, however, eluted from phosphocellulose columns at higher ionic strength (0.4 M) and exhibited considerable charge dispersity, suggesting it was a proteolytic fragment (Fig. 2). A difference was also seen upon heating of cytosol to 20-37°C. In tumor, epididymis, testis and seminal vesicles the 3.5 S form was extremely labile showing a complete loss of binding properties in a few minutes. In ventral prostate cytosol smaller fragments were produced (fragment B in Table 1) by the action of serine-type proteases (Lea et al., 1979a). Interconversion between the 3.5 S and 5 S receptor forms was not observed in these experiments. Heating of tumor cytosol at 37°C for periods up to 30 min had no effect on the 5 S form compared to a 70-90% destruction seen in other tissues.

Dissociation of receptor-^{3}H-DHT complex was followed for 3 days after adding a 1000-fold excess of cold steroid to labeled tumor cytosol. Bound ^{3}H-DHT was measured at different time intervals using a charcoal assay (Wilson et al., 1978). The receptor-DHT complex dissociated with an estimated half life of 200 hr at 0°C.

Tumor receptor concentration as quantitated by the recovery of labeled receptor from phosphocellulose columns was 100-220 fmol/mg cytosol protein. This is 2-5 times the level observed in other androgen dependant tissues of the male reproductive tract.

Discussion

This investigation has shown that the Dunning tumor cytosol receptors are identical with respect to charge, size and symmetry, to receptors found in normal androgen dependant tissues. Two salt stable forms of receptor were characterized. The predominant form had a molecular weight of 118,000 Daltons compared to 56,000 Daltons for the less abundant form. These two forms could not be interconverted by heating and do not participate in a simple monomer-dimer equilibrium. The 3.5 S form is probably derived from the larger receptor by the action of proteolytic enzymes (Wilson and French, 1979). The relative abundance of the large and small receptor (approximately 9:1) is also seen in testis, epididymis and, quite often, in seminal vesicles.

The dorsal prostate was suggested as the site of origin of the R 3327 tumor (Dunning, 1963). The absence of Prostatein, a secretory protein specific for the rat ventral prostate (Lea et al., 1979b), strongly supports this assumption. The predominance of the small receptor form found in dorsal prostate cytosol may reflect a higher level of proteolytic activity compared with tumor cytosol. Still higher protease levels were observed in the ventral prostate (Anderson and Müntzing, 1972; Lea et al., 1979a; Wilson and French, 1979) and also in transplantable adenocarcinomas derived from this gland (Müntzing et al., 1979).

No biological function for proteases in receptor transformation has been established, but proteases could play a role in receptor processing and in the termination of the androgenic response by destruction of the hormone-receptor complex. The stability of the tumor cytosol receptor may reflect a defect in this mechanism which may have implications for tumor growth.

Acknowledgements

We wish to thank Dr. N.H. Altman and M. Stevens of the Papanicolaou Cancer Research Center, Miami, USA, for supplying the tumor-bearing Copenhagen-Fisher rats.

References

Anderson, M. and Müntzing, J. (1972): *Invest. Urol., 9,* 401.
Dunning, W.I. (1963): *Nat. Canc. Inst. Monogr., 12,* 351.
Lea, O.A., Petrusz, P. and French, F.S. (1979b): *J. Biol. Chem., 254,* 6196.
Lea, O.A., Wilson, E.M. and French, F.S. (1979a): *Endocrinology, 105,* in press.
Müntzing, J., Kirdani, R.Y., Murphy, G.P. and Sandberg, A.A. (1979): *Invest. Urol., 17,* 37.
Siegel, L.M. and Monty, K.J. (1966): *Biochim. Biophys. Acta, (Amst.), 112,* 346.
Wilson, E.M. and French, F.S. (1979): *J. Biol. Chem., 254,* 6310.
Wilson, E.M., Lea, O.A. and French, F.S. (1978): In: *Receptors and Hormone Action, Vol II,* p. 491. Editors: B.W. O'Malley and L. Birnbaumer. Academic Press, New York.

Prostatic cancer: diagnostic and prognostic methods

F.H. SCHRÖDER

Department of Urology, Erasmus University, Rotterdam, The Netherlands

Incidence of prostatic cancer

Prostatic cancer accounts for roughly 9% of all cancer deaths in males. This makes prostatic cancer the second to third most frequent cause of death due to malignant disease in males. Due to large numbers of patients dying from other diseases in the involved age group the incidence of clinical cases is about twice as high as the mortality and amounted to about 50 per 100,000 men in 1974 in the U.S.A. (Silverberg and Holleb, 1974). If prostatic carcinoma is made the subject of a systematic search at the time of post mortem examinations the incidence rises to 28.9-100% for the age groups 50-90 yrs (Franks, 1977).

Clinical prostatic cancer is the tip of the ice-berg. Considering the tremendous difference between the mortality, clinical incidence and autopsy incidence of this tumor it becomes evident that most prostatic carcinomas will not kill their host and will also not lead to symptomatic disease.

The key problem of this tumor at the present time is that no reliable method exists to differentiate between cancers that will progress, cause symptoms and kill and the ones that will not do so. Clearly, case finding studies and clinical treatment trials make little sense if it does not become possible to differentiate harmless and life-threatening disease which unfortunately has the same histological appearance.

Diagnosis of prostatic cancer

The diagnosis of prostatic cancer can only be made by histological or cytological examination of a prostate found to be suspicious for prostatic cancer by rectal examination or other means. Sometimes prostatic cancer is diagnosed by detection of metastases or their symptoms. The search for a primary tumor will then lead to the prostate.

Symptoms

Most prostatic carcinomas remain non symptomatic until obstructive symptoms of urination or pain caused by metastases occur (Fergusson, 1973). The initial symptoms and the distribution of the clinical stages of 82 patients

TABLE 1.

Presenting symptoms and local extent (stage) of 82 prostatic carcinomas. Four cases were found to have unilateral edema of legs and 2 had palpable lymphnodes (inguinal)

Presenting symptoms	82 Patients
Urinary symptoms of 'prostatism'	58
Retention of urine	7
Backache (bone metastases)	14
Edema of leg	4
Paraplegia (bone metastases)	1
Abdominal mass	1

Clinical examination	Staging
Tx	8
T1	1
T2	7
T3	15
T4	48
Unknown	3

(From Fergusson, 1973)

is shown in Table 1. It can be seen that symptoms of prostatism still most frequently lead to the diagnosis of prostatic cancer. Unfortunately these symptoms are really no early symptoms. Early symptoms of localized disease unfortunately do not exist. The second most frequent symptom is pain or neurological disorder due to bone metastases. Only 10 of 82 patients had tumors that were confined to the prostate. Most prostatic carcinomas (90%) are detected in a locally wide spread or metastatic stage (Whitmore, 1973).

Rectal examination

Rectal examination is the single most important step in the diagnosis of prostatic cancer. This technique identifies irregularities and changes in the consistency of the prostate. In the hands of most clinicians 40-50% of suspicious lesions found by rectal examination turn out to be carcinomas when biopsied (Jewett, 1956; Schröder and Kowohl, 1971). Table 2 shows this histological diagnosis of 60 patients whose prostates were suspicious for carcinoma on rectal examination. In this series 40% of the patients turned out to have biopsies positive for carcinoma. Other differential diagnoses are listed. Prostatic stones, tuberculous prostatitis and other conditions which can mimic prostatic carcinoma were not found in this series.

Rectal examination is also useful in determining the local extent of the tumor. Significant errors are, however, made especially in the sense of

TABLE 2.

Histological diagnosis of 60 prostates suspicious for prostatic carcinoma on rectal examination

Histological diagnosis	No.	%
Carcinoma	24	40.0
Prostatitis	6	10.0
Granulomatous prostatitis	5	8.3
BPH	19	31.7
Technical failures	6	10.0
Total	60	100.0

(From Schröder and Kowohl, 1971)

TABLE 3.

Comparison of local tumor extent by rectal (T) and histological (P) examination in 484 patients. % staging error

	Total	P1 No.	P1 %	P2 No.	P2 %	P3 No.	P3 %	PX No.	PX %
Total	484	15	–	170	–	286	–	13	–
T0	55	15	27.3	18	32.7	20	36.4	2	3.6
T1-2	262	–	–	123	47.0	137	52.3	2	0.7
T3	152	–	–	23	15.1	125	82.3	4	2.6
TX	15	–	–	6	40.0	4	26.7	5	33.3

(From Schröder, 1980)

understaging lesions apparently confined to the prostate. Table 3 indicates the findings obtained on rectal examination (T category) and on histological examination of the radical prostatectomy specimens (P category) of 484 patients. The T_0 category was confirmed in only 27.3%, the T_1, T_2 category in 47.0% and the T_3 category in 82.3% of the cases examined. The staging errors made by rectal examination are 69.1% for T_0, 52.3% for T_1, T_2 and 15.1% for the T_3 categories, respectively (Schröder, 1980).

Still, in spite of these errors, survival is strongly dependent on local tumor extension as determined by rectal examination. This is shown below in more detail under Tumor Extent.

Diagnosis of metastases

The most common sites of metastatic disease are regional and juxta-regional

TABLE 4.

Lymphnode metastases and local tumor extent

Author	Category + LN metastases				
	T0	T1,2	T3	T3 + seminal vesicle vesicles	T4
Flocks et al. (1953, 1973)			7.0	35.0	
Whitmore (1973)				50.0	
Mackenzie (1959)					
Ardouino,			12.9	–	91.0
Glucksman (1962)					
Kopecky (1970)	12.0				
McCullough (1974)			25.0	51.0	82.0	82.0
McCullough, McLoughlin (unpublished)			11.0	67.0	
Whitmore et al. (1972)			25.0	55.0	
Castellino et al. (1973)			44.0	56.0	

(From Schröder,1978)

lymphnodes. Table 4 indicates the incidence of metastic lymphnodes in correlation to the local extent of the tumor. These data were obtained in patients undergoing diagnostic lymphadenectomies. Roughly, the incidence of lymphnode metastases increases from 25% in tumors confined to the prostate to 50% in tumors extending through the prostatic capsule and 80% in tumors that have reached the seminal vesicles (Schröder, 1978). Barzell et al. (1977) have found that tumor volumes of more than 3 cm^3 in lymphnodes have a strong negative impact on the prognosis, and that small lymphnode metastases do not seem to influence the prognosis if they are removed.

Lymphnode metastases are commonly evaluated by pedal lymphangiography, an examination which consists of the slow injection of a contrast medium into the lymphvessels. Unfortunately, this technique is associated with a large number of false negative and false positive results and has been abandoned by many clinicians. Instead of this, the operative exploration of the lymphnodes for determination of the N category is used in many centers. Bones and lungs are the next common sites of metastases associated with prostatic carcinoma.

Early detection of metastases is of the greatest importance because different treatment modalities have to be used in metastatic and non metastatic patients. The latter can be considered potentially curable.

Radioisotope bone scanning is the most useful technique in identification and localization of bone metastases. ^{99}Te-Polyphosphate is most commonly used at the present time and produces sensitive and fast results. Bone scanning is more sensitive but also more unspecific than X-ray examinations.

TABLE 5.

Serum acid phosphatase activities determined by radioimmuno assay (RIA) and enzyme assay in normal male controls, patients with prostatic carcinoma and other disorders

Prostatic cancer		Acid phosphatase			
Group	No. patients	RIA > 8.0 ng/.1 ml		Enzyme assay > 0.2 SU/1.0 ml	
		No.	%	No.	%
Controls	50	0	0	0	0
Prostatic CA					
Stage I	24	8	33	3	12
Stage II	33	26	79	5	15
Stage III	31	22	71	9	29
Stage IV	25	23	92	15	60
BPH	36	2	6	0	0
Other CA	83	9	11	7	8
Gastrointestinal disorders	20	1	5	0	0
Post total prostatectomy	28	1	4	0	0

(From Foti et al., 1977)

Bone scanning does not detect osteolytic processes which fortunately rarely occur without being associated with osteoblastic lesions (Fitzpatrick et al., 1978). Old fractures and degenerative bone changes cannot be differentiated from metastases by bone scans. The high rate of false positive bone scan studies can however be markedly reduced by adding X-ray studies and biopsies of the suspicious areas to the diagnostic procedure. In this way the high accuracy of bone scanning in detecting occult lesions can be combined with the better specificity of X-ray and biopsy procedures.

Lung metastases are detected by chest X-rays and planigrams.

Markers

Acid phosphatase was the first marker enzyme ever used in any human cancer (Gutman et al., 1936). Recent development of radioimmunological techniques, immunochemical techniques and counter electrophoresis has opened new dimensions not only for the diagnosis of metastases but also for the diagnosis of small primary tumors. Recently, the evaluation of serum acid phosphatase in 113 patients with prostatic malignancy detected high values in 33%, 79%, 71% and 92% of patients with stage I, II, III and IV tumors respectively. Problems are the definition of the normal values, false positive findings associated with other disorders and the cost of the assay (Foti et al., 1977). Some additional data are summarized in Table 5, which also shows the greater sensitivity of the radioimmunoassay as compared to one of the enzyme assays which is commonly used in clinical laboratories. It can be seen, that other carcinomas, intestinal disorders and benign prostatic hyperplasia (BPH) were associated with elevated acid phosphatase values in 5-11% of the cases studied. The high rate of positive studies in the tumors confined to the prostate may, after more extensive study, qualify this new parameter as a screening test for prostatic carcinoma. It is not yet known whether prostatic acid phosphatase as determined by radioimmunoassay or related techniques will be a useful marker to monitor the clinical course of the disease. Van der Werf-Messing et al. (1976) have shown that an elevation of previously normal serum acid phosphatase is the earliest sign of metastases after irradiation treatment. Studies of acid phosphatase in bone marrow aspirates may even improve these results (Belville et al., 1979). Other markers of possible usefulness are alkaline phosphatase (Wajsman et al., 1978), LDH isoenzyme V/I ratio, urinary cholesterol, urinary ketosteroids, carcinoembryonic antigen (CEA), N-acetylneuraminic acid (NANA) (Moss et al., 1979), spermine-spermidine ratio and others.

Prognostic factors

The absence of reliable prognostic parameters which allow identification of potentially lethal carcinomas is one of the major gaps in our knowledge of this tumor. Once a clinically progressive course is taken by any prostatic cancer the prognosis can be predicted with some approximation by the use of information concerning the extent of the disease, its grade of malignancy and tumor markers.

Tumor extent (T-category)

For the description of the extent of the primary tumor and its metastases the use of the TNM system (tumor, nodes, metastases) is recommended. The extent of the primary tumor, the T category, correlates significantly with survival in most series of patients published. Figure 1 presents an example. Survival correlates significantly with the T categories in this series of 469 patients treated by total perineal prostatectomy (Schröder, 1980).

Independent of the type of treatment used, the 5 years survival figures for the different T categories are roughly T_0 = identical with life expectancy, T_1, T_2 = 70-80%, T_3, T_4 = 40-60%. Patients with metastases usually die within 3 years after diagnosis. Approximately 50% die of unrelated causes. Tumor extension is an important parameter for treatment decisions (VACURG, 1967).

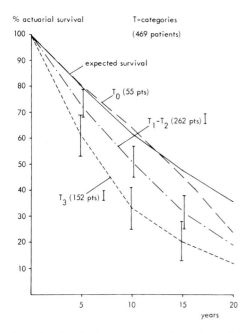

Fig. 1. Survival and expected survival of 469 patients with prostatic carcinoma treated by total prostatectomy. Survival correlates significantly with tumor extent (T-categories). (From Schröder, 1980)

Grade of malignancy

Morphological features of the prostatic cancer cell or structures of the tissue could turn out to have the prognostic relevance so urgently needed for the identification of potentially dangerous tumors. A good correlation between survival and such morphological parameters has been found by many investigators. The problem remains that some patients categorized as having 'well differentiated' lesions will die within a short period of time of their disease and others with apparently aggressive tumors will live for a very long time. The most frequently used systems for histological grading of prostatic cancer are those of Gleason (1977) and Mostofi (1975). A disadvantage of these techniques is that the extreme groups contain relatively few patients and that most patients fall into intermediate groups with tumors which may behave either way. In the system of Mostofi nuclear pleomorphism was found to be the parameter that would predict death from prostatic carcinoma with the greatest accuracy.

This is demonstrated in Figure 2. The survival and expected survival of 259 patients with prostatic carcinoma treated by radical prostatectomy is considered in the groups with slight, moderate and marked nuclear pleomorphism in the histological specimens. The differences observed are even

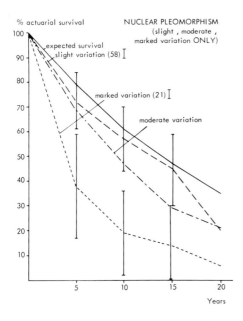

Fig. 2. Survival and expected survival in 259 patients with prostatic carcinoma treated by radical prostatectomy. Data are separated into groups with slight, moderate and marked nuclear pleomorphism. (From Schröder, 1980).

more significant if one considers the deathrate from prostatic carcinoma in similar groups. These data are presented in Table 6. It can be seen that there is a highly significant increase of disease related mortality with the grade of malignancy as determined by the parameter of nuclear pleomorphism.

If one combines both parameters, the local extent (T category) and the grade of malignancy (nuclear pleomorphism), an even more significant prognostic parameter can be obtained. Table 7 presents an example. Small tumors which are well differentiated are listed on the left side of this table. It can clearly be seen that less than 10% of these patients die of prostatic carcinoma with metastases. It remains unclear as to how far the natural history or the treatment effect is reflected by these data. The moderately and poorly differentiated tumors are listed towards the right side of the table. 20-45% of these patients die of their disease in spite of total prostatectomy.

Similar data can also be obtained by determining the grade of malignancy by cytological means (Esposti, 1971), which are less involving and less dangerous for the patient. The accuracy of this procedure, however, has not been determined as well as that of histological examination and needs to be further investigated.

The combination of the grade of malignancy and local tumor extent

TABLE 6.

Disease related mortality and grade of malignancy (nuclear pleomorphism)

Nuclear variation	No. patients	No. dead patients	Dead from CA. prost.	
			No. patients	%
Slight	58	38	4	10
Moderate	223	157	45	29 (28)*
Marked	65	47	24	51 (60)*

*Moderate or marked *only.*

TABLE 7.

Correlation between tumor extent and grade of malignancy as prognostic parameters in patients following radical prostatectomy. Identification of risk groups

T and P categories	Nuclear pleomorphism								
	Slight			Moderate			Marked		
	No. patients	No. dead	CA. %	No. patients	No. dead	CA. %	No. patients	No. dead	CA. %
T0	10	0	0	23	6	26.1	5	2	40.0
P1	6	0	0	4	0	0	0	0	0
T1-2	33	3	9.1	125	18	14.4	31	10	32.3
P2	28	2	7.1	72	7	9.7	14	2	14.3
T3	15	1	6.7	73	21	28.8	27	12	44.4
P3	22	1	4.6	146	38	26.0	51	22	43.1

allows identification of prognostic groups of patients. Unfortunately, these parameters are not yet sufficiently reliable to identify patients, who may not require treatment at all. Still, considering the large discrepancy between autopsy incidence and clinical incidence respectively mortality, large numbers of patients with potentially not life-threatening tumors do exist and are probably treated unnecessarily. Establishing a reliable prognostic marker which allows differentiation between such groups of tumors still remains the most urgent problem to be solved in the field of prostatic carcinoma.

Markers

Elevated serum acid phosphatase levels determined by routine enzyme assays decrease in patients responding to endocrine management of the prostatic carcinoma. A rise in serum acid phosphatase in a patient with previously

152   F.H. Schröder

normal values indicates, with very high reliability, the presence of metastases. Our knowledge about the application of immunological assays for prostatic acid phosphatase in the follow-up of patients is still very limited. The usefulness of monitoring the course of the disease and the response to treatment of prostatic carcinoma patients has not yet been sufficiently established. Some preliminary results are very promising.

The role of the other markers mentioned above and that of steroid receptors in prostatic cancer tissue as well as peripheral steroid levels in monitoring the non-specific response of the host remains experimental for the moment.

References

Barzell, W., Bean, M.A., Hilaris, B.S. and Whitmore, W.F., Jr. (1977): *J. Urol., 118,* 278.
Belville, W.D., Cox, H.D., Mahan, D.E., Stutzman, R.E. and Bruce, A.W. (1979): *J. Urol., 121,* 442.
Esposti, P.L. (1971): *Scand. J. Urol. Nephrol., 5,* 199.
Fergusson, J.D. (1973): In: *XVIe Congrès de la Société Internationale d'Urologie, Paris, Tome 1,* p. 53.
Fitzpatrick, Z.M., Constable, A.R., Sherwood, T., Stephenson, J.J., Chisholm, G.D. and Donovan, E.P.N.O. (1978): *Brit. J. Urol., 50,* 555.
Foti, A.G., Cooper, J.F., Herschman, H. and Malvaez, R.R. (1977): *New Engl. J. Med., 279,* 1357.
Franks, L.M. (1977): In: *Urologic Pathology: The Prostate,* p. 23. Editor: M. Tannenbaum. Lea and Febiger, Philadelphia.
Gleason, D.F. (1977): In: *Urologic Pathology: The Prostate,* p.17 Editor: M. Tannenbaum. Lea and Febiger, Philadelphia.
Gutman, E.G., Sproul, E.E. and Gutman, A.B. (1936): *Amer. J. Cancer, 28,* 485.
Jewett, H.J. (1956): *J. Amer. Med. Ass., 160,* 838.
Moss, A.J. Jr., Bissada, N.K., Boyd, C.M. and Hunter, W.C. (1979): *Urology, XIII,* 182.
Mostofi, F.H. (1975): *Cancer Chemother. Rep., 1,* 111.
Schröder, F.H. (1978): *Med. Welt, 29,* 1206.
Schröder, F.H. (1980): *Scand. J. Urol. Nephrol., Suppl.,* in press.
Schröder, F.H. and Kowohl, K. (1971): *Urologe A, 10,* 170.
Silverberg, E. and Holleb, A.I. (1974): *CA (A Cancer Journal for Clinicians), 24,* 2.
Veterans Administration Co-operative Urological Research Group (1967): *SGO, 124,* 1011.
Wajsman, Z., Chu, T.M., Bross, D., Saroff, J., Murphy, G.P., Johnson, D.E., Scott, W.W., Gibbons, R.P., Prout, G.R. and Schmidt, J.D. (1978): *J. Urol., 119,* 244.
Van der Werf-Messing, B., Sourek-Zikova, V. and Blonk, D.I. (1976): *Int. J. Radiat. Oncol. (Biol. Phys.), 1,* 1043.
Whitmore, W.F., Jr. (1973): *Cancer, 32,* 1104.

Prostatic secretion protein, an androgen-sensitive protein in rat and human prostate*

Å. POUSETTE[1], P. BJÖRK[2], K. CARLSTRÖM[3], B. FORSGREN[2], B. HÖGBERG[2] and J.-Å. GUSTAFSSON[1]

[1] *Department of Chemistry and Department of Medical Nutrition, Karolinska Institutet, Stockholm;* [2] *Leo Research Laboratories, Helsingborg;* [3] *Hormone Laboratory, Sabbatsberg Hospital, Stockholm, Sweden*

The prostatic secretion protein (PSP) or estramustine-binding protein (EMBP) was discovered when investigating the mechanism of action of estramustine phosphate (Estracyt) (Forsgren et al., 1978). This drug was introduced in 1966 as a therapeutic agent in the treatment of prostatic carcinoma (Jönsson et al., 1977). The mechanism of action of estramustine phosphate is complex. Studies in man and in animals have shown that the drug decreases testosterone and gonadotropin levels in serum, causes atrophy of the testes and accessory sex organs, reduces the uptake of zinc by the prostate, depresses the 5α-reductase, arginase and acid phosphatase activities in the prostate, and affects lipid and carbohydrate metabolism (Gustafsson et al., 1977). Although the observed effects in many respects are similar to estrogenic effects, several experimental and clinical results indicate that estramustine phosphate affects normal and neoplastic tissue in a way that cannot solely be attributed to its anti-gonadotropic or weak estrogenic properties. The main metabolite of estramustine phosphate was found to be estramustine, and in order to analyze this compound, estramustine of high specific radioactivity was synthesized. Using autoradiographic techniques after injection of ^{3}H-estramustine in male rats, a high uptake was observed especially in the prostate (Appelgren et al., 1978). Radioactivity was localized in the epithelial cells as well as in the lumina of the ventral prostate. These data indicated that estramustine was taken up into the epithelial cells of the prostate and secreted into the lumina of the ductuli.

In vivo as well as in vitro studies showed that estramustine was bound to a protein in the prostate gland. This protein was called prostatic secretion protein. Estramustine was shown to bind to the protein with a K_d of about 10^{-8} M, and the binding was shown to be relatively specific with regard to the ligand-binding site (Forsgren et al., 1980). The steroid-PSP complex had an M_r of 46,000 as estimated by gel filtration and an isoelectric point of about 5. The protein was purified to homogeneity using chromatography on

*This study was supported by grants from the Swedish Cancer Society and from Leo Research Council.

DEAE-cellulose, Sephadex G-100 Superfine, Octyl-Sepharose CL-4B and polyacrylamide gel electrophoresis.

Following analysis by polyacrylamide gel electrophoresis in the presence of sodium dodecyl sulfate, the protein was found to consist of 2 subunits with M_r values of about 20,000 and 18,000, respectively. After reduction of disulfide bridges, the protein decomposed into 3 components with M_r values of about 12,000, 11,000 and 8,000, respectively (Forsgren et al., 1979). Amino acid analysis showed that the protein is a glycoprotein. Antibodies against the protein were raised in rabbits, and a radio-immunoassay was developed to quantitate the protein. Using this method, it was shown that estramustine-binding protein was predominantly found in the accessory sexual glands of the male rat. It was estimated that the prostatic secretion protein constituted about 18% of the total protein in rat ventral prostate. PSP was also present in the dorsal and lateral lobes of the prostate and in the seminal vesicles, coagulating glands, epididymes and preputial glands of the male rat. Preliminary studies also show that it is present in the secretion fluid from the prostate gland.

Prostatic secretion protein is an androgen-sensitive protein, e.g. the amount of the protein is decreased following testectomy and is restored after administration of testosterone propionate. An immunologically similar protein is also present in prostate from mouse, rabbit, boar and man. Also in these species, we have found a high tissue specificity of the protein (Pousette et al., 1980).

In cytosol from human prostate, estramustine is bound to a protein immunologically similar to rat PSP and with a K_d of about 35 nM. The estramustine-protein complex in human prostate cytosol has an isoelectric point of about 5, a characteristic in common with the complex in rat prostate cytosol.

Since the estramustine-binding protein is almost exclusively found in the male sex accessory glands and is secreted into the reproductive tract, it may be suggested that it plays a role in maintaining normal male fertility. Furthermore, the androgen dependence of this protein may make it a unique indication of hormonal action on the prostate. It is therefore possible that quantitation of the estramustine-binding protein could be used as a predictive test when selecting therapy in cases of prostatic carcinoma.

References

Appelgren, L.-E., Forsgren, B., Gustafsson, J.-Å., Pousette, Å. and Högberg, B. (1978): *Acta Pharmacol. (Kbh.), 43,* 368.

Forsgren, B., Björk, P., Carlström, K., Gustafsson, J.-Å., Pousette, Å. and Högberg, B. (1979): *Proc. Nat. Acad. Sci. (Wash.), 76,* 3149.

Forsgren, B., Gustafsson, J.-Å., Pousette, Å. and Högberg, B. (1980): *Cancer Res.,* submitted for publication.

Forsgren, B., Högberg, B., Gustafsson, J.-Å. and Pousette, Å. (1978): *Acta Pharm. Suecica, 15,* 23.

Gustafsson, A., Nilsson, S., Persson, B., Tisell, L.-E., Wiklund, O. and Ohlson, R. (1977): *Invest. Urol., 15,* 220.

Jönsson, G., Högberg, B. and Nilsson, T. (1977): *Scand. J. Urol. Nephrol., 11,* 231.

Pousette, Å., Björk, P., Carlström, K., Forsgren, B., Gustafsson, J.-Å. and Högberg, B. (1980): *Acta Chem. Scand., 334,* 155.

156

Radioimmunoassay of human prostate-specific acid phosphatase in the diagnosis and follow-up of therapy of prostatic cancer*

P. VIHKO

Departments of Anatomy and Clinical Chemistry, University of Oulu, Oulu, Finland

Since the original findings of Gutman et al. (1936) and of Huggins and Hodges (1941) that serum acid phosphatase (EC 3.1.3.2) activity is markedly increased in patients with prostatic carcinoma, determination of this enzyme activity has been widely used to detect prostatic carcinoma and to monitor the effects of therapy (Gittes and Chu, 1976). When the assay of serum acid phosphatase is based on the measurement of its catalytic activity, serum phosphatases of non-prostatic origin contribute to the results (Yam, 1974). Another factor complicating these measurements is the great instability of the catalytic activity of the enzyme (Woodard, 1951; Vihko, 1978). Many potential errors limit the clinical usefulness of the measurement of the catalytic activity of this enzyme, which is considered to be one of the most promising tumor markers.

Shulman et al. (1964) and Ablin et al. (1970) first reported the possible immunological specificity of acid phosphatase of the human prostate. Their results suggested that an immunological assay could be developed, which would specifically detect prostatic acid phosphatase. The radioimmunoassay technique for the enzyme protein combines the specificity of the immunologic analysis with the sensitivity of current radioisotopic technology.

Because circulating acid phosphatase is a mixture of isoenzymes originating from several tissues (Yam, 1974), it is essential to pay great attention to the purity of the antigen and tracer used if one is to have an organ-specific determination of serum acid phosphatase. We have previously described a specific and sensitive radioimmunoassay (RIA) for human prostatic acid phosphatase (PAP) in serum (Vihko et al., 1978a). The antigen we used was purified to homogeneity from human prostatic tissue (Vihko et al., 1978b), and subsequently used to raise monospecific antibodies, which had no crossreactivity with acid phosphatases originating from other human tissues, particularly those having the same electrophoretic mobility. We have further developed the RIA for the determination of serum prostate-specific acid phosphatase and studied its application to the diagnosis and follow-up of therapy of prostatic carcinoma.

This investigation was partially supported by a grant from the Finnish Cancer Foundation.

Material and methods

RIA procedure

In short, RIA of human prostatic acid phosphatase is performed as follows: (1) incubation of 0.2 ml of serum with 0.2 ml of diluted antiserum (1:30,000) for 1 hr; (2) addition of 0.2 ml of an iodinated tracer (50,000 cpm) and incubation of the mixture for 3 hr; (3) separation of bound and free radioactivity by precipitation with antirabbit γ-globulin-PEG solution for 15 min; (4) counting of radioactivity in the bound fraction. The concentrations of acid phosphatase in sera were calculated with the aid of standards of 0, 0.5, 1, 3, 10, 15 and 30 $\mu g/l$ of the purified enzyme.

Other techniques

Assay of the catalytic activity of acid phosphatase was made by the method described by Bessey et al. (1946) using p-nitrophenylphosphate as substrate and L(+)-tartrate as inhibitor.

Serum specimens

The group of normal males consisted of 199 young (aged 20-50 yrs) and 195 older (aged 51-75 yrs) volunteers. Subjects who had previously experienced any form of urinary difficulty or urogenital disease were excluded. Only subjects with normal prostate size, as judged by rectal palpation, were accepted.

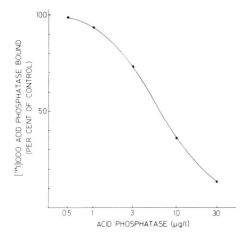

Fig. 1. Radioimmunoassay of human prostatic acid phosphatase. Indicated amounts of prostatic acid phosphatase were added to acid phosphatase-free sheep serum and incubated with the antiserum 1 + 3 hr. Bound and free antigen fractions were separated by precipitation with antirabbit γ-globulin-PEG-solution. (Vihko et al., 1980).

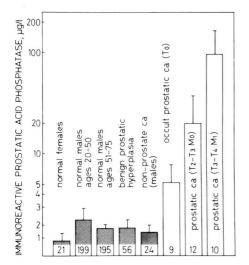

Fig. 2. Immunoreactive prostatic acid phosphatase in sera of healthy females (n = 21), normal males aged 20-50 (n = 199), normal males aged 51-75 (n = 195), patients with histologically proven benign prostatic hyperplasia (n = 56), nonprostate carcinoma (n = 24), occult prostatic carcinoma (n = 9), prostatic carcinoma (n = 12) and patients with metastatic prostatic carcinoma (n = 10).

Our patient group consisted of men attending the Division of Urology, Department of Surgery, Oulu University Central Hospital, for treatment or observations in connection with either benign prostatic hyperplasia (n = 56), carcinoma of the prostate (n = 22) or some other carcinomas (n = 24). Occult prostatic carcinomas (n = 9) were incidental histopathological findings after an operation for prostatic hyperplasia. For the diagnosis and primary classification of the disease, patients were examined by rectal palpation of the prostate, isotopic bone scan, X-ray bone studies and prostate biopsy. The patients with prostatic carcinoma were either treated with polyestradiol phosphate, or castration, or both. During the follow-up period, the patients were seen 0.5, 1, 3, 6, 9 and 12 months after starting treatment. Serum samples for RIA were taken before rectal palpation of the prostate, and stored at $-20°C$ before assay.

Results

Characteristics of the RIA

Figure 1 shows a standard curve for the RIA of PAP. With antiserum dilution of 1:30,000 and using 0.2 ml of serum samples, the lowest measurable acid phosphatase level was 0.2 $\mu g/l$. Dilution of aliquots of the samples with acid phosphatase-free sheep serum allowed quantification of concentrations many fold higher than the standard upper limit (30 $\mu g/l$) of the assay. Within- and

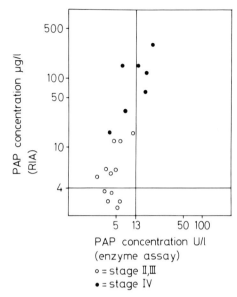

Fig. 3. Measurements of immunoassayable prostatic acid phosphatase and catalytic activity of prostatic acid phosphatase in diagnosis of prostatic carcinoma (stages II, III, IV). Upper limit for reference range of immunoassayable prostatic acid phosphatase was 4 μg/l (= mean + 3 SD) and for total catalytic activity of acid phosphatase 13 U/l.

between-assay variation coefficients were between 7 and 9% and 6 and 11%, respectively, and nonspecific binding was 5%.

Concentrations of prostate-specific acid phosphatase in serum

Figure 2 shows the concentrations of immunoreactive prostatic acid phosphatase, measured by the present RIA, in serum samples from healthy women and men, patients suffering from benign prostatic hyperplasia, patients with nonprostatic carcinoma and patients with prostatic carcinoma. The mean concentrations ± 1 SD, μg/l for normal healthy men and for patients with benign prostatic hyperplasia were 1.94 ± 0.66 (n = 394) and 1.71 ± 0.76 (n = 56), respectively. Values for patients with prostatic carcinoma were up to more than 100 times higher. (T_0 (= occult prostatic ca), 5.02 ± 2.59, n = 9; T_2-T_3 M_0, 19.85 ± 16.82, n = 12; T_3-T_4 M_1, 94.3 ± 66.17, n = 10). In the present group of stage II-III patients (VACURG, 1967) prior to institution of any form of therapy, serum radioimmunoassayable PAP exceeded the upper limit of our reference range of 4 μg/l (mean + 3 SD) in 7/12 patients, whereas the measurement of catalytic activity, both total and tartrate-labile, gave normal results in all stage II-III patients. In stage IV patients, the catalytic activity was elevated in 4/7, whereas immunoassayable PAP was elevated in all patients of this group (Fig. 3).

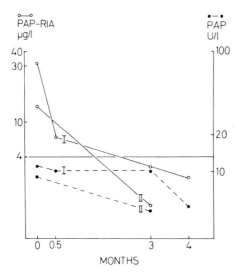

Fig. 4a

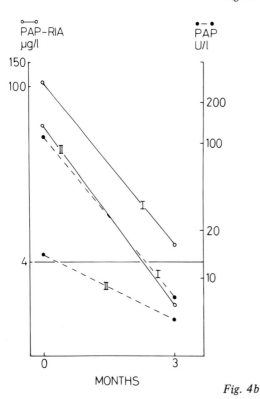

Fig. 4b

Fig. 4. (a) Effect of endocrine therapy on prostatic acid phosphatase concentrations in sera of patients with prostatic carcinoma, over 4 months. Patient I = $T_3 M_0$, patient II = $T_2 M_0$. (b) As in (a), but for 3 months. Patient I = $T_4 M_1$ and patient II = $T_4 M_0$.

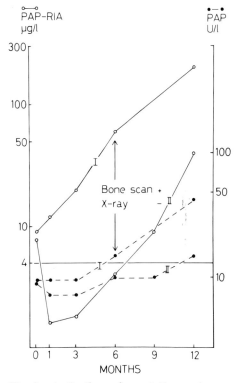

Fig. 5. Activation of prostatic carcinoma during endocrine treatment of patients with prostatic carcinoma. Follow-up of concentrations of prostatic acid phosphatase of patients I (= $T_3 M_0$) and II (= $T_2 M_0$).

As seen in Figures 4a and 4b, after the initiation of therapy, a favorable response was reflected by the results of both methods, but the per cent changes in immunoassayable PAP were larger and occurred earlier than those obtained by the measurement of the catalytic activity.

In the course of therapy, clinical signs of activation of the disease were preceded by an increase in immunoassayable PAP (Fig. 5).

Conclusions

The levels of immunoreactive prostate-specific acid phosphatase in sera of healthy men were < 4 μg/l (mean + 3 SD), serum concentrations of this phosphatase in patients with benign prostatic hyperplasia were identical to those in healthy reference subjects. The concentration of serum immunoreactive prostatic acid phosphatase seems to reflect the dissemination of prostatic carcinoma. The measurement of the immunoreactive enzyme was more sensitive than the measurement of the catalytic activity for the detection of elevated enzyme levels in stages II-IV of prostatic carcinoma.

162 *P. Vihko*

Favorable effects of the various forms of endocrine treatment were detected earlier by the measurement of immunoassayable PAP than by the measurement of catalytic activity. Activation of the disease during various forms of endocrine treatment of prostatic carcinoma (stages II-IV) was more efficiently revealed by RIA than by measurement of catalytic activity. The per cent changes of radioimmunoassayable PAP were larger than those found by the measurement of catalytic activity.

References

Ablin, R.J., Bronson, P., Soanes, W.A. and Witebsky, E. (1970): *J. Immunol., 104,* 1329.
Bessey, O.A., Lowry, O.H. and Brock, M.J. (1946): *J. Biol. Chem., 164,* 321.
Gittes, R.F. and Chu, T.M. (1976): *Semin. Oncol., 3,* 123.
Gutman, E.B., Sproul, E.E. and Gutman, A.B. (1936): *Amer. J. Cancer, 28,* 485.
Huggins, C. and Hodges, C.V. (1941): *Cancer Res., 1,* 293.
Shulman, S., Marnrod, L., Gondor, M.J. and Soanes, W.A. (1964): *J. Immunol., 94,* 474.
The Veterans Administration Co-operative Urological Research Group (1967): *Surg. Gynec. Obstet., 124,* 1011.
Vihko, P. (1978): *Clin. Chem., 24,* 1783.
Vihko, P., Kontturi, M. and Korhonen, L.K. (1978b): *Clin. Chem., 24,* 466.
Vihko, P., Kostama, A., Jänne, O., Sajanti, E. and Vihko, R. (1980): *Clin. Chem., 26/11.*
Vihko, P., Sajanti, E., Jänne, O., Peltomen, L. and Vihko, R. (1978a): *Clin. Chem., 24,* 1915.
Woodard, H.O. (1951): *J. Urol., 65,* 688.
Yam, L.T. (1974): *Amer. J. Med., 56,* 604.

Diagnosis of prostate cancer using a radioimmunoassay for prostatic acid phosphatase in serum*

O.A. LEA and P.Å. HØISAETER

Hormone Laboratory and Department of Surgery, University of Bergen, Bergen, Norway

Determination of prostatic acid phosphatase, PAP, (orthophosphoric mono-ester phosphohydrolase, acid optimum, EC 3.1.3.2.) in serum has a long standing recognition as a useful aid in the detection of prostatic cancer. Measurement of PAP by conventional enzyme assay is, however, subject to a number of potential errors (Yam, 1974). The enzymatic activity is difficult to distinguish from that of other acid phosphatases of nonprostatic origin. Lack of stability of the catalytic activity is another complicating factor. The introduction of immunological methods seems to circumvent some of these problems (Cooper et al., 1978; Lee et al., 1978; Vihko et al., 1978). This paper describes our experience in developing and evaluating a specific radioimmunoassay.

Material and methods

Clinical measurements of PAP (tartrate inhibited acid phosphatase) in serum were carried out in the Laboratories of Clinical Biochemistry, Haukeland Sykehus, Bergen, according to Bergmeyer (1970). Sera received in the Hormone Laboratory, University of Bergen, from patients undergoing evaluation for various endocrinological disorders, were used as reference material for this study.

Acid phosphatase was isolated from hypertrophied prostatic tissue removed at surgery, as outlined in Table 1. Rabbits were immunized using a primary injection of 250 μg pure protein in approximately 20 intradermal sites. Antigen was emulsified in saline-Freund's complete adjuvant (1:1). At subsequent 6-week intervals the rabbits received subcutaneous booster injections using 200 μg PAP emulsified in Freund's incomplete adjuvant. 1-2 weeks following each booster injection the rabbits were bled from an ear vein. Antisera obtained appeared monospecific when tested by immunodiffusion and bidimensional (crossed) immunoelectrophoresis against purified antigen and prostate cytosol.

*This work was supported by the Norwegian Cancer Society (Landsforeningen mot Kreft), Oslo, Norway.

Radioiodination was carried out using the Chloramine T method of Greenwood et al. (1963). 2.5 µg pure PAP was reacted with 1 mCi carrier-free [125]I (Institute for Nuclear Energy, Kjeller, Norway). A yield of 40-50% was achieved using a reaction time of 1 min. Specific activity ranged from 160 to 200 Ci/µg PAP. Labelled protein could be used for periods up to 3 weeks when stored at 0-4°C.

Tris-HCl buffer, 50 mM, pH 7.4 containing 0.05% sodium azide and 0.1% bovine serum albumin, was used throughout as a diluent and assay buffer. Sheep anti-rabbit immunoglobulins covalently coupled to cellulose (Organon Teknika B.V., Oss, Holland) served as second antibody.

Radioimmunoassay procedure

In each tube 100 µl sample was mixed with 200 µl buffer containing 40-70,000 cpm ^{125}I-PAP. Then 200 µl antiserum diluted 1:40,000 was added and the mixture allowed to incubate overnight at room temperature. One ml of a 1:100 suspension of second antibody in buffer was then added and the tube rotated end over end in a 'Rotamixer' (Heto, Birkeroed, Denmark) for a minimum of 3 hr. Following centrifugation at 2000 g the pellet was washed 3 times with assay buffer and then counted in a Packard automated gamma counter. Calibration plots were constructed based on the binding of iodinated trace in the presence of 7 different concentrations of unlabelled PAP in the range 0.2-25 ng/100 µl.

Results

Data relevant to the performance of the purification procedure is summarized in Table 1. The final PAP preparation was homogeneous when analyzed by agarose gel electrophoresis in 1% gels. In SDS-polyacrylamide gel electrophoresis (7% gels) according to Weber and Osborne (1969) PAP migrated as a single band. A molecular weight of 54,000 Daltons was estimated by this method which is in excellent agreement with values published for the monomeric enzyme (Luchter-Wasyl and Ostrowski, 1974). Electrophoresis in 5, 7, 9 and 11% polyacrylamide gels under nondenaturing conditions (Rodbard and Chrambach, 1971) caused PAP to split up in several enzymatically active bands reminiscent of a polymeric series.

A typical standard calibration curve for the radioimmunoassay is presented in Figure 1 as a plot of relative binding of trace, B/B_0, vs PAP concentration. Binding of trace alone (B_0) usually ranged from 30-38% of added ^{125}I-PAP. The fact that parallel standard curves were obtained using crude cytosol or pure antigen (Fig. 1) confirms the specificity of the assay system.

Sera from various sources, together with some common proteins listed in Table 2, had an inhibitory effect on the binding of ^{125}I-PAP to antiserum.

TABLE 1.

Purification of prostatic acid phosphatase

Purification step	Cumulative recovery (%)	Specific activity (U*/mg protein)
Cytosol	100.0	6.4
Ion exchange chromatography on DEAE-Sepharose CL 6B	77.7	17.9
Affinity chromatography on Concanavalin A-Sepharose 4 B	62.1	159
Gel filtration on LKB Ultrogel AcA 44	46.0	234
Gel filtration repeated in presence of 1.0 M KCl	40.0	261

*One unit hydrolyzes 1 μmol p-nitrophenylphosphate per min at pH 5.0 and 25°C.

TABLE 2.

Influence of proteins from various sources on assay system expressed in PAP equivalents

Source	ng/100 μl Mean	± SD	No. observations
Serum, men > 50 yrs	1.10	0.35	54
Serum, women	0.67	0.24	15
Serum, pregnant women (3rd trimester)	1.59	0.51	10
Serum, patients with cancer of the testis	1.05	0.40	37
Serum, horse	0.85	0.06	4
Serum, male rats	0.85	0.22	4
Cytosol, rat ventral prostate	0.15	0.04	4
Bovine serum albumin, 1 mg/ml	0.031	0.026	4
Bovine serum albumin, 50 mg/ml	0.31	0.15	8
Human serum albumin, 50 mg/ml	0.06	0.05	4
Bovine γ-globulin, 20 mg/ml	0.60	0.17	4

Sera from rat and horse caused a 25% reduction in binding which is equal to the displacement produced by 0.85 ng PAP in the assay system. This is, most likely, a totally nonspecific effect since in the rat, prostatic proteins showed no immunological crossreactivity with human PAP (Table 2). Sera from men above 50 years of age and with no evidence of neoplastic disease, produced an inhibition comparable to 1.1 ng PAP/100 μl. This figure should be regarded as a normal background or blank value. Based on the individual variation in blank value an upper limit of 1.8 ng/100 μl (mean + 2x SD) was established. Serum PAP values above this limit are considered significant and

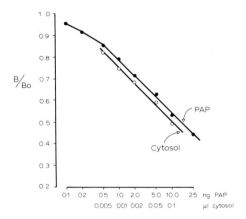

Fig. 1. Standard calibration curves obtained using purified PAP (●——●) or human prostate cytosol (○——○).

are referred to as elevated or positive. Female sera showed somewhat lower
values but this difference was not statistically significant. The highest blank
values were found in sera from pregnant women in the 3rd trimester (Table
2).

Blank values could be reduced numerically if the standard reference curve
was based on measurements in the presence of 100 μl normal female serum.
This modification did not significantly alter the slope of the standard curve
when plotted as in Figure 1. The normal range (or blank value) was then
reduced to 0.32 ± 0.42 ng/100 μl (mean ± SD, 22 observations). Besides
introducing a new variable this modification also caused a number of sera to
receive negative values which created computational and statistical problems.
More important, the ability of the method to discriminate between normal
and elevated PAP values was not improved.

Data on the precision of the assay system are presented in Table 3.
Reproducibility was within 16% (7 observations) when measured on a pool
of PAP-positive sera. No loss in PAP content of this pool was observed after
storage for 6 months at −20°C.

In a double blind study 127 samples from patients with various urological
disorders were analyzed. Thirty-six patients suffered from prostatic cancer
and received various forms of treatment. Elevated PAP values were found in
50% (18/36) of the prostatic cancer group compared to only 6% (2/36) using
the standard enzyme assay. The remaining patients including 37 patients
with testis cancer, showed normal PAP values.

PAP values in patients with prostatic cancer, grouped according to the
clinical classification, are presented in Figure 2. Elevated PAP values were
found in 25% (1/4) of patients with stage I (occult) carcinoma and in 50%
(4/8) of those with stage II. 62% (8/13) and 45% (5/11) of patients with
stage III and IV, respectively, were classified as PAP positive.

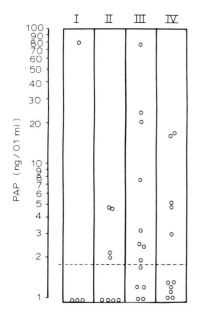

Fig. 2. Distribution of prostatic acid phosphatase concentration in sera from cancer patients classified according to clinical stage (I-IV). Broken line: upper normal limit.

Histological classification of primary tumour differentiation has so far been obtained from 40 patients. Significant PAP values were found in 50% (9/18) of patients with poorly differentiated tumours, compared to 63% (5/8) and 64% (9/14) of medium and highly differentiated tumours, respectively.

Discussion

The purification procedure presented for prostatic acid phosphatase is comparatively simple, reproducible, gives high yields and employs only commercially available chromatography media. The final PAP preparation was homogeneous by acceptable criteria and showed a specific enzyme activity comparable to the highest reported in the literature (Torchilin, 1977; Van Etten and Saini, 1977). The immunization protocol used produced monospecific antibodies which could be used for radioimmuno-assay in a final dilution of 1:100,000.

The double antibody radioimmunoassay presented is fast and simple to carry out. An assay can be completed in 24 hr. Sensitivity, reproducibility and specificity were satisfactory. A normal range of 0.4-1.8 ng/100 μl was established in elderly men without evidence of prostatic disease. These values

TABLE 3.

Precision of the radioimmunoassay

Range (mg/100 μl)	Mean	±SD*	No. observations
0-2	1.00	0.20	64
2-10	3.8	0.30	31
> 10	63.8	6.2	13

*SD obtained by duplicate analysis.

probably reflect a nonspecific interference of serum proteins with the antigen-antibody reaction. The normal range for PAP reported by Cooper et al. (1978), using a solid phase radioimmunoassay, is approximately 4 times higher than our values. This difference could be explained by a higher specificity being obtained with the present method due to a more extensive purification of antigen. If differences in experimental design are taken into consideration our values are in general agreement with the normal range reported by Vihko et al. (1978) using a double antibody radioimmunoassay.

Our assay correctly classified 50% of an arbitrary selection of cancer patients which is far better than the 6% score obtained with the conventional enzyme assay. Particularly notable and encouraging is the high incidence of elevated PAP values detected in patients with intraprostatic stage I and II carcinomas. In the more advanced stages III and IV, 62% and 45%, respectively, were correctly classified. The score for advanced metastatic carcinoma (stage IV) was unexpectedly low, especially when compared to the results of Cooper et al. (1978). In the present study most patients in this category were on oestrogen treatment which is known to inhibit prostate function, and may thus explain the low PAP blood levels.

The present results show that there is no correlation between tumour differentiation and the presence of immunoreactive PAP in serum. Half the patients with poorly differentiated carcinomas were PAP positive compared to 63% and 64% for medium and highly differentiated tumours, respectively. This seems to indicate that the ability of cancer cells to produce PAP is of little consequence for the PAP blood level. Disruption of acinar structure and organization within the prostate gland caused by the cancerous cells could be the main factor responsible for the leakage of secretory proteins into the general circulation.

References

Bergmeyer, H.U. (1970): In: *Methoden der Enzymatische Analyse*, p. 818. Verlag Chemie, Weinheim.

Cooper, J.F., Foti, A., Herschman, H. and Finkle, W. (1978): *J. Urol., 119,* 388.

Greenwood, F.C., Hunter, W.M. and Glover, J.S. (1963): *J. Biochem., 89,* 114.

Lee, C.L., Wang, M.C., Murphy, G.P. and Chu, T.M. (1978): *Cancer Res., 38,* 2871.

Luchter-Wasyl, E. and Ostrowski, W. (1974): *Biochim. Biophys. Acta (Amst.), 365,* 349.

Rodbard, D. and Chrambach, A. (1971): *Anal. Biochem., 40,* 95.

Torchilin, V.P., Galka, M. and Ostrowski, W. (1977): *Biochim. Biophys. Acta (Amst.), 483,* 331.

Van Etten, R.L. and Saini, M.S. (1977): *Biochim. Biophys. Acta (Amst.), 484,* 487.

Vihko, P., Sajanti, E., Jänne, O., Peltonen, L. and Vihko, R. (1978): *Clin. Chem., 24,* 1915.

Weber, K. and Osborne, M. (1969): *J. Biol. Chem., 244,* 4406.

Yam, L.T. (1974): *Amer. J. Med., 56,* 604.

Prostatic carcinoma: correlation of hormonal pattern in plasma and urine with local extent of tumour, presence of metastases, grade of differentiation and primary response to hormonal treatment*

S. RANNIKKO[1], A.-L. KAIRENTO[2], S.-L. KARONEN[2] and H. ADLERCREUTZ[2]

[1]II Department of Surgery and [2]Department of Clinical Chemistry, University of Helsinki, Helsinki, Finland

Because of the hormonal dependence of the normal development and function of the prostatic gland, and because of a favourable effect of hormonal treatment in most cases, the hormone status of a patient with prostatic cancer is likely to play a role in the growth and differentiation of the tumour and may correlate with the response to endocrine treatment.

A large number of studies have been performed on differences in plasma levels and urinary excretion of gonadotropic and sex hormones between normal men and patients with benign prostatic hyperplasia or prostatic cancer (Marmorston et al., 1965; Harper et al., 1976; Sköldefors et al., 1976, 1978; Bartsch et al., 1977, 1979; Hammond et al., 1977, 1978). However, the results are rather controversial and the range of individual values, even within the same study, is large. Therefore, it is not possible at present to demonstrate a typical hormonal pattern in a patient with prostatic cancer. In addition, very little information is available in the literature on the relationship between the hormonal status and the extent, differentiation grade and treatment response of prostatic carcinoma.

In order to study the correlation of hormonal pattern in prostatic cancer with local extent of tumour, presence of metastases, grade of differentiation and the primary response to hormonal treatment 18 hormones or groups of hormones were assayed in plasma and urine of patients classified according to the TNM classification system (UICC, 1974). The results indicate that a low plasma testosterone/oestrogen ratio is typical for patients with less differentiated advanced prostatic carcinoma and that assay of plasma testosterone (T), 17β-oestradiol (E_2), and prolactin (PRL) aid in the evaluation of the prognosis in this disease.

*The development of many of the methods used in this study was supported by the Ford Foundation, New York. Part of the expenses was defrayed by a grant from the Leo Research Foundation, Helsingborg, Sweden.

Material and methods

Subjects

The series consisted of 32 men with histologically or cytologically confirmed prostatic carcinoma. The mean age of patients was 68.0 ± 7.0 yrs. Fifteen patients were under 70 yrs of age and 17 patients were 70 yrs or more. Eight patients had an intracapsular (T1-2) tumour, in 24 patients the tumour extended outside the prostatic capsule (T3-4). Seventeen patients had metastases (M1) at the time of diagnosis. Eight patients had well differentiated (G1) and 24 patients moderately or poorly differentiated (G2-3) carcinoma. The primary response to hormonal treatment (orchiectomy and/or polyoestradiol phosphat-Estradurin®) (Leo, Helsingborg, Sweden) in 22 patients was estimated good on the basis of subjective changes and objective findings.

The differences between the mean ages in the TNM classification and treatment response groups were not statistically significant.

Methods

Blood samples for hormone analyses were obtained between 07.30 and 09.30 a few days before orchiectomy or start of the oestrogen therapy. The samples, from the cubital vein, were collected in heparinized tubes and the plasma stored at −20°C until analyzed. Urine, for hormone analyses, was collected during the 24 hr before taking the blood sample. Urine samples were analyzed immediately. Regular quality control samples were included in all series of assays. The laboratory participates in two international and one national quality control programme for hormone analyses. All analyses were done in duplicate. As a rule the analysis was repeated if the difference between the duplicates exceeded 10% calculated from the mean value.

The plasma FSH, LH, PRL, T, oestrone (E_1), E_2, and progesterone were determined by radioimmunoassay (RIA), plasma cortisol by fluorometry. Urinary 17-ketosteroids, 11-deoxy-17-ketosteroids (androsterone, etiocholanolone, dehydroepiandrosterone), 17-ketogenic steroids, pregnanediol and pregnanetriol were assayed by gas chromatography, urinary oestrogens by a colorimetric method.

The given mean values are geometric means. Statistical comparisons were made using the t test of De Jonge (1964).

Results

Statistically significant differences between the 2 age groups (< 70 and ⩾ 70 yrs) were found in the mean plasma LH level, which was higher ($p < 0.05$) in the older age group, and also in the mean urinary outputs of 11-deoxy-17-

TABLE 1.

Plasma hormone levels (geometric mean) in patients with carcinoma of the prostate, by local extent of the tumour (T classification)

	T classification		
	T 1-2 (n = 8)	T 3-4 (n = 24)	
Prolactin (mIU/1)	197.0	257.0	NS
Testosterone (nmol/l)	19.9	17.1	NS
Oestrone (pmol/l)	162.0	175.0	NS
17β-oestradiol (pmol/l)	56.6	79.9	NS
Oestrone + 17β-oestradiol (pmol/l)	245.0	272.0	NS

TABLE 2.

Hormone ratios (geometric mean) in patients with carcinoma of the prostate, by local extent of the tumour (T classification)

	T classification		
	T 1-2 (n = 8)	T 3-4 (n = 24)	
P-testosterone / P-17β-oestradiol	1.3	0.8	NS
P-testosterone / P-(oestrone + 17β-oestradiol)	0.3	0.3	NS
P-testosterone / P-prolactin	0.1	0.07	NS

ketosteroids which were lower in the older age group ($p < 0.05$-0.01). The mean excretion of 17-ketogenic steroids was also significantly lower in the older age group ($p < 0.025$).

There were no statistically significant differences in the mean plasma hormone levels (Table 1) and in the mean hormone ratios (Table 2) between the T1-2 and T3-4 groups. The mean urinary excretion of 17-ketosteroids, etiocholanolone and dehydroepiandrosterone, and also of 17-ketogenic steroids was significantly lower in the locally more extended group (T3-4) ($p < 0.005$-0.05) (Table 3).

The mean plasma level of E_2 was significantly higher ($p < 0.05$) in the M1 category than in the M0 category (Table 4). There were no differences in the urinary hormone excretion. In addition, the mean ratios of plasma T to E_2

TABLE 3.

Urinary hormone excretion (geometric mean) in patients with carcinoma of the prostate, by local extent of the tumour (T classification)

	T classification		
	T 1-2 (n = 8)	T 3-4 (n = 24)	
17-KS (μmol/24 hr)	33.5	20.5	$p < 0.005$
Androsterone (μmol/24 hr)	2.6	2.1	NS
Etiocholanolone (μmol/24 hr)	4.9	2.8	$p < 0.025$
DHEA (μmol/24 hr)	0.9	0.3	$p < 0.05$
17-KGS (μmol/24 hr)	36.4	26.3	$p < 0.025$

TABLE 4.

Plasma hormone levels (geometric mean) in patients with carcinoma of the prostate, by presence of metastases at the time of diagnosis (M classification)

	M classification		
	M0 (n = 15)	M1 (n = 17)	
Prolactin (mIU/l)	211.0	263.0	NS
Testosterone (nmol/l)	19.6	16.3	NS
Oestrone (pmol/l)	143.0	202.0	NS
17β-oestradiol (pmol/l)	59.6	87.1	$p < 0.05$
Oestrone + 17β-oestradiol (pmol/l)	216.0	303.0	NS

(No differences in urinary hormone excretion).

TABLE 5.

Hormone ratios (geometric mean) in patients with carcinoma of the prostate, by presence of metastases at the time of diagnosis (M classification)

	M classification		
	M0 (n = 15)	M1 (n = 17)	
$\dfrac{\text{P-testosterone}}{\text{P-17}\beta\text{-oestradiol}}$	1.2	0.7	$p < 0.025$
$\dfrac{\text{P-testosterone}}{\text{P-(oestrone + 17}\beta\text{-oestradiol)}}$	0.3	0.2	$p < 0.05$
$\dfrac{\text{P-testosterone}}{\text{P-prolactin}}$	0.09	0.06	NS

174   *S. Rannikko et al.*

TABLE 6.

Plasma hormone levels (geometric mean) in patients with carcinoma of the prostate, by differentiation grade of the tumour (G classification)

	G classification		
	G1 (n = 8)	G2-3 (n = 24)	
Prolactin (mIU/l)	240.0	236.0	NS
Testosterone (nmol/l)	19.9	17.0	NS
Oestrone (pmol/l)	123.0	191.0	NS
17β-oestradiol (pmol/l)	54.4	80.6	NS
Oestrone + 17β-oestradiol (pmol/l)	191.0	285.0	$p < 0.025$

(No differences in urinary hormone excretion).

TABLE 7.

Hormone ratios (geometric mean) in patients with carcinoma of the prostate, by differentiation grade of the tumour (G classification)

	G classification		
	G1 (n = 8)	G2-3 (n = 24)	
$\dfrac{\text{P-testosterone}}{\text{P-17}\beta\text{-oestradiol}}$	1.3	0.8	NS
$\dfrac{\text{P-testosterone}}{\text{P-(oesterone + 17}\beta\text{-oestradiol)}}$	0.4	0.2	$p < 0.025$
$\dfrac{\text{P-testosterone}}{\text{P-prolactin}}$	0.08	0.07	NS

and to E_1 plus E_2 were significantly lower ($p < 0.025$ and 0.05) in the M1 category (Table 5).

The mean plasma level of E_1 plus E_2 was significantly higher ($p < 0.025$) in the G2-3 group as compared with the G1 category (Table 6). The mean ratio of plasma T to E_1 plus E_2 was significantly lower ($p < 0.025$) in the G2-3 category (Table 7).

Generally, in addition to the significant differences mentioned above, a common trend was observed with respect to the stage and differentiation grade of the tumour: the more advanced or less differentiated the tumour, the higher the mean plasma levels of PRL, E_1 and E_2, and the lower the mean ratios of plasma T to E_2, to E_1 plus E_2 and to PRL.

TABLE 8.

Plasma hormone levels (geometric mean) in patients with carcinoma of the prostate, by primary response to hormonal treatment

	Primary response		
	Good (n = 22)	Poor (n = 10)	
Prolactin (mIU/l)	220.0	279.0	NS
Testosterone (nmol/l)	19.4	14.6	$p < 0.05$
Oestrone (pmol/l)	157.0	209.0	NS
17β-oestradiol (pmol/l)	66.2	90.1	NS
Oestrone + 17β-oestradiol (pmol/l)	238.0	311.0	NS

(No differences in urinary hormone excretion).

TABLE 9.

Hormone ratios (geometric mean) in patients with carcinoma of the prostate, by primary response to hormonal treatment

	Primary response		
	Good (n = 22)	Poor (n = 10)	
$\dfrac{\text{P-testosterone}}{\text{P-17}\beta\text{-oestradiol}}$	1.1	0.6	$p < 0.025$
$\dfrac{\text{P-testosterone}}{\text{P-(oestrone + 17}\beta\text{-oestradiol)}}$	0.3	0.2	$p < 0.025$
$\dfrac{\text{P-testosterone}}{\text{P-prolactin}}$	0.09	0.05	$p < 0.025$

In relation to the primary response to the hormonal therapy a significantly higher ($p < 0.05$) mean plasma T level was observed in patients with good response compared with those with poor response (Table 8). There were no differences in urinary hormone excretion. The mean ratios of plasma T to E_2, to E_1 plus E_2 and to PRL were significantly higher ($p < 0.025$) in patients with good response (Table 9).

It was also observed that in patients with poor response the ratio of plasma T (nmol/l) to E_2 (pmol/l) was $\leqslant 0.3$ and the ratio of plasma T (nmol/l) to PRL (mIU/l) $\leqslant 0.1$, whereas among patients with good response there were two groups of cases, those with ratios $\leqslant 0.3$ and $\leqslant 0.1$, respectively, and those with higher ratios (Fig. 1).

Discussion

When a large number of comparisons are made, statistically significant differences emerge also by chance. This means that not too much attention should be paid to single significant associations unless such associations support each other and result in a biologically meaningful picture of the hormonal alterations.

Because the urinary oestrogen excretion did not change in the more malignant metastatic tumour cases and these had higher plasma oestrogen values, a decreased metabolic clearance rate of oestrogens perhaps due to increased sex hormone binding globulin (SHBG) level is a likely explanation. Because the testosterone levels were not significantly different this would mean a decreased ratio of biologically active androgen to biologically active oestrogen in the more advanced cases which agrees with the finding of significantly decreased plasma testosterone oestrogen ratios in these subjects. Whether these changes have anything to do with the differentiation or progress of the cancer or if they are secondary to the disease cannot be judged from the present study.

The findings that patients with high plasma T and low PRL and oestrogens show a good response to treatment is logical on the basis of available literature. Very early studies demonstrated (Huggins et al., 1939, 1941; Huggins and Clark, 1940) that both normal and cancerous prostate show androgen dependence. It has also been well demonstrated that prolactin stimulates prostate function and development. There seem to be many mechanisms for this action but the final result is higher androgen activity in the prostate (Grayhack et al., 1955; Farnsworth, 1972). Oestrogens may act in the opposite way by inhibiting LH release and T production or by increasing plasma concentration of SHBG which in turn has been shown to decrease the available androgens at tissue level (Lasnitzki and Franklin, 1972). Endocrine therapy by orchiectomy and/or oestrogen treatment with the aim to decrease the androgen activity in the prostatic cancerous tissue has therefore the best effect in those subjects where the androgen effect in the tissue is expected to be high due to high circulating T and low E_2 and PRL levels. However, it does not appear to be possible by hormonal assays to predict prognosis for those with both low T/E_2 and T/PRL ratios. It is possible that assays of hormone receptors in prostatic tissue, for these subjects, will give the necessary information to be used for predicting prognosis and establishing therapy.

It may be concluded that of all 18 hormone determinations carried out, the plasma prolactin, testosterone and 17β-oestradiol assays may be of value in the evaluation of responsiveness of prostatic carcinoma to hormonal

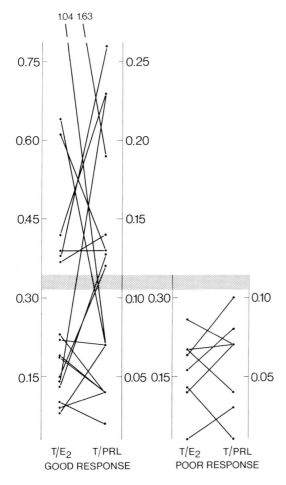

Fig. 1. Testosterone/oestradiol (T/E_2) and testosterone/prolactin (T/PRL) ratios in 26 ιbjects with prostatic carcinoma in relation to primary response to treatment.

treatment, and that the prostatic cancer patients with high ratios of plasma testosterone to oestradiol and to prolactin could be selected for primary hormonal treatment.

Acknowledgements

We are grateful to the National Institute of Arthritis, Metabolism and Digestive Diseases, National Pituitary Agency, U.S.A., for supplying the hormones LH, FSH and prolactin and the corresponding antisera. We would also like to thank all the technicians in the Department of Clinical Chemistry who carried out the numerous analyses involved in this study, and the members of the nursing staff at the Second Department of Surgery for their pleasant co-operation.

178   *S. Rannikko et al.*

References

Bartsch, W., Becker, H., Pinkenburg, F.-A. and Krieg, M. (1979): *Acta Endocr. (Kbh.)*, *90*, 727.

Bartsch, W., Horst, H.-J., Becker, H. and Nehse, G. (1977): *Acta Endocr. (Kbh.)*, *85*, 650.

De Jonge, H. (1964): *Inleiding tot de Medische Statistiek, Deel 2.* 2nd ed., p. 486-487. Verhandeling van het Nederlands Instituut voor Praeventieve Geneeskunde, Leiden.

Farnsworth, W.E. (1972): In: *Prolactin and Carcinogenesis*, p. 217. Editors: A.R. Boynes and K. Griffiths. Alpha Omega Alpha Publishing, Cardiff.

Grayhack, J.T., Bunce, P.L., Kearns, J.W. and Scott, W.W. (1955): *Bull. Johns Hopk. Hosp.*, *96*, 154.

Hammond, G.L., Kontturi, M.J., Määttälä, P., Puukka, M. and Vihko, R. (1977): *Clin. Endocr.*, *7*, 129.

Hammond, G.L., Kontturi, M., Vihko, P . and Vihko, R. (1978): *Clin. Endocr.*, *9*, 113.

Harper, M.E., Peeling, W.B., Cowley, T., Brownsey, B.G., Phillips, M.E.A., Groom, G., Fahmy, D.R. and Griffiths, K. (1976): *Acta Endocr. (Kbh.)*, *81*, 409.

Huggins, C. and Clark, P.J. (1940): *J. Exp. Med.*, *72*, 747.

Huggins, C.B., Masina, M.H., Eichelberger, L. and Wharton, J.D. (1939): *J. Exp. Med.*, *70*, 543.

Huggins, C., Stevens, R.E., Jr. and Hodges, C.V. (1941): *Arch. Surg.*, *43*, 209.

Lasnitzki, I, and Franklin, H.R. (1972): *J. Endocr.*, *54*, 333.

Marmorston, J., Lombardo, L.J., Jr., Myers, S.M., Gierson, H., Stern, E. and Hopkins, C.E. (1965): *J. Urol.*, *93*, 287.

Sköldefors, H., Blomstedt, B. and Carlström, K. (1978): *Scand. J. Urol. Nephrol.*, *12*, 111.

Sköldefors, H., Carlström, K. and Furuhjelm, M. (1976): *J. Steroid Biochem.*, *7*, 477.

UICC (Union Internationale Contre le Cancer) (1974): *TNM Classification of Malignant Tumours.* Geneva.

Endocrine treatment of prostatic disease*

H. BECKER

Clinic of Urology, University of Hamburg, F.R.G.

Prostatic disease includes benign prostatic hypertrophy (BPH) and prostatic carcinoma. Both diseases will be the subject of this presentation, inflammatory disease of the prostate will not be taken into consideration. Benign prostatic hypertrophy and prostatic cancer are androgen dependent, neither disease has been found in men over 40 castrated before puberty (Moore, 1944). There are some differences in metabolism of androgens at the cellular level of BPH and prostatic cancer which have been recently detected by more sensitive and accurate biochemical methods.

Benign prostatic hypertrophy

BPH is very common in men older than 40 years of age. In autopsy studies an incidence of BPH in 80.1% (165 out of 206) was found and in men over 80 yrs of age this number increased to 95.5% (64 of 67) (Harbitz and Haugen, 1974). Similar results were obtained by Moore (1944) and Pradhan and Chandra (1975), who found the first nodule in the prostate of a 35-year-old man. The first attempts to treat BPH by endocrine therapy were based on the observation that its development depends on hormonal stimulation. White in 1895 and Cabot in 1896 were the first to employ bilateral orchiectomy for the treatment of patients suffering from BPH, they saw an improvement in micturition and a reduction of the prostate growth after the operation. Huggins and Stevens (1940) derived from their studies after castration of patients with BPH that the development of BPH is under the control of the testes. Various treatment models followed based on the assumption that BPH develops in consequence of a hormonal imbalance of estrogens and androgens with age. An increasing estrogen: androgen ratio in urine with age was demonstrated by Kaufmann (1968). Clinical trials to treat BPH with estrogens/androgens or a mixture of both did not lead to successful results (Geller, 1974).

The introduction of very sensitive biochemical methods enabled several laboratories to study the metabolism and action of hormones at the cellular level of the animal and human prostate. Siiteri and Wilson (1970) demonstrated an accumulation of 5α-dihydrotestosterone (DHT) in BPH

*Supported by the DFG, Sonderforschungsbereich 34 (Endokrinologie).

180   H. Becker

TABLE 1.

Endogenous testosterone, 5α-dihydrotestosterone and 5α-androstan-3α,17β-diol in homogenates of human benign prostatic hypertrophy and normal prostate measured by RIA

| | Androgen levels (ng/g tissue) | |
	BPH	Normal prostate
Testosterone	0.3 ± 0.1 (11)	0.2 ± 0.1 (7)
5α-Dihydrotestosterone	4.5 ± 1.4 (14)	1.6 ± 1.0 (6)*
5α-Androstan-3α,17β-diol	0.6 ± 0.7 (14)	1.7 ± 0.3 (3)**

*Significantly different from BPH, p < 0.05.
**Significantly different from BPH, p < 0.05.
(From Krieg et al., 1979)

compared to normal prostate. Further, it was shown by in vitro and in vivo application of testosterone, that this androgen is metabolized in the prostate of several animals (Aliapoulios et al., 1965; Anderson and Liao, 1968; Baulieu et al., 1968; Bruchovsky and Wilson, 1968; Shimazaki et al., 1969; Tveter and Aakvaag, 1969; Buric et al., 1972) as well as in human benign prostatic hypertrophy (Farnsworth and Brown, 1963; Shimazaki et al., 1965; Geller and Baron, 1969; McMahon and Thomas, 1970; Pike et al., 1970; Siiteri and Wilson, 1970; Giorgi et al., 1971; Becker et al., 1972). After in vivo injection of ^{3}H-testosterone an accumulation of radioactivity was detected in BPH compared to skeletal muscle (Becker et al., 1972). This accumulation was mainly due to the metabolized androgen 5α-dihydro-testosterone, which was bound to a specific receptor protein. This specific androgen receptor protein could be determined by various procedures in BPH cytosol and nuclei (Voigt and Krieg, 1978). By the agar gel electro-phoresis technique, according to Wagner (1972), the androgen receptor protein of BPH can be separated from the Sex Hormone Binding Globulin (SHBG) in plasma.

Determination of endogenous androgen levels in BPH and normal prostate demonstrated significantly higher amounts of DHT and diminished 5α-androstan-3α,17β-diol levels in BPH (Krieg et al., 1979). Geller et al. (1976) also found significantly lower 5α-androstan-3α,17β-diol concentrations in BPH compared to normal prostate. Incubation studies of surgically removed BPH tissue with ^{3}H-testosterone showed similar results, 5α-dihydro-testosterone was the main metabolite, whereas the amount of 5α-androstan-3α,17β-diol formed was diminished when compared to normal prostates removed from young men who had been involved in fatal accidents (Krieg et al., 1978).

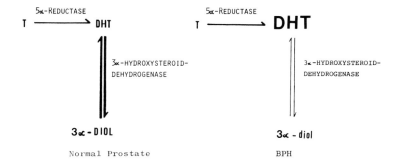

Fig. 1. Testosterone metabolism in normal prostate and in BPH.

As BPH starts at the age of 40 yrs we looked for alterations of hormonal parameters in the plasma of normal men with and without benign prostatic hypertrophy between 36 and 65 yrs of age. No significant difference in hormone and SHBG blood levels between the 'normal' and the 'BPH' group within this age range could be detected. On the other hand, a significant increase of FSH and a decrease of 5α-androstan-3α,17β-diol with age was seen in the normal group. A distinct increase of DHT with age was seen in the BPH group, which was not so pronounced in the normal group (Bartsch et al., 1979).

The interpretation of this blood hormone pattern with increasing age and the metabolism in the BPH tissue is that the decrease of the 3α-hydroxysteroid dehydrogenase activity leads to an intracellular increase of 5α-dihydrotestosterone (Fig. 1) and to a long-lasting stimulation of the prostatic cells.

What conclusions for a treatment concept can be drawn from these metabolic findings? The aim of endocrine treatment for BPH should be the reduction of the intracellular binding of DHT to the receptor protein, which will lead to decreased stimulation of the prostate cells. This can be done by:
1. diminution of testosterone in plasma by (a) castration, (b) application of gestagens or (c) application of estrogens;
2. inhibition of the 5α-reductase activity;
3. displacement of DHT from the receptor protein;
4. activation of the 3α-hydroxysteroid dehydrogenase activity.

As mentioned above castration was performed in 1895 by White, in 1896 by Cabot and in 1940 by Huggins and Stevens with good results. Treatment with progestational drugs which act by reducing the gonadotrophin excretion of the hypophysis has been introduced with several drugs. Cyproterone acetate, chlormadinone acetate, delatutine, 19-nor-delatutine and megastrol acetate were used and showed a good clinical effect in many cases (Geller, 1974). It is, however, very difficult to make an objective assessment of the results of this treatment.

Treatment with estrogens reduces testosterone levels. However, this hormone itself seems to be involved in the pathogenesis of BPH, as demonstrated by the existence of estrogen receptors in BPH cytoplasm (Jungblut et al., 1971; Hawkins et al., 1975). Clinical trials with estrogens did not show a significant alteration of the symptoms or of the prostate enlargement (Heckel, 1944; Roberts, 1966).

Inhibition of the 5α-reductase activity was demonstrated by Altwein et al. (1974) after adding progesterone and gestonorone capronate (Depostate®) to an in vitro system in which the metabolism of ³H-testosterone in BPH was investigated.

5α-dihydrotestosterone is displaced from the receptor protein by antiandrogens. Cyproterone acetate acts, beside its progestational qualities, as an antiandrogen. After application of 50 mg per day orally Scott and Wade (1969) and Vahlensieck and Godde (1968), who used 100 mg per day, saw good results in patients suffering from BPH. Treatment with flutamide (SCH 13521) – a non-steroidal antiandrogen, which is given orally – led to improvement of micturition and urine flow, but no alteration of residual urine, prostate enlargement and histology when compared to a control group treated by placebo (Caine et al., 1975).

Activation of the 3α-hydroxysteroid dehydrogenase activity would be the most physiological treatment, if we could find a drug with such effect. This treatment would lead to a reduction of the intracellular concentration of 5α-dihydrotestosterone and would probably not influence the potency of the patients, which is a side effect of the hitherto endocrine clinical trials.

It should be mentioned that, at this moment, surgical removal of the prostate adenoma, by transurethral resection or the open way, is the main therapeutical procedure as most of the patients are in good condition. Patients in poor condition may undergo cryosurgery of their prostate without general anesthesia.

Another question is preventation therapy for BPH. Further investigations into the hormonal metabolism and influence on the various tissue compartments of benign prostatic hypertrophy, e.g. stromal, muscular and epithelial portions, will lead probably to a better explanation of pathogenesis and to a rational treatment of BPH.

Prostatic carcinoma

Huggins and Hodges (1941) were the first to show that prostatic carcinoma growth is under the influence of androgens. This finding led to the introduction of hormonal therapy in patients with prostatic cancer. Bilateral orchiectomy or treatment with estrogens causes a rapid reduction of plasma testosterone. The metabolism of androgens and the mode of action at the cellular level in prostatic cancer is qualitatively similar, but quantitatively different when compared to the situation in the BPH and the normal

TABLE 2.

Receptor concentration in prostatic cancer and in BPH

	No.	5α-DHT receptor protein fmol/mg protein
Prostatic carcinoma	14	30.9*
Highly differentiated	6	21.7
Cribriform and/or low differentiated	8	37.8**
Benign prostatic hypertrophy	14	12.3

*Significantly different from BPH, p < 0.04.
**Significantly different from highly differentiated prostatic cancer, p < 0.05.
(From Krieg et al., 1978)

prostate. Krieg et al. (1979) found in prostatic cancer significantly higher testosterone levels compared to BPH and to normal prostate. On the other hand they found that DHT was elevated in BPH but not significantly compared to prostatic cancer, whereas in normal prostate DHT levels were significantly lower compared to both prostatic tumors. Habib et al. (1976) also found a higher testosterone amount in cancer than in BPH.

In incubation studies of homogenates from prostatic cancer, BPH and normal prostates with tritiated androgens, Krieg et al. (1978) demonstrated that testosterone remained mainly unaltered in prostatic cancer, with the formation of 5α-dihydrotestosterone and 5α-androstan-3α,17β-diol being 15% lower than in BPH and normal prostate. This diminished reduction of testosterone in prostatic cancer tissue had also been found by Shimazaki et al. (1965), and Giorgi et al. (1971, 1972). Kliman et al. (1978) likewise found a significant higher DHT concentration in BPH compared to prostatic cancer after incubation with ^{3}H-testosterone, and the metabolism of testosterone to DHT in metastases was again significantly lower than in the primary prostatic tumor. No significant differences were seen in the accumulation studies between BPH, prostatic cancer and metastases. From their studies they suggested a limited role for 5α-dihydrotestosterone formation in cancer specimens, especially in the metastases, where the DHT content was smallest. The authors conclude that probably testosterone itself may play a direct role for the intranuclear action and that autonomous deoxyribonucleic acid production requires only a small amount of testosterone or 5α-dihydrotestosterone. This alteration of the androgen metabolism in prostatic cancer compared to BPH may explain to some extent the resistance of some prostatic cancers to endocrine treatment. Jenkins and McCaffery (1974) demonstrated differences in the amount of conversion of testosterone to DHT depending on the tumor differentiation. One well differentiated carcinoma converted testosterone in the same manner as BPH, whereas in the outer part of this carcinoma and in poorly differentiated tumors the conversion was much lower. They also showed that estrogen application reduced testosterone metabolism drastically.

As it is well known that only 70-80% of patients with prostatic cancer respond to endocrine therapy (Holland and Grayhack, 1976), many groups have studied the androgen receptor content to find out if it is possible to predict which patients will respond to endocrine manipulation. It was thought that patients with a positive androgen receptor might respond with a good remission of their tumor growth whereas patients without an androgen receptor would not be influenced by hormonal therapy. Unfortunately this theory could not be confirmed. On the contrary Krieg et al. (1978) demonstrated a significantly higher cytosolic 5α-DHT receptor protein content in cribriform or cribriform and poorly differentiated tumors compared to highly differentiated prostatic carcinoma. This was a surprising finding, as it is known that the prognosis of cribriform and poorly differentiated prostatic cancer is bad compared to that of highly differentiated tumors. 5α-DHT receptor proteins could be detected in all of the prostatic cancer specimens investigated. Tveter et al. (1971) found a cytosolic androgen receptor in an advanced prostatic tumor and its metastasis, and in 1975 they showed that no qualitative differences exist between androgen receptors in neoplastic and non-neoplastic prostatic tumors (Attramadal et al., 1975). In an investigation of 7 prostatic carcinomas Wagner et al. (1975) found that in 3 cases the androgen receptor was absent, in 3 cases an androgen and an estradiol receptor were found and only in 1 case was a 5α-DHT receptor alone found.

Bilateral orchiectomy reduces the testosterone level in plasma rapidly to amounts between 0.2 and 0.5 μg/l, values normally found in women (Young and Kent, 1968; Robinson and Thomas, 1971; Mackler et al., 1972; Shearer et al., 1973; Bartsch et al., 1977). These small testosterone values are produced mainly in the adrenal cortex. Treatment with estrogens reduce the testosterone levels also, the extent depending on the dose of the administered estrogen. Robinson and Thomas (1971) and Shearer et al. (1973) have shown that 3 mg stilbestrol per day suppresses plasma testosterone levels to values found after orchiectomy.

The indication for endocrine treatment in prostatic cancer is at that stage where the tumor has penetrated the capsule and invaded the surrounding organs and has set up metastases. From histological studies it is known that in clinical stage C lymph node metastases could be detected in 50 to 75% of cases (McLaughlin et al., 1976; Bruce et al., 1977; Wilson et al., 1977). Radical prostatectomy and radiotherapy may cure patients with a localized prostatic cancer but not those in an advanced stage.

The benefit of endocrine treatment in prostatic cancer was described in 1950 by Nesbit and Baum, who found a survival rate of 44% after 5 yrs of patients without metastases treated by orchiectomy combined with diethylstilbestrol, whereas the untreated control group showed a survival rate of

TABLE 3.

Treatment concept in stage C prostatic carcinoma

Radiotherapy: 6000 R
Subcapsular orchiectomy

Additional endocrine therapy (randomized)

1.	Diethyldioxystilbendiphosphate	(Honvan®)	3 x 120 mg per day
2.	Prednisolone	(Decortin®)	3 x 5 mg per day
3.	Natriureticum	(Baycaron®)	2 x 25 mg per day
4.	Cyproterone acetate	(Androcur®)	300 mg i.m. every 2 weeks
5.	Placebo		

10%. Patients with metastases showed, after castration alone or combined with diethylstilbestrol, a 5-year survival rate of 20% compared to 6% in the untreated group. As the first study of the Veterans Administration Co-operative Urological Research Group (VACURG) demonstrated a high incidence of cardiovascular deaths in the estrogen treated patients, the dose of diethylstilbestrol was reduced in their second study. In patients with stage C, receiving 5 mg diethylstilbestrol, a greater number of cardiovascular deaths occurred compared to those patients taking placebo or the lower estrogen dose. In patients with stage D an increased risk of cardiovascular death was not seen with the higher estrogen dose. On the other hand it could be shown that patients receiving 1 or 5 mg diethylstilbestrol had significantly fewer cancer deaths than patients taking placebo or 0.2 mg diethylstilbestrol. Patients with stage C receiving 1 or 5 mg diethylstilbestrol showed a reduced conversion rate to stage D compared to those receiving placebo or 0.2 mg diethylstilbestrol (Byar, 1973). Based on the recommendations of this VACURG study II, many clinicians today perform a delayed treatment, and start with endocrine manipulation when bone pain occurs or laboratory parameters show tumor progress.

Five-year survival rates up to 50% in stage C call for further efforts for the improvement of endocrine treatment. In 1968 we started to treat advanced prostatic cancer in a randomized prospective study. All patients with stage C and D underwent orchiectomy and received additionally either 360 mg diethylstilbendiphosphate (Honvan®), or 3 x 5 mg prednisolone (Decortin®), or 2 x 25 mg of a natriureticum (Baycaron®), or, at two weekly intervals, 300 mg cyproterone acetate (Androcur®) i.m. or placebo (Klosterhalfen et al., 1973, 1975). In stage C, local radiotherapy with 6000 rad was performed, the rationale of this additional radiotherapy was the fact that about 20-30% of the prostatic cancers do not respond to endocrine manipulation. The 5-year survival rate based on 209 patients with stage C prostatic carcinoma showed no better results compared to other studies. 105 (50.2%) patients died during the first 5 years, 56 patients (26.8%) died of

TABLE 4.

5-year follow-up

Patients	209	=	100%
Patients died	105	=	50.2%
Death on tumor	56	=	26.8%
Death on poorly differentiated prostatic cancer	48 of 156	=	30.8%
Death on highly differentiated prostatic cancer	8 of 53	=	15.1%

TABLE 5.

Remission and survival time after hypophysectomy in metastasizing prostatic cancer

Histology of prostatic cancer	No. of patients	Remission in months after hypophysectomy	Survival time after hypophysectomy in months
Well differentiated	3	4	9
Well differentiated	2	0	9
Poorly differentiated	10	6	12
Poorly differentiated	4	0	2½

their tumor. Patients with poorly differentiated prostatic cancer died of their tumor more frequently (48 of 156 = 30.8%) than patients with highly differentiated prostatic cancer (8 of 53 = 15.1%). As the number of patients is as yet too small, and there are too many variables which influence tumor growth, we cannot at this moment recommend any of these 5 additional treatment principles. It should be mentioned that in the groups receiving cyproterone acetate and prednisolone fewer patients died of their tumor.

The inefficiency of endocrine treatment alone, or combined with radiotherapy, in about 50% of the patients may be related to a high incidence of metastases. Taking into consideration the findings of Kliman et al. (1978) that metastases have an altered metabolism of androgens, and secondly that our own results using metastases from a patient who showed a tumor progression after 4 yrs of endocrine treatment, where we estimated high receptor protein amounts, it may be derived that a more aggressive endocrine treatment could be necessary. Up to now hypophysectomy or adrenalectomy have only been performed in patients who relapsed after a first remission under endocrine treatment. In 22 patients with metastatizing prostatic cancer who relapsed under endocrine therapy a transnasal-transsphenoidal hypophysectomy was performed in our neurosurgical depart-

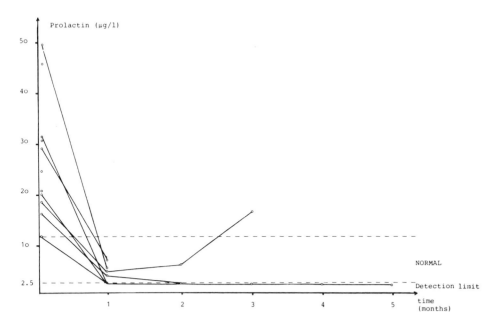

Fig. 2. Prolactin levels in serum during administration of SH 3.1072 B.

ment. Two patients died immediately after the operation when this method was introduced. From 19 patients, who were controlled regularly, 13 (= 68.5%) showed a good remission, which lasted on an average 5.5 (3 to 8) months. The survival time of these patients with a good remission was 11.5 months, whereas in patients without remission it was 4.8 months. When we compared remission and survival time with the primary histological differentiation of the tumor it could be shown that patients with poorly differentiated prostatic cancer showed better results (Klosterhalfen et al., 1980). This unexpected result may probably be explained by a higher receptor protein content in the metastatic tissue which is stimulated by very small testosterone levels in plasma. It should be mentioned that this conclusion is speculative, but I think it is urgently necessary to find the minimum androgen levels which stimulate the various differentiated prostatic cancer cells and the meaning of the androgen and estrogen receptor proteins in the primary tumor and in metastases.

The factor which causes remission after hypophysectomy was assumed to be prolactin in addition to androgens. Jacobi et al. (1978) demonstrated a decreased uptake of testosterone into the carcinomatous tissue under antiprolactin treatment with bromocriptine. In a clinical trial we treated patients with metastatic prostatic cancer suffering from bone pain with lisuride hydrogen maleate (SH 3.1072 B) – an ergot derivative which lowers prolactin in plasma. In these 10 patients an increased prolactin plasma level

TABLE 6.

Results after antiprolactin treatment with SH 3.1072 B

Patient	Age (yrs)	Additional endocrine treatment	Prolactin in serum (μg/l)	Prolactin in serum after SH 3.1072 B (μg/l)	Bone pain	Serum phos- phatases	Survival time after SH 3.1072 B
W.B.	65	P, CyAc	12	< 2.5	↓	↑	alive 9 months
H.F.	69	H	18	4.2 – 4.7	↓	↑	3 months
G.G.	63	Est., CyAc	32	< 2.5	↓	↑	3 months
U.H.	60	H	31	–	–	–	10 days
G.H.-P.	61	CyAc	14	No control. Because of side effects therapy not continued.			
W.M.	76	H, CyAc	30	< 2.5	↓	↑	2 months
E.O.	57	H	29	7.0	–	↑	1 month
H.R.	56	CyAc	24	–	–	–	10 days
C.S.	60	CyAc	16	< 2.5	↓	↑	4 months
K.S.	76	H	46	–	–	–	12 days
H.S.	70	CyAc	21	< 2.5	↓	↑	alive 3 months
R.V.	52	H	49	< 5.2	–	normal	2 months

CyAc = Cyproterone acetate; Est = Estracyt®; p = Prednisolone; H = Honvan®.

was found due to treatment with diethylstilbendiphosphate and cyproterone acetate. Therapy with SH 3.1072 B led to a reduction of the prolactin levels to non measurable amounts (Fig. 2). Four of the 10 patients died within 2 weeks after starting lisuride therapy, 1 patient discontinued this treatment because of side effects. In 5 patients we saw a significant relief of pain, which was demonstrated by a reduced intake of analgesic drugs, but no objective tumor remission could be seen, and alkaline and acid serum phosphatases showed no alteration under antiprolactin treatment (Kloster- halfen et al., 1979). Clinical trials with bromocriptine did not give better results (Coune and Smith, 1975). The influence of prolactin in an earlier stage of prostatic cancer needs further investigation, as there are some findings which show that prolactin might be elevated in cribriform prostatic cancers. These elevated prolactin levels in plasma were obtained with a bioassay (the pigeons crop test) but not with radioimmunoassay (Bartsch et al., 1977b).

Antiandrogens, which act in the peripheral cell may play a greater role in the future concept of advanced prostatic cancer. Good results have been obtained after administration of cyproterone acetate (Geller et al., 1968, Smith et al., 1973, Wein and Murphy, 1973) or flutamide (SCH-13521) (Stolear and Albert, 1974). Both act by intracellular inhibition of androgen binding, with cyproterone acetate acting additionally as a progestational hormone to inhibit gonadotrophin secretion. All those androgens which could not be influenced by orchiectomy or suppression of the adrenal cortex will be inhibited by antiandrogens.

Conclusion

The testes are the source of 95% of androgens. As most of the prostatic cancers are in an advanced stage when the disease is detected it seems logic to eliminate these androgens as no other curative treatment exists at this moment. In our opinion, bilateral orchiectomy is the best way to reduce testosterone in plasma, because it shows no side effects compared with other medical treatment. Testosterone levels are decreased rapidly and surely after castration, whereas it is not sure that the older patients who receive drugs as an alternative to orchiectomy take their drugs constantly. To inhibit the remaining androgens in plasma, further investigations are necessary to find more active antiandrogens or combined drugs like estramustine phosphate (Estracyt®) (Jönsson et al., 1977), a cytotoxic drug which is bound to estrogen and which is assumed to act in prostatic cancer after separation from the hormone. Further studies on the receptor proteins and androgen metabolism in the primary cancer and in the metastases will probably lead to a better understanding of the tumor and bring us perhaps other treatment concepts with better results.

References

Aliapoulios, M.A., Chamberlain, J., Jagarinec, N. and Ofner, P. (1965): *Biochem. J., 98,* 15P.
Altwein, J.E., Rubin, A., Klose, K., Knapstein, P. and Orestano, F. (1974): *Urologe A, 13,* 41.
Anderson, K.M. and Liao, S. (1968): *Nature (Lond.), 219,* 277.
Attramadal, A., Tveter, K.J., Weddington, S.C., Djöseland, O., Naess, O., Hansson, V. and Torgersen, O. (1975): *Vitam. and Horm., 33,* 247.
Bartsch, W., Becker, H., Pinkenburg, F.-A. and Krieg, M. (1979): *Acta Endocr. (Kbh.), 90,* 727.
Bartsch, W., Horst, H.-J., Becker, H. and Nehse, G. (1977): *Acta Endocr. (Kbh.), 86,* 650.
Bartsch, W., Steins, P. and Becker, H. (1977): *Europ. Urol., 3,* 47.
Baulieu, E.E., Lasnitzki, I. and Robel, P. (1968): *Nature (Lond.), 219,* 1155.
Becker, H., Kaufmann, J., Klosterhalfen, H. and Voigt, K.D. (1972): *Acta Endocr. (Kbh.), 71,* 589.

Bruce, A.W., O'Cleirachain, F., Morales, A. and Awad, S.A. (1977): *J. Urol., 117*, 319.
Bruchovsky, N. and Wilson, J.D. (1968): *J. Biol. Chem., 243*, 2012.
Buric, L., Becker, H., Petersen, C. and Voigt, K.D. (1972): *Acta Endocr. (Kbh.), 69*, 153.
Byar, D.P. (1973): *Cancer, 32*, 1126.
Cabot, A.T. (1896): *Ann. Surg., 24*, 265.
Caine, M., Perlberg, S. and Gordon, R. (1975): *J. Urol., 114*, 564.
Coune, A. and Smith, P. (1975): *Cancer Chemother. Rep., 59*, 209.
Farnsworth, W.E. and Brown, J.R. (1963): *J. Amer. Med. Ass., 183*, 436.
Geller, J. (1974): In: *The Treatment of Prostatic Hypertrophy and Neoplasia*, Chapter 2, p. 27. Editor: J.E. Castro. Medical and Technical Publishing Co Ltd., Lancaster.
Geller, J., Albert, J., Lopez, D., Geller, S. and Niwayama, G. (1976): *J. Clin. Endocr., 43*, 656.
Geller, J. and Baron, A. (1969): *51st Meeting of the Endocrine Society, Abstr. 288*, p. 144.
Geller, J., Vazakas, G., Fruchtman, B., Newman, H., Nakao, K. and Loh. A. (1968): *Surg. Gynec. Obstet., 127*, 748.
Giorgi, E.P., Stewart, J.C., Grant, J.K. and Scott, R. (1971): *Biochem. J., 123*, 41.
Giorgi, E.P., Stewart, J.C., Grant, J.K. and Shirley, I.M. (1972): *Biochem. J., 126*, 107.
Habib, F.K., Lee, I.R., Stitch, S.R. and Smith, P.H. (1976): *J. Endocr., 52*, 327.
Harbitz, T.B. and Haugen, D.A. (1974): *Acta Path. Microbiol. Scand. (A), Suppl. 224*, 1.
Hawkins, E.F., Nijs, M., Brassinne, C. and Tagnon, H.J. (1975): *Steroids, 26*, 458.
Heckel, N.J. (1944): *J. Clin. Endocr., 4*, 166.
Holland, J.M. and Grayhack, J.T. (1976): In: *Scientific Foundation of Urology, Vol. II*, Chapter 44, p. 338. Editors: D.I. Williams and G.D. Chisholm. William Heinemann Medical Books, London.
Huggins, C. and Hodges, C.V. (1941): *Cancer Res., 1*, 293.
Huggins, C. and Stevens, R. (1940): *J. Urol., 43*, 705.
Jacobi, G.H., Sinterhauf, K., Kurth, K.H. and Altwein, J.E. (1978): *J. Urol., 119*, 240.
Jenkins, J.S. and McCaffery, V.M. (1974): *J. Endocr., 63*, 517.
Jönsson, G., Högberg, B. and Nilsson, T. (1977): *Scand. J. Urol. Nephrol., 11*, 231.
Jungblut, P.W., Hughes, S.F., Görlich, L., Gowers, U. and Wagner, R.K. (1971): *Hoppe-Seyler's Z. Physiol. Chem., 352*, 1603.
Kaufmann, J. (1968): *Z. Urol., 61*, 229.
Kliman, B., Prout, G.R., Jr., MacLaughlin, R.A., Daly, J.J. and Griffin, P.P. (1978): *J. Urol., 119*, 623.
Klosterhalfen, H., Becker, H. and Burchardt, P. (1975): In: *Hormonal Therapy of Prostatic Cancer*, p. 193. Editors: U. Bracci and F. Di Silverio. Cofese Edizioni, Palermo.
Klosterhalfen, H., Becker, H. and Krieg, M. (1979): *Cancer Treatm. Rep., 63*, Abstr. 392, 1220.
Klosterhalfen, H., Becker, H., Lotzin, C. and Kautzky, R. (1980): *Urologe A, 19*, in press.
Klosterhalfen, H., Burchardt, P. and Wartke, U. (1973): *Urologe A, 12*, 304.
Krieg, M., Bartsch, W., Herzer, S., Becker, H. and Voigt, K.D. (1977): *Acta Endocr. (Kbh.), 86*, 200.
Krieg, M., Bartsch, W., Janssen, W. and Voigt, K.D. (1979): *J. Steroid Biochem., 11*, 615.
Krieg, M., Grobe, I., Voigt, K.D., Altenähr, E. and Klosterhalfen, H. (1978): *Acta Endocr. (Kbh.), 88*, 397.
Mackler, M.A., Liberti, J.P., Smith, M.J.V., Koontz, W.W. Jr. and Prout, G.R. Jr. (1972): *Invest. Urol., 9*, 423.
McLaughlin, A.P., Saltzstein, S.L., McCullough, D.L. and Gittes, R.F. (1976): *J. Urol., 115*, 89.
McMahon, M.J. and Thomas, G.H. (1970): *J. Endocr., 48*, 20.
Moore, R.A. (1944): *Surgery, 16*, 152.
Nesbit, R.M. and Baum, W.C. (1950): *J. Amer. Med. Ass., 43*, 1317.

Pike, A., Peeling, W.B., Harper, M.E., Pierrepoint, C.G. and Griffith, K. (1970): *Biochem. J., 120,* 443.

Pradhan, B.K. and Chandra, K. (1975): *J. Urol., 113,* 210.

Roberts, H.J. (1966): *J. Amer. Geriat. Soc., 14,* 657.

Robinson, M.R.G. and Thomas, B.S. (1971): *Brit. Med. J., 4,* 39.

Scott, W.W. and Wade, J.C. (1969): *J. Urol., 101,* 81.

Shearer, R.J., Hendry, W.F., Sommerville, J.F. and Fergusson, J.D. (1973): *Brit. J. Urol., 45,* 668.

Shimazaki, J., Kurihara, H., Ito, Y. and Shida, K. (1965): *Gunma J. Med. Sci., 14,* 313.

Shimazaki, J., Matsushita, J., Furuya, N., Yamanaka, H. and Shida, K. (1969): *Endocr. Jap., 16,* 453.

Siiteri, P.K. and Wilson, J.D. (1970): *J. Clin. Invest., 49,* 1737.

Smith, R.B., Walsh, P.C. and Goodwin, W.E. (1973): *J. Urol., 110,* 106.

Stolear, B. and Albert, D.J. (1974): *J. Urol., 111,* 803.

Tveter, K.J. and Aakvaag, A. (1969): *Acta Endocr. (Kbh.), 85,* 683.

Tveter, K.J., Unhjem, V., Attramadal, A., Aakvaag, A. and Hansson, V. (1971): *Advanc. Biosci., 7,* 193.

Vahlensieck, W. and Godde, S. (1968): *Münch. Med. Wschr., 110,* 1573.

Voigt, K.D. and Krieg, M. (1978): In: *Current Topics in Experimental Endocrinology, Vol. 3,* p. 173. Academic Press, Inc., New York, San Francisco, London.

Wagner, R.K. (1972): *Hoppe Seyler's Z. Physiol. Chem., 353,* 1235.

Wagner, R.K., Schulze, K.H. and Jungblut, P.W. (1975): *Acta Endocr. (Kbh.), Suppl. 193,* 52.

Wein, A.J. and Murphy, J.J. (1973): *J. Urol., 109,* 68.

White, J.W. (1895): *Ann. Surg., 22,* 1.

Wilson, C.S., Dahl, D.S. and Middleton, R.G. (1977): *J. Urol., 117,* 197.

Young, H.H. and Kent, J.R. (1968): *J. Urol., 99,* 788.

OVARIAN FUNCTION AND DISEASE

Normal ovarian function

G.T. ROSS

The Clinical Center, National Institutes of Health, Bethesda, MD, U.S.A.

After the menarche, the hallmarks of normal ovarian function are cyclic production of a single oocyte and of sufficient sex steroid hormone to provide for implantation and early maintenance of the conceptus should the oocyte become fertilized. The only completely unequivocal test for these functions is pregnancy, but testing fertility is not always a practical method for evaluating ovarian function. However, over the past 2 decades, extensive studies have been made of the functional correlates of changes in blood and urine hormone levels during spontaneous and induced ovulatory menstrual cycles. Results of these studies have established that sex steroid hormones, produced by the follicle destined to ovulate and by the corpus luteum to which it gives rise, pace hormonal events and coordinate interactions of hypothalamic-pituitary-ovarian and genital organs during ovulatory cycles. Consequently, appropriately timed measurements of gonadotropins and of sex steroid hormones provide the basis for practical and rational tests of normal ovarian function in women after the menarche. Some of the evidence which supports this contention will be reviewed here.

Blood hormone levels throughout spontaneous ovulatory menstrual cycles

Remarkably similar patterns of cyclic changes in levels of gonadotropins and sex steroids have been reported when these hormones were measured in specimens of mixed venous blood collected once daily throughout presumptively ovulatory menstrual cycles in normal women (Ross et al., 1970; Franchimont, 1971; Johansson et al., 1971; Thorneycroft et al., 1971; Abraham et al., 1972; Sherman and Korenman, 1974). Blood levels of luteinizing hormone (LH) rose minimally but progressively throughout the follicular phase prior to a 'mid-cycle' preovulatory surge or peak. After the peak, levels progressively declined throughout the luteal phase.

Late in the luteal phase, levels of follicle stimulating hormone (FSH) began to rise. This elevation persisted throughout the first half of the follicular phase of the following cycle, declined to a low point just prior to a mid-cycle peak coincident with that for LH. After the mid-cycle peak, FSH levels progressively declined to reach a nadir late in the luteal phase, and then began to rise again.

When concentrations of estrogens, progestogens, and androgens were measured in aliquots of the same specimens, the following patterns were observed: from low levels during the menses, estradiol levels rose rapidly during the second half of the follicular phase of the cycle to reach a maximum just prior to or coincident with the LH peak. This maximal level declined immediately after the LH peak, rose again early in the luteal phase to reach a maximum in mid-luteal phase, after which levels declined again to very low menstrual levels (Thorneycroft et al., 1971; Abraham et al., 1972; Sherman and Korenman, 1974). Although absolute values differed, concentrations of androstenedione (Abraham, 1974) and 17OH progesterone (Ross et al., 1970; Abraham et al., 1972; Thorneycroft et al., 1971) followed patterns similar to that for 17β-estradiol. In contrast, concentrations of progesterone, which remained at relatively low levels throughout the follicular phase, began to rise either slightly before or coincident with the mid-cycle LH peak and reached a mid-luteal phase maximum before declining to low levels around menses.

The low frequency changes in gonadotropins described above have been shown to be reproduced by appropriate manipulation of the sex steroid hormone milieu. Thus, blood levels of FSH declined when estrogen levels were increased and rose when an estrogen antagonist was given concomitantly to normal women during the early follicular phase (Vaitukaitis et al., 1971). Depending upon the timing, magnitude and duration of increased estrogen levels, both negative and positive feedback on LH levels could be demonstrated (Vande Wiele et al., 1970; Yen et al., 1974a, b, c). LH discharges were elicited in amenorrheic women who bled following administration of progesterone (Goldenberg et al., 1973), and levels of both LH and FSH rose in amenorrheic women given clomiphene, an estrogen antagonist (Ross et al., 1970).

Recently March et al. (1979) have adduced evidence consistent with a role of progesterone in regulating the mid-cycle LH and FSH surges.

When the interval between samples was reduced to less than 1 hr, patterns of high frequency pulses in blood LH and FSH levels were seen to be imposed upon the low frequency patterns described above (Midgley and Jaffe, 1971). Both frequency and amplitude of these pulses varied with time in cycle: higher frequency and lower amplitude pulses were characteristic of the follicular phase while lower frequency and higher amplitude were characteristic of pulses occurring during the luteal phase (Santen and Bardin, 1973; Yen et al., 1974a, b, c). When sufficient quantities of the hormone in hypothalamic extracts which stimulate pituitary gonadotropin secretion (GnRH) became available for clinical studies, the amplitude of induced pulses was shown to be influenced by dose of GnRH and by time in cycle (Yen et al., 1972; Nillius and Wide, 1972). The amplitude of pulses induced by a fixed dose of GnRH increased progressively from early to middle to late follicular phase and decreased progressively from early to middle to late luteal phase. Furthermore, Yen et al. (1974a, b, c) and Jaffe and Keye (1974) showed that estradiol modulated pituitary gonadotropin secretion in response to exogenous GnRH.

Cyclic changes in pulsatile secretion of gonadotropins and sex steroid hormone modulation of pituitary responses to GnRH, taken together, imply that steroid hormones might act at the level of the hypothalamus or the pituitary or at both sites to regulate gonadotropin secretion during ovulatory cycles. Although measurements of GnRH levels in peripheral and pituitary portal blood are technically complicated, unequivocal evidence for a pituitary site of action has been adduced from studies in subhuman primate models. Although frequency and amplitude of spontaneous GnRH pulses have not been measured, studies in rhesus monkeys have shown that pulsatile secretion occurs (Carmel et al., 1976). Nakai et al. (1978) have shown that spontaneous cycles and feedback effects of estrogens on gonadotropin secretion were eliminated by electrolytic destruction of the arcuate nuclei in the hypothalamus of sexually mature female rhesus monkeys. Ferin et al. (1979) have shown that similar changes result from transection of the pituitary stalk. In both models, feedback responses to estrogens (Nakai et al., 1978; Ferin et al., 1979) and ovulatory cycles with hormonal patterns consistent with those seen in spontaneous cycles (Knobil et al., 1979) were resumed after intravenous infusions of *fixed doses* of GnRH for 6 min out of each hour of every day for 30 to 60 days. Neither lower dose pulses nor continuous infusions of GnRH were effective in restoring the functional integrity of the pituitary ovarian axis.

In these 'open loop' models, where endogenous hypothalamic function had been eliminated, the evidence that ovarian steroid hormones acted directly upon pituitary cells was unequivocal. However, the possibility of a hypothalamic site of action of sex steroid hormones has not been excluded. Indeed, the demonstration of an obligatory role of pulsatile GnRH secretion for the expression of sex steroid hormone effects is consistent with the concept of a hypothalamic site of action of these hormones.

Relation of follicle growth to hormone levels during ovulatory menstrual cycles

In the light of the determinant role of ovarian steroid hormone secretion in setting the cadence of events in ovulatory cycles, it is important to recall that only one follicle in only one ovary ovulates normally during each cycle in women. How does the growth of the ovulating follicle correlate with hormonal events during the cycle?

Consider the morphologic changes first. The changes in cellular components of normal follicles associated with follicular growth and atresia throughout the preovulatory phase of the cycle have been characterized by McNatty et al. (1979a, b, c) who studied these phenomena in follicles recovered from surgically removed ovarian tissue. Criteria based upon numbers of granulosa cells and progression of the first meiotic division of the oocyte nucleus in vivo and in vitro were used to classify follicles as normal or atretic. Normal follicles contained more granulosa cells than atretic follicles, and the first meiotic division was completed in vitro more often in oocytes from normal than from atretic follicles (McNatty et al., 1979c). In a sample of more than 200 follicles examined by these criteria, they concluded that granulosa cell proliferation progressed at a normal rate in only one or two of the antral follicles which were 4 mm in diameter, the size of the largest extant normal follicle at the outset of the follicular phase of the cycle (McNatty et al., 1979a). Rates of granulosa cell proliferation correlated with hormonal composition of the antral fluid in follicles of all sizes, and concentrations of estrogens were higher in follicles with normal rates of granulosa cell proliferation.

In addition to numbers of granulosa cells and hormonal composition of antral fluid, the mass of theca and the volume of antral fluid were determined for these follicles. As numbers of granulosa cells and volume of antral fluid increased, the theca hypertrophied (McNatty et al., 1979c). Since thecal hypertrophy also occurs in association with atresia when granulosa cell proliferation is inhibited (Hillier and Ross, 1979), correlation of the two phenomena may not be obligatory.

Turning now to the functional correlates of hormonal changes in the cycle, McNatty et al. (1979a, b, c) compared the in vitro steroidogenic capabilities of granulosa cells and theca cells from normal and atretic follicles. In vitro, theca from normal follicles synthesized more estradiol than theca from atretic follicles, suggesting an interaction of the two components in estrogen synthesis by the chosen follicle. Moreover, in vitro granulosa cells from normal follicles synthesized 17β-estradiol de novo whereas granulosa cells from atretic follicles did not. Since both theca and granulosa cells of normal follicles have the capacity to synthesize more 17β-estradiol than these components from atretic follicles, it would seem reasonable to suppose that the normal follicles could be the major source of blood estradiol during the cycle. Moreover, since only one normal follicle persists in the late follicular phase, it should be the principal source of rising estradiol blood levels just prior to ovulation.

Comparisons of sex steroid hormone levels in venous effluent from the two ovaries and in peripheral venous blood throughout ovulatory cycles have shown that both ovaries produce estrogens, androgens, and progestogens throughout the cycle (Mikhail, 1970; Baird and Fraser, 1975; McNatty et al., 1976). However, once it could be determined by gross inspection that a dominant preovulatory follicle had been selected, levels of estrogens, androgens, and progestogens rose dramatically in the venous effluent from the ovary containing that follicle. Indeed, rising steroid hormone levels occurred coincident with the rapid preovulatory growth of that follicle late in the follicular phase, indicated in the data of Block (1951) and of McNatty et al. (1979b). Recently Goodman et al. (1977) have shown that electrolytic destruction of the dominant follicle complex was followed by a dramatic decline in serum estrogen levels. Channing and Coudert (1976) have reported that removal of the granulosa cells from the dominant follicle produced no acute change in ovarian venous estradiol concentrations and suggested that the estrogens were produced by thecal cells of the dominant follicle complex. Thus, while the cellular sites of its production remain to be defined, it seems likely that rapidly rising levels of 17β-estradiol in peripheral blood late in the follicular phase reflect the secretory activity and normal progression of preovulatory growth of the dominant follicle.

After ovulation, levels of estrogens, androgens, and progestogens are higher in venous blood from the ovary containing the corpus luteum (Mikhail, 1970; Baird and Fraser, 1975). Moreover, surgical ablation of the corpus luteum in women (Czapo et al., 1973) and in rhesus monkeys (Goodman and Hodgen, 1977) is followed by rapidly declining levels of these steroids in peripheral blood. Hence, the corpus luteum is the principal source of ovarian sex steroid hormones during the luteal phase of the cycle. Baird et al. (1975) discussed the role of the corpus luteum in determining cycle intervals. They pointed out that growing follicles are the sole source of estrogens in species where surrogate follicles could be recruited rapidly after destruction of a dominant follicle. They proposed that this phenomenon would not occur in species where estrogens and progestogens produced by the corpus luteum inhibit pituitary gonadotropin secretion to make extant antral follicles atretic and to inhibit postantral growth of new follicles.

Goodman and Hodgen (1977) adduced evidence consistent with Baird's hypothesis by examining perturbations in cycle length following removal of the corpus luteum with and without systemic replacement therapy with progesterone. If no replacement treatment was given, removal of the corpus luteum advanced the onset of menses and the initiation of a new follicular phase. In contrast, systemic replacement of progesterone prevented onset of menses and delayed initiation of a new cycle in direct relation to the duration of systemic replacement therapy. Some delay following implantation of progesterone into the ovary contralateral to the ovary from which the corpus luteum had been removed, suggested a local as well as a systemic action of progesterone in determining length of the follicular phase.

Collectively, results of these ablative experiments are consistent with the concept that the dominant follicle and its successor, the corpus luteum, are the source of sex steroid hormones which modulate pituitary responses to GnRH and pace the ovulatory cycle. If this concept be valid, then destruction of the dominant follicle or the corpus luteum should interrupt the sequence of events during the remainder of the cycle in progress. Goodman et al. (1977) and Goodman and Hodgen (1977) have studied these relationships. Daily measurements of gonadotropin levels in cycles in which the dominant follicle or corpus luteum were destroyed showed that the expected sequence of normal events in the remainder of the cycle in progress was interrupted. Moreover, in each case a new cycle was initiated, and ovulation occurred about 13 days later. If sex steroid hormones secreted by the dominant follicle coordinate preovulatory interactions of the ovary and the pituitary, then knowledge about changes in steroid hormone levels might provide useful information concerning the progression of follicle growth prior to ovulation.

The models of ovulation induction with exogenous gonadotropins in women with anovulatory infertility provide evidence of the utility of such information. From this experience it is clear that both FSH and LH or hCG in appropriate quantities, given in the proper sequence, are required for the production of an oocyte, its fertilization and implantation. To determine the adequacy of the stimulus and to minimize the likelihood of inducing multiple rather than single ovulations, repeated measurements of blood or urinary estrogen levels are required. While failure of urinary or blood estrogen levels to rise can be equated with inadequate stimulation, multiple ovulations are more likely to occur when blood or urinary estrogen concentrations exceed the range of values seen in women responding with ovulation of a single follicle. From a large, carefully studied experience in which urinary estrogen excretion was used to monitor responses, Brown (1978) showed that the total quantity of FSH required for adequately stimulating the preovulatory maturation of a single follicle varied from person to person but was relatively consistent from cycle to cycle for an individual. Furthermore, for a given woman adequate quantities usually did not differ from inadequate quantities by more than 30% and frequently did not differ by more than 10%.

Thus measurements of blood or urinary estrogens can be used to monitor the progress of follicular maturation prior to ovulation. Furthermore, chemical measurements of urinary pregnanediol, evaluation of endometrial morphology and more recently measurements of blood progesterone levels have been used to assess corpus luteum function (Ross and Hillier, 1978).

In summary then, measures of sex steroid hormone levels provide reliable indirect evidence for the extent to which both the gametogenic (ovulation) and steroidogenic (sex steroid hormone production) aspects of ovarian function are normal after the menarche.

Conclusions

The foregoing discussion demonstrates that progression of follicle growth to the point of the choice of an ovulatory follicle is the central event in normal ovarian function after the menarche. After that event has occurred, sex steroid hormones produced by this follicle signal the preovulatory surges of LH and FSH. After ovulation, sex steroid hormones produced by the corpus luteum derived from the dominant follicle pace events leading to the termination of the cycle in progress and initiation of the next cycle. Since the patterns of change in hormone levels reflected the progress of this sequence of events in the dominant follicle, assessment of levels of sex steroid and gonadotropic hormones becomes the basis for evaluating ovarian function in clinical practice.

Acknowledgements

The author is grateful to Dr. Kenneth McNatty for permission to quote from papers in press at the time this manuscript was prepared and to Mrs. Ollie S. Monger for skillful assistance in preparing the manuscript.

References

Abraham, G.E. (1974): *J. Clin. Endocr. Metab., 39,* 340.
Abraham, G.E., Odell, W.D., Swerdloff, R.S. and Hopper, K. (1972): *J. Clin. Endocr. Metab., 34,* 312.
Baird, D.T., Baker, T.G., McNatty, K.P. and Akal, P. (1975): *J. Reprod. Fertil., 45,* 611.
Baird, D.T. and Fraser, I.J. (1975): *Clin. Endocr., 4,* 259.
Block, E. (1951): *Acta Endocr. (Kbh.), 8,* 33.
Brown, J.B. (1978): *Aust. N.Z. J. Obstet. Gynaec., 18,* 46.
Carmel, P.W., Araki, S. and Ferin, M. (1976): *Endocrinology, 99,* 243.
Channing, C.P. and Coudert, S.P. (1976): *Endocrinology, 98,* 590.
Czapo, A.I., Pulkinnen, M.O. and Weist, W.G. (1973): *Amer. J. Obstet. Gynec., 115,* 759.
Ferin, M., Rosenblatt, H., Carmel, P.W., Antunes, J.L. and Vande Wiele, R.L. (1979): *Endocrinology, 104,* 50.
Franchimont, P. (1971): *Secrétion Normale et Pathologique de la Somatotropine et des Gonadotropines Humaines.* Masson, Paris.
Goldenberg, R.L., Grodin, J.M., Vaitukaitis, J.L. and Ross, G.T. (1973): *Amer. J. Obstet. Gynec., 115,* 1993.
Goodman, A.L. and Hodgen, G.D. (1977): *J. Clin. Endocr. Metab., 45,* 837.
Goodman, A.L., Nixon, W.E., Johnson, A.K. and Hodgen, G.D. (1977): *Endocrinology, 100,* 155.
Hillier, S.G. and Ross, G.T. (1979): *Biol. Reprod., 20,* 261.
Jaffe, R.B. and Keye, W.R., Jr. (1974): *J. Clin. Endocr. Metab., 39,* 850.
Johansson, E.D.B., Wide, L. and Gemzell, C.A. (1971): *Acta Endocr. (Kbh.), 68,* 501.
Knobil, E., Plant, T.M., Wildt, L. and Belchetz, P. (1979): *61st Annual Meeting of the Endocrine Society,* p. 70 (Abstract).
March, C.M., Goebelsmann, U., Nakamura, R.M. and Mishell, D.R., Jr. (1979): *J. Clin. Endocr. Metab., 49,* 507.
McNatty, K.P., Baird, D.T., Bolton, A., Chambers, P., Corker, C.S. and McLean, H. (1976): *J. Endocr., 71,* 77.
McNatty, K.P., Makris, A., Degrazia, C., Osathanondh, R. and Ryan, K.J. (1979a): *J. Clin. Endocr. Metab., 49,* 687.
McNatty, K.P., Smith, D.M., Makris, A., Osathanondh, R. and Ryan, K.J. (1979b): *J. Clin. Endocr. Metab.,* in press.
McNatty, K.P., Smith, D.M., Osathanondh, R. and Ryan, K.J. (1979c): *Biochim. Biophys. Acta (Amst.),* in press.
Mikhail, G. (1970): *Gynec. Invest., 1,* 5.
Midgley, A.R., Jr. and Jaffe, R.B. (1971): *J. Clin. Endocr. Metab., 33,* 962.
Nakai, Y., Plant, T.M., Hess, D.L., Keogh, E.J. and Knobil, E. (1978): *Endocrinology, 102,* 1008.
Nillius, S.F. and Wide, L. (1972): *J. Obstet. Gynaec. Brit. Cwlth, 79,* 865.

Ross, G.T., Cargille, C.M., Lipsett, M.B., Rayford, P.L., Marshall, J.R., Strott, C.A. and Rodbard, D. (1970): *Rec. Progr. Hormone Res., 26,* 1.

Ross, G.T. and Hillier, S.G. (1978): *Clin. Obstet. Gynaec., 5,* 391.

Ross, G.T., Hillier, S.G., Zeleznik, A.J. and Knazek, R.A. (1979): In: *Research on Steroids, Vol. VIII,* p. 185. Editors: A. Klopper, L. Lerner, H.J. van der Molen and F. Sciarra. Academic Press, London.

Santen, R.J. and Bardin, C.W. (1973): *J. Clin. Invest., 52,* 2617.

Sherman, B.M. and Korenman, J.G. (1974): *J. Clin. Endocr. Metab., 38,* 89.

Thorneycroft, I.H., Mishell, D.R., Stone, S.C., Kharma, K.M. and Nakamura, R.M. (1971): *Amer. J. Obstet. Gynec., 111,* 1947.

Vaitukaitis, J.L., Bermudez, J.A., Cargille, C.M., Lipsett, M.B. and Ross, G.T. (1971): *J. Clin. Endocr. Metab., 32,* 503.

Vande Wiele, R., Bogumil, J., Dyrenfurth, I., Ferin, M., Jewelewicz, R., Warren, M., Rizkallah, T. and Mikhail, G. (1970): *Rec. Progr. Hormone Res., 26,* 63.

Yen, S.S.C., VandenBerg, G., Rebar, R. and Yehara, Y. (1972): *J. Clin. Endocr. Metab., 35,* 931.

Yen, S.S.C., VandenBerg, G. and Siler, T.M. (1974a): *J. Clin. Endocr. Metab., 39,* 170.

Yen, S.S.C. VandenBerg, G., Tsai, C.C. and Parker, D. (1974b): In: *Biorhythms and Human Reproduction,* p. 203. Editors: M. Ferin, F. Halberg, R.M. Richart and R.L. Vande Wiele. John Wiley and Sons, New York.

Yen, S.S.C., VandenBerg, G., Tsai, C.C. and Siler, T. (1974c): In: *Biorhythms and Human Reproduction,* p. 219. Editors: M. Ferin, F. Halberg, R.M. Richart and R.L. Vande Wiele. John Wiley and Sons, New York.

Oestrogen synthesis by isolated human ovarian cells *

J.R.T. COUTTS, J.M. GAUKROGER, A.D.T. GOVAN and M.C. MAC-NAUGHTON

Department of Obstetrics and Gynaecology, Royal Maternity Hospital, Glasgow University, Glasgow, U.K.

The ovary is one of the major steroid secreting glands of the body and contains a number of potential steroid secreting organs. Graafian follicles and corpora lutea are the major ovarian sources of steroid biosynthesis. Each of these structures contains at least 2 cell types which possess all the requirements of steroid secreting cells — theca and granulosa cells. Although a great deal of data has been reported during the past decade establishing the secretory patterns of the ovary at different stages of development and in different environments (Coutts, 1976), the exact biosynthetic roles and steroidogenic capacities of the individual cell types have not been clearly established.

Falck (1959) demonstrated that within the Graafian follicle the 2 cell types had a complementary role and that both were required for normal functioning. This symbiotic relationship between the theca and granulosa cells was the basis of the 2 cell theory for follicular oestrogen formation (Short, 1962). This hypothesis proposed that one cell type produced a precursor which was aromatised by the other cell type. Almost 2 decades later the situation, particularly in human ovarian follicles is not clear. Knowledge of the steroidogenic capacities of the cells of the human corpus luteum is even more fragmentary than that for follicular cells.

This paper describes attempts using isolated human theca and granulosa cells from both Graafian follicles and corpora lutea to determine the biosynthetic pathway(s) to oestradiol in the human ovary.

Material and methods

Ovarian material

Human Graafian follicles and corpora lutea were obtained throughout the menstrual cycle from women having laparotomy and oophorectomy for conditions which did not affect their reproductive cycle, e.g. fibroids,

*This work was supported by a grant G977/564/C from the British M.R.C.

carcinoma in situ etc. The stage of the cycle was dated on the basis of endometrial histology, ovarian histology, menstrual history and the plasma levels of circulating steroid hormones.

Isolation of ovarian cells

The theca and granulosa cells from Graafian follicles and corpora lutea were isolated using a physical scraping method (Gaukroger et al., 1977) which was an adaptation of that described by Ryan and Petro (1966). After crude separation of theca and granulosa cells, they were further purified by centrifugation through a Nybolt mesh (John Stanier and Co. Ltd., Manchester) of an appropriate pore size to allow passage of one cell type whilst retaining the other.

Isolated cell preparations

Aliquots from all cell preparations were analysed histologically. Using the methods described above, pure homogeneous preparations of follicular granulosa and theca cells and luteal granulosa cells were obtained. Theca lutein cell preparations were contaminated by up to 40% of granulosa lutein cells. However, where simultaneous experiments using granulosa and theca lutein cells from the same corpus luteum were performed, any metabolic activity due to the contaminating granulosa cells could be quantitated and the theca values corrected for it. The estimated % contamination of the theca lutein cell preparations by granulosa cells was probably an overestimate since disruption of some granulosa cells at the Nybolt mesh would result in the appearance in the theca lutein preparation of granulosa cell nuclei which although inactive steroidogenically, would appear histologically as contamination.

All cell preparations prepared by these methods were viable both histologically and steroidogenically.

Incubation studies

Isolated cell preparations (200,000 cells/flask) were incubated under conditions suitable for steroidogenesis in Krebs bicarbonate buffer pH 7.4 (10 ml) with either [4-^{14}C] labelled androstenedione or testosterone (1 μCi each: 5 μg). Incubations were performed in the presence or absence, as indicated in the text, of 1 mM NADPH$_2$ (Boehringer Ltd.) and 20 mIU/ml of FSH or LH. After 6 hr the incubations were terminated by the addition of acetone. A mixture of ^{3}H labelled potential metabolites was then added and the metabolites formed were isolated, identified and characterised by chromatography and sequential derivative formation to constant isotope ratio. Figure 1 is a flow sheet of the experimental methodology.

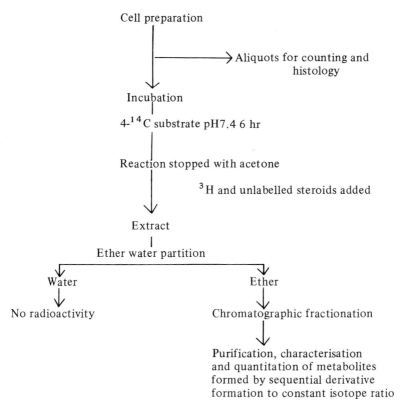

Cell preparation

→ Aliquots for counting and histology

Incubation

4-^{14}C substrate pH7.4 6 hr

Reaction stopped with acetone

^{3}H and unlabelled steroids added

Extract

Ether water partition

Water

No radioactivity

Ether

Chromatographic fractionation

Purification, characterisation
and quantitation of metabolites
formed by sequential derivative
formation to constant isotope ratio

Fig. 1. Flow diagram of methods used for steroidogenic studies with isolated human ovarian cells

Results

Table 1 shows the metabolites isolated following incubation of [4-^{14}C] androstenedione with granulosa cells from medium (0.6-0.9 diameter) and large (> 1.0 cm diameter) follicles. Qualitatively the results were very similar but the substrate was metabolised to a greater extent by the larger follicle. Table 2 shows a comparison of the metabolites isolated following incubation of granulosa cells from a large follicle with androstenedione and testosterone. The results showed similar metabolic patterns from the 2 substrates, both in extent of metabolism and in the pattern of metabolites formed, oestradiol being the major product. However, despite the presence of NADPH$_2$ which should have favoured conversion of androstenedione to testosterone the former appeared if anything to be the more efficient precursor for oestradiol.

Incubations of Δ^4A with follicular granulosa cells in the presence and absence of the gonadotrophins FSH and LH showed an apparent stimulation

TABLE 1.

Metabolism of [4-^{14}C]androstenedione by follicular granulosa cells

Metabolite*	Medium follicle (0.8 cm)	Large follicle (> 1.0 cm)
	% of total metabolites	
Testosterone	23.55	1.81
19-OH-Testosterone	n.d.	0.30
Oestrone	5.25	17.86
Oestradiol	71.20	43.21
19-OH Androstenedione	0.97	36.22
Dihydrotestosterone	n.d.**	0.60
% Metabolism of substrate	3.19	5.99

*Incubations performed in presence of 1 mM NADPH$_2$.
** n.d. = not detectable.

TABLE 2.

Comparison of metabolites formed by follicular granulosa cells (large follicle) from [4-^{14}C] androstenedione and [4-^{14}C] testosterone

Metabolite*	Substrate	
	Testosterone	Androstenedione
Testosterone	—	1.81
19-OH-Testosterone	7.83	0.30
Oestrone	18.32	17.86
Oestradiol	49.39	43.21
19-OH-Androstenedione	0.34	36.22
Androstenedione	20.56	—
Dihydrotestosterone	3.56	0.60
% Metabolism of substrate	5.84	5.99

*Both substrates incubated in the presence of 1 mM NADPH$_2$.

of the whole pathway by both FSH and LH for large follicles whilst the granulosa cells of medium follicles were stimulated by FSH but not LH.

Incubations of follicular theca cells with androstenedione and testosterone (Table 3) showed that the theca cells were much less efficient in metabolising C19 androgens (particularly in aromatisation) than were the granulosa cells. Theca cell metabolism of these substrates was unaffected by incubation in the presence of LH or FSH.

Both granulosa and theca lutein cells on incubation with androstenedione and testosterone showed only relatively small capacities for metabolism.

TABLE 3.

Comparison of the metabolites formed from [4-^{14}C] testosterone by follicular theca and granulosa cells

Metabolite*	Theca cells	Granulosa cells
	% of total metabolites	
Androstenedione	77.88	20.56
19-OH-Testosterone	3.74	7.83
Oestrone	4.64	18.32
Oestradiol	9.42	49.39
19-OH-Androstenedione	0.51	0.34
Dihydrotestosterone	3.80	3.56
% Metabolism of substrate	0.63	5.84

*Incubated in the presence of 1mM NADPH$_2$.

TABLE 4.

Metabolism of [4-^{14}C] testosterone by corpus luteum cells

Metabolite*	Granulosa cells	Theca cells**
	% of total metabolites	
Androstenedione	56.25	80.70
19-OH-Androstenedione	n.d.***	n.d.
Oestrone	5.76	n.d.
Oestradiol	23.15	n.d.
19-OH-Testosterone	10.45	1.31
Dihydrotestosterone	n.d.	17.99
% Metabolism of substrate	(0.78)	(0.38)

*Incubated in the presence of 1 mM NADPH$_2$.
**Result corrected for granulosa cell contamination.
***n.d. = not detectable.

However, qualitatively the relative patterns of metabolism of the 2 cell types were similar to their follicular equivalents since only in the granulosa lutein cells was the aromatase present. The theca cells in fact appeared largely capable only of interconversion of the 2 substrates and 5$\propto$ reduction whilst the granulosa cells were capable of oestradiol formation at least from testosterone (Table 4).

Discussion

The incubation studies with isolated human ovarian cells reported in this paper lend evidence to support the 2 cell hypothesis for ovarian steroidogenesis. In both the follicle and the corpus luteum the theca cells are relatively inefficient at metabolism of C19 androgens compared to the granulosa cells. Since our previous work has shown that C19 androgens are elaborated mainly by the theca cells the 2 cell hypothesis would hold with the theca cells being responsible for production of androgens which are then aromatised largely by the granulosa cells.

From the results it appears likely that this situation exists not only in the Graafian follicle but also in the corpus luteum since only the granulosa lutein cells could aromatise the substrate.

The formation of DHT by the human follicular theca cells is of interest since it has been reported (Schwarzel et al., 1973) that this compound inhibits follicular growth.

The granulosa cells of large Graafian follicles responded to both FSH and LH producing increased total synthesis of oestradiol whilst the equivalent cells of medium sized follicles only responded to FSH. This discrepancy in response to gonadotrophin stimulation probably reflects the fact that pre-ovulatory granulosa cells develop receptors for LH (Channing and Kammerman, 1973) thus enabling them to respond when the pre-ovulatory rise in LH occurs.

From the data obtained on incubation with androstenedione and/or testosterone, it appears that aromatisation may proceed using either of these C19 steroids as precursor. However, the ability of the follicular granulosa cells to metabolise androstenedione (Table 2) to such an extent under conditions which should have favoured utilisation of testosterone (presence of excess $NADPH_2$) suggests that the substrate of choice for aromatisation may be androstenedione.

The data from granulosa lutein cells on the other hand favours testosterone as the immediate precursor of oestradiol (Table 4).

References

Channing, C.P. and Kammerman, S. (1973): *Endocrinology, 92,* 531.
Coutts, J.R.T. (1976): *Clin. Obstet. Gynaec., 3,* 63.
Falck, B. (1959): *Acta Physiol. Scand., 47, Suppl. 163,* 1.
Gaukroger, J.M., Govan, A.D.T., Macnaughton, M.C. and Coutts, J.R.T. (1977): *J. Endocr., 73,* 20.
Ryan, K.J. and Petro, Z. (1966): *J. Clin. Endocr., 26,* 46.
Schwarzel, W.C., Kruggel, W.G. and Brodie, H.J. (1973): *Endocrinology, 92,* 866.
Short, R.V. (1962): *J. Endocr., 24,* 59.

The excretion of two new phenolic compounds during the human menstrual cycle and in pregnancy

K.D.R. SETCHELL[1], A.M. LAWSON[1], M. AXELSON[2] and
H. ADLERCREUTZ[3]

[1] *Division of Clinical Chemistry, Clinical Research Centre, Harrow, Middlesex, U.K.;* [2] *Department of Chemistry, Karolinska Institutet, Stockholm, Sweden; and* [3] *Department of Clinical Chemistry, Meilahti Hospital, Helsinki, Finland*

Two previously unidentified phenolic compounds have recently been shown to exhibit significant patterns of excretion in urine during the menstrual cycle and in pregnancy of the vervet monkey (*Cercopithecus aethiopus pygerthrus*) (Setchell et al., 1980). These compounds, of related but undetermined structure, were designated as compounds 180/442 and 180/410 (since these are the principal ions in the mass spectra of the trimethylsilyl ether derivatives) and their excretion in the vervet monkey was shown to increase in the luteal phase of the cycle, reaching maximum excretion prior to corpus luteum maturity.

During pregnancy the excretion of 180/442 and 180/410 was characterised by maximum levels during the first trimester but decreased as gestation proceeded (Setchell et al., 1980).

In the course of the last 7 yrs both of these compounds have been consistently detected in the urine of other subhuman primate species and of humans during routine gas chromatography-mass spectrometry (GC-MS) analysis of steroid extracts. The recent observations from our studies of the vervet monkey have led us to initiate a thorough investigation of the physiological behaviour of these new compounds in humans. In view of the close similarity between steroid metabolism and excretion during the menstrual cycle of the vervet monkey and that of the human (Setchell et al., 1980), our first objective was to determine whether a similar pattern of excretion of these phenolic compounds occurred in humans. More fundamentally and obviously of prime importance, is the question of the chemical structure of both compounds, particularly since our early data would appear to indicate that they are unusual structures and imply the presence of a new class of physiological compound.

A highly specific and sensitive GC-MS method has been developed using selected ion monitoring for the semi-quantification of both compounds 180/410 and 180/442. This communication will report on some of the preliminary physiological findings regarding their excretion in the urine of women during the menstrual cycle and pregnancy, of male subjects, and of infants.

Results and discussion

Determination of the unknown phenolic compounds

A method was developed for the extraction, isolation and specific measurement of these unknown phenolic compounds in urine. An outline of this method is shown in Figure 1 and has been described in detail elsewhere (Setchell et al., 1980). Quantification of these compounds was based upon selected ion monitoring GC-MS of their trimethylsilyl (TMS) ether derivatives. Following the addition of a known and constant amount of an internal standard (5α-androstane-3β,17β-diol) the peak height response obtained from the ion m/z 436, specific to this compound, was compared with the responses obtained for the characteristic ions of the phenolic compounds (m/z 442 and m/z 410); all 3 ions were monitored simultaneously by accelerating voltage switching. As the absolute ion responses for 180/442 and 180/410 for given concentrations of these compounds were not known, absolute quantitation could not be achieved. However, by applying a correction factor (x 0.1) to the m/z 442 and m/z 410 responses, to account

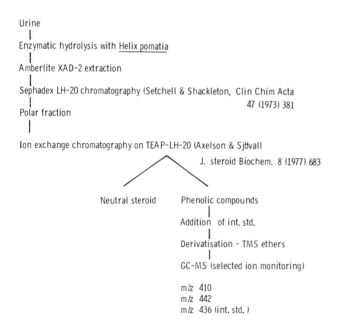

Fig. 1.   Scheme for measurement of unknown phenolic compounds in urine.

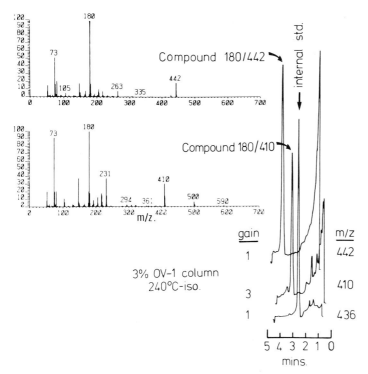

Fig. 2. Selected ion monitoring GC-MS analysis of trimethylsilyl ether derivatives of a polar phenolic fraction of human urine. Ions m/z 442, m/z 410 and m/z 436 were simultaneously monitored using accelerating voltage switching. Sensitivity of each ion response is indicated by the gain setting; gas chromatographic conditions are shown. Internal standard is 5β-androstane-3β,17β-diol. The complete mass spectrum obtained by scanning the peaks confirmed specificity of the assay.

for the difference between the proportions of the total ionisation carried by these ions and the ion for the internal standard, semi-quantitative values for the amounts of the compounds were obtained. Although these may not be accurate they allowed the urinary excretion of the phenolic compounds to be compared from day-to-day.

A typical selected ion monitoring recording obtained from a human female urine sample submitted to the procedure, is shown in Figure 2, and the complete mass spectra of these two compounds indicate the homogeneity of the peaks and allow confirmation of the specificity of the assay. The mass spectra, with their characteristic base peaks at m/z 180, are identical to those obtained from vervet monkey urine, details of which have been discussed previously (Setchell et al., 1980).

Menstrual cycle

The glass capillary column gas chromatographic analysis of a typical

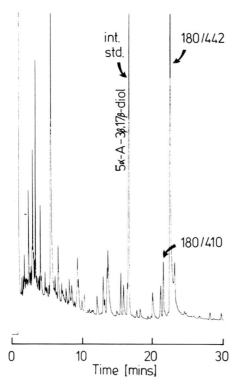

int.
std.

180/442

5α-A-3β.17β-diol

180/410

0   10   20   30
Time [mins]

Fig. 3. Gas chromatogram of trimethylsilyl ether derivatives of the polar phenolic fraction from human urine collected during the mid-luteal phase of menstrual cycle. Gas chromatography was carried out using a 20 metre open-tubular glass capillary column coated with silicone OV-1 and temperature programmed operation from 170°C to 265°C with increments of 2°C/min. This chromatogram is representative of approximately 60 µl of urine injection on the column.

trimethylsilylated polar phenolic fraction, from a urine collected during the mid-luteal phase of the cycle, is shown in Figure 3. The relatively large amounts of these compounds which are present in urine, in this case the equivalent of only 60 µl of urine was injected on column, permits quantification to be readily carried out by gas chromatography alone, although this is a more time consuming procedure.

The cyclic behaviour in the daily excretion of compounds 180/442 and 180/410 has already been demonstrated and reported for the vervet monkey when gas chromatography was used for quantification (Setchell et al., 1980). Using the described GC-MS method the excretion of these phenolic compounds has been measured in daily urine collections obtained from a number of women throughout the complete menstrual cycle. To enable an assessment of the time of ovulation, the urinary excretion of oestrone-glucuronide, oestradiol-3-glucuronide, oestriol-16α-glucuronide, in addition to the total oestrone, oestradiol and oestriol, were measured using radio-

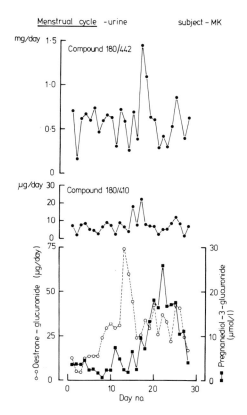

Fig. 4. Typical excretion of compounds 180/442 and 180/410 during human menstrual cycle. Excretion of oestrone-glucuronide and pregnanediol-3∝-glucuronide measured by radioimmunoassay are also represented.

immunoassay procedures described in the literature (Samarajeewa and Kellie, 1975; Lehtinen and Adlercreutz, 1977; Baker et al., 1979; Collins et al., 1979). In a number of isolated samples the urinary and plasma luteinising hormone (LH) concentrations were determined. To allow the detection of the luteal phase of the cycle, pregnanediol-3∝-glucuronide excretion was measured by radioimmunoassay (Baker et al., 1976) in all samples and in some cases plasma progesterone concentrations were determined.

A typical example of the urinary excretion of compounds 180/442 and 180/410, during a normal menstrual cycle and their relationship to the excretion of oestrone-glucuronide and pregnanediol-3∝-glucuronide is shown in Figure 4. Ovulation in this subject occurred on day 13 of the cycle and is characterised by the expected increase in oestrone-glucuronide excretion, at which time the excretion of the 180/442 and 180/410 compounds is low. This was a conspicuous feature of all the normal menstrual cycles so far

212   K.D.R. Setchell et al.

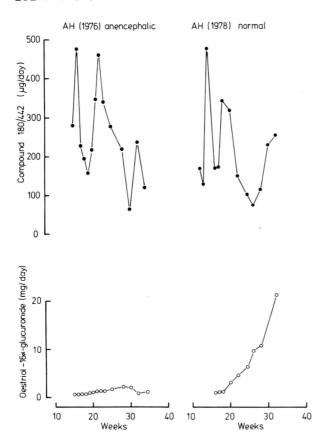

Fig. 5.   Excretion of oestriol-16α-glucuronide (mg/day) measured by radioimmunoassay and of compound 180/442 (μg/day) during 2 pregnancies of a woman who first gave birth to an anencephalic fetus and 2 yrs later a normal infant.

studied. During the early to mid-luteal phase of the cycle, when progesterone production by the developing corpus luteum increases and a corresponding increase in urinary pregnanediol-3α-glucuronide occurs, there is a marked elevation in the excretion of these phenolic compounds with levels being 3-4 fold greater than in the follicular or ovulatory period. Levels of the unknowns have been shown to decrease rapidly before maximum progesterone secretion occurs. This significant increase in excretion of compounds 180/442 and 180/410 in the luteal phase has been a consistent observation for all normal menstrual cycles so far studied and could suggest that they may have an important role to play in the hormonal control of the menstrual cycle.

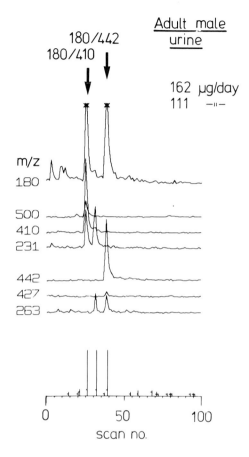

Fig. 6.   Computer reconstructed ion current chromatograms obtained from repetitive magnetic scanning GC-MS analysis of a urine sample from normal adult male subject (age 25 yrs). Ions selected were characteristic of the 2 phenolic compounds and their identification is based upon a coincidence in the peaking of these ions. Daily excretion of compounds 180/442 and 180/410 is indicated.

Pregnancy

Having demonstrated relatively high levels of compound 180/442 in early pregnancy of the vervet monkey (Setchell et al., 1980) it was not surprising to find a similar trend in human pregnancy. Figure 5 shows the excretion of this compound in a pregnant woman who gave birth to an anencephalic fetus and then two years later, after a normal pregnancy, delivered a normal infant. This unique example, apart from illustrating that greater amounts of this phenolic compound are excreted in early pregnancy, also indicates that the source of production in pregnancy is not fetal or under the influence of the fetal hypophyseal-pituitary-adrenal axis. In anencephaly when the functional role of the fetal hypothalamic-pituitary-adrenal axis is impaired, oestrogen production and excretion is low, as was observed in this example (Fig. 5). The excretion of compound 180/442 was found to be almost identical in the normal and abnormal pregnancies, indicating that its source of production is maternal, rather than fetal.

It is most probable that the relatively high amount of compound 180/442 in early pregnancy is a continuation of its peak level in the luteal phase of the cycle. If fertilisation does not occur the amounts excreted decrease, regression of the corpus luteum occurs and the next cycle is initiated. This, however, remains to be confirmed as does the implication that these compounds have any physiological role.

At the present time circumstantial evidence suggests the major source of these compounds to be ovarian and not adrenal as was suggested in the earlier report of their presence in the vervet monkey (Setchell et al., 1980). The finding of a smaller amount of compound 180/442 (119 μg/day) in the urine of one postmenopausal woman and the much reduced amounts in the urine of ovariectomised women. (30-60 μg/day) provides some evidence to support this statement.

Males

Both compounds have been identified in the urine from adult males in slightly lower amounts than in female urine. Figure 6 shows computer reconstructed ion current chromatograms of the ions characteristic of compounds 180/442 and 180/410, obtained following the repetitive magnetic scanning GC-MS analysis of an adult male urine. Furthermore, although these compounds were detected in the urine of infants (male) the amounts excreted were much lower than in adults, being less than 10 μg/day at the age of 1 year, and almost undetectable in the first week of life.

As yet there is insufficient evidence to indicate the origin of these compounds in males. Oestrogens, which are produced primarily by the ovaries in women, are also present in men in comparable concentrations to the follicular phase of the ovarian cycle and in greater concentrations than in postmenopausal women. Thus by analogy the occurrence of compounds 180/442 and 180/410 in males may indicate that there are different sites of production in men and women.

Structural characteristics of phenolic compounds

A number of the physico-chemical characteristics of these polar phenolic compounds have been described previously (Setchell et al., 1980). The important structural features of each compound which have been determined using GC-MS are listed in Table 1. The mass spectra of the trimethylsilyl ether derivatives and their chemical behaviour do not support a classical type of steroid structure. If this is the case they may

TABLE 1.

Principal structural features of compounds 180/442 and 180/410

	Compound 180/442	Compound 180/410
Molecular weight	298	302
Elemental composition	$C_{18}H_{18}O_4$	$C_{18}H_{22}O_4$
Structural characteristics	Aromatic ring (phenol group)	Aromatic ring (phenol group)
	Dihydroxy compound	Tetrahydroxy compound
	2 other oxygen atoms	
	(C = O based upon i.r. spectrum)	

comprise a class of endogenous compound not previously described. Other instrumental techniques, including nuclear magnetic resonance spectroscopy, together with wet chemical methods, are currently being applied in an attempt to elucidate their structure*.

*Note added in proof
Recent structural elucidation studies have provided definitive evidence that the structures of the two unknowns belong to a class of compound defined as lignans. The structures are 2,3-bis-(3'-hydroxybenzyl)-butyrolactone (180/442) and 2,3-bis-(3'-hydroxybenzyl)-butane-1,4-diol (180/410) and the evidence which led to the identification is reported elsewhere (Setchell, K.D.R., Lawson, A.M., Mitchell, F.L., Adlercreutz, H., Kirk, D.N. and Axelson, M. *Nature*, 1980).

References

Axelson, M. and Sjövall, J. (1977): *J. Steroid Biochem.*, 8, 683.
Baker, T.S., Chester, Z., Cooley, G., Jennison, K.M., Kellie, A.E., Samarajeewa, A.E. and Steele, S.J. (1976): *J. Endocr.*, 71, 51.
Baker, T.S., Jennison, K.M. and Kellie, A.E. (1979): *Biochem. J.*, 177, 729.
Collins, A.P., Collins, P.O., Kilpatrick, M.J., Manning, P.A., Pike, J.A. and Tyler, J.P.P. (1979): *Acta Endocr. (Kbh.)*, 90, 336.
Lehtinen, T. and Adlercreutz, H. (1977): *J. Steroid Biochem.*, 8, 99.
Samarajeewa, P. and Kellie, A.E. (1975): *Biochem. J.*, 151, 369.
Setchell, K.D.R., Bull, R. and Adlercreutz, H. (1979): *J. Steroid Biochem.*, in press.
Setchell, K.D.R. and Shackleton, C.H.L. (1973): *Clin. Chim. Acta, 47*, 381.

Gap communicating junctions in theca interna cells of mouse ovarian follicles

G. FAMILIARI and P.M. MOTTA

Istituto di Anatomia Umana Normale, Facoltà di Medicina e Chirurgia, Università di Roma, Rome, Italy

Ultrastructural observations on the theca interna have been reported in the mouse (Byskov, 1969; Hiura and Fujita, 1977), but no comprehensive account of the ultrastructure of the theca interna in this species has been published.

Ultrastructural studies of the mammalian ovary have also indicated that cellular populations within several ovarian compartments exhibit membrane specialization implicated in cell-to-cell communication (Motta et al., 1971; Van Blerkom and Motta, 1979). By freeze-fracture methods these specializations termed 'gap junctions' have been identified between granulosa cells (Albertini et al., 1975), corpus luteum cells (Albertini and Anderson, 1975) and ovarian interstitial cells (Lawrence Jr. and Burden, 1976). In addition, heterocellular gap junctions have been observed between cumulus cells and the oocyte (Anderson and Albertini, 1976).

In this paper, the theca interna has been studied by transmission electron microscopy and freeze-etching methods in a variety of developing and atretic follicles with particular reference to the occurrence and development of intercellular junctions.

Material and methods

Electron microscopy

Ovaries of sexually mature mice were fixed in glutaraldehyde at 2.5% in cacodylate buffer 0.1 M pH 7.3, washed in cacodylate buffer 0.1 M pH 7.3 and post-fixed in osmium tetroxide at 1% in the same buffer. The fixative, the buffer wash solution and the post-fixative, contained 1% of lanthanum nitrate (Revel and Karnowski, 1967). Dehydrated in a graded acetone series, the blocks were embedded in Epon 812. Thin sections were cut on a LKB ultramicrotome and stained with uranyl acetate (Watson, 1958) and lead citrate (Reynolds, 1963) before viewing in an electron microscope Zeiss EM9A.

Freeze-fracture

Tissue processed for freeze fracture, was fixed in glutaraldehyde at 2.5% in cacodylate buffer 0.1 M pH 7.3, washed in cacodylate buffer, and infiltrated with 30% glycerol in the same buffer. Small tissue fragments were frozen in the liquid phase of freon 22, cooled and stored with liquid nitrogen.

Samples were then fractured at $-115°C$ and shadowed with platinum and carbon in a Balzer apparatus (Balzers High Vacuum Corp., Balzers, Liechtenstein). Replicas were cleaned in a clorox solution, mounted on copper grids and observed in an electron microscope Zeiss EM9A.

Results

In primordial and primary follicles, the theca interna consisted of a few layers of concentric arranged fibroblasts and small bundles of collagen fibers. Intercellular junctions as zonulae adherentes and gap junctions were rarely observed. When present they appeared very small.

In growing follicles the theca interna layer often showed three different cell types: (1) fibroblast-like cells; (2) steroid-secreting cells; (3) transitional elements. The intercellular junctions (zonulae adherentes and gap junctions) were relatively numerous at this time.

In Graafian and preovulatory follicles the theca interna cells generally assumed a clear polyhedral shape and were larger than those observed in previous stages. Their cytoplasm was filled with organelles considered characteristic for steroid cells (smooth endoplasmic reticulum, mitochondria with villiform and/or tubular cristae and lipid droplets).

Fibroblast-like cells and intermediary stages were also observed. In this stage of follicular development the gap junctions increased in number and in length assuming, in some cases, the typical aspect of annular structures. The other junctions were apparently reduced.

In atretic (Graafian and preovulatory) follicles the steroidogenic cells of the theca interna survived and appeared mixed up with several fibroblasts. Numerous cells among these showed signs of cytolysis. Gap junctions and zonulae adherentes were still present between preserved cells and often appeared numerous.

In all the follicles studied, gap junctions and zonulae adherentes were always present not only between two differentiated theca interna (steroidogenic) cells, but also between two immature elements and/or closely related mature and immature cells.

Occasional solitary cilia were also observed in the variable population of the theca interna cells (Figs 1a and b; 2a and b; 3a and b).

Discussion

Gap communicating junctions may have a role in the cellular differentiation of the theca interna and possibly also coordinate the hormonal activity of

218   G. Familiari and P.M. Motta

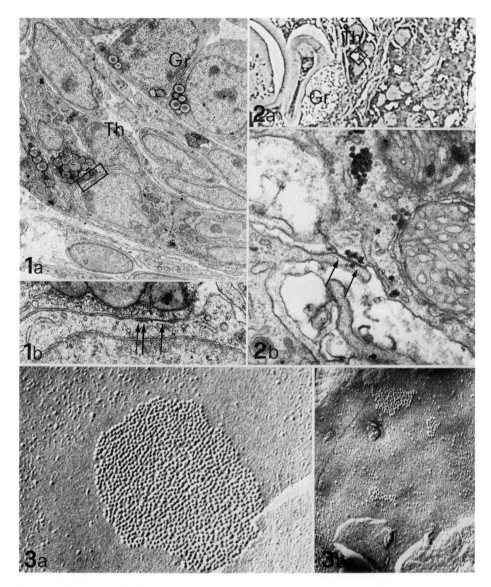

Fig. 1. Growing follicle. Lanthanum nitrate. Th = theca interna, Gr = granulosa cells. Gap junction (arrow) and zonula adherens (double arrow) between differentiating steroidogenic cells. (a = x2800, b = x21000). (b) is boxed area of (a).

Fig. 2. Atretic follicle. Lanthanum nitrate. Th = theca interna, Gr = granulosa cells. Gap junction (arrows) between mature thecal cells. (a = x280, b = x42000).

Fig. 3. Growing follicle. Freeze-fracture. P face view of typical gap junctions occurring between thecal cells (arrows) (a = x110000, b = x75000).

this cellular population which also seems to persist during follicular atresia.

In these cases in fact the theca interna cells, which already assumed a steroidogenic function, are called 'interstitial gland cells' of thecal origin (Motta and Van Blerkom, 1979).

Closely related to the coordination role among theca interna cells (differentiation and hormonal production) is perhaps the occurrence of a single cilium in a few among these cells.

The intriguing possibility that this organelle may be associated to some function (chemoreceptor?) should not be completely ruled out if gap junctions are regarded as selective channels for transferring intercellular signals (Loewenstein, 1974).

References

Albertini, D.F. and Anderson, E. (1975): *Anat. Rec., 18,* 171.

Albertini, D.F., Fawcett, D.W. and Olds, P.J. (1975): *Tissue and Cell, 7,* 389.

Anderson, E. and Albertini, D.F. (1976): *J. Cell Biol., 71,* 680.

Byskov, A.G.S. (1969): *Z. Zellforsch., 100,* 285.

Hiura, M. and Fujita, H. (1977): *Arch. Histol. Jap., 40,* 95.

Lawrence, I.E., Jr. and Burden, H.W. (1976): *Amer. J. Anat., 147,* 81.

Loewenstein, W.R. (1974): In: *Cell Membranes: Biochemistry, Cell Biology and Pathology,* Chapter IV, p. 105, Editors: G. Weissmann and R. Claiborne. HP Publishing Co. Inc., New York.

Motta, P.M., Takeva, Z. and Nesci, E. (1971): *Acta Anat. (Basel), 80,* 537.

Motta, P.M. and Van Blerkom, J. (1979): In: *Human Ovulation. Mechanisms, Prediction, Detection and Induction,* Chapter II, p. 17. Editor: E.S.E. Hafez. North-Holland Publishing Co., Amsterdam-New York.

Reynolds, E.S. (1963): *J. Cell Biol., 17,* 208.

Revel, J.P. and Karnowski, M.J. (1967): *J. Cell Biol., 33,* C7.

Van Blerkom, J. and Motta, P.M. (1979): In: *The Cellular Basis of Mammalian Reproduction,* Chapter I, p. 5. Urban and Schwarzenberg, Baltimore-Munich.

Watson, M.L. (1958): *J. Biophys. Biochem. Cytol., 4,* 475.

Steroidogenesis in perfused human corpus luteum tissue: the effects of flow rate and serum concentration in perfusion fluid*

J.S.G. BIGGS, FRANCES J. THOMAS and S. MIKLOSI

Department of Obstetrics and Gynaecology, University of Queensland, Royal Brisbane Hospital, Brisbane, Australia

The significance of changes in blood flow in the stimulation of endocrine tissues has been the subject of several recent studies (L'Age et al., 1970; Lee and Novy, 1978; Caffrey et al., 1979). The opportunity to pursue similar investigations in the human is limited and there is need for continuing development of 'in vitro' methods in study of this area.

Studies of function of human corpus luteum have mostly been of a static nature (Hammerstein et al., 1964; Marsh et al., 1976); such methods have given little ability to manipulate flow rates or observe changes in steroidogenesis due to alterations in supply of substrates or the addition of gonadotrophins or other potentially stimulatory or suppressive substances. Some preliminary work on short-term changes in an organ culture system was described by Biggs and Baker (1978), but the problems of frequent sampling in a closed system limit its usefulness in examining dynamic effects.

Several methods for flow perfusion of endocrine tissues have been described using the terms 'continuous flow incubation', 'superfusion' and 'perifusion'. These methods were extended to the corpus luteum of the rat (Hashimoto et al., 1975) and pig (Watson and Leask, 1975). The present paper describes application of the flow perfusion method to the human corpus luteum and reports on the effects of changes of flow rate and serum concentration of perfusion fluid.

Material and methods

Corpora lutea

Corpora lutea of the menstrual cycle were obtained at operation for reasons unrelated to the present study. Glands were removed intact and cut into 1 mm slices. Central clot and outer fibrous connective tissue were removed and the luteal tissue cut into pieces measuring approximately 1 x 1 x 4 mm.

*Supported by a National Health and Medical Research Council (Australia) grant to Dr. Biggs.

Dissection took place in frequently-changed medium consisting of Eagle's minimum essential medium with Earle's salts and Hepes Buffer, to which were added kanamycin (40 μg/ml), fungizone (2 μg/ml) and glutamine (2.0 mM) (MEM).

The tissue was divided into portions of about 100-150 mg and perfused for periods of 6-24 hr.

Flow incubation system

The flow system was adapted from that described by Lowry and McMartin (1974). The perfusion chambers consisted of disposable polypropylene filter units (Swinnex, 25 mm, Millipore, U.S.A.), with nylon mesh filters.

Perfusion fluid consisting of MEM with or without 5% newborn calf serum was placed in a covered glass container at 37°C and aerated with 5% CO_2 in oxygen. Fluid passed via an 8-channel variable-speed peristaltic pump to a heating coil and the perfusion chamber, which were maintained at 37°C. Fluid was then passed through teflon tubing to a 10 place fraction collector. Absorption of steroids in the perfusion chambers and efferent tubing system was found to be negligible.

The system was allowed to run for 1-2 hr before an experiment was commenced. In the first study, flow rates of approximately 5, 10, 20 and 40 ml/hr were each applied to tissue portions from 2 corpora lutea for at least an hour, with fluid collections every 15 min. Hormone production rates, expressed as μg/g of tissue/hr are the means of 4-6 collections. In the second study, portions of a corpus luteum were perfused with MEM, and then with successively higher concentrations of calf serum, each for 1 hr. The flow rate was kept constant at 9.0 ml/hr.

Radioimmunoassays

Progesterone was assayed by the method of Abraham et al. (1971, 1975) with minor modifications. Solvent extraction with ether was carried out where the culture medium contained calf serum, but otherwise the assay was applied directly to the samples. Progesterone antiserum (# 334) was kindly supplied by Dr. R.I. Cox, C.S.I.R.O. Division of Animal Production, Prospect, Australia. Sensitivity of the standard curve was 9 pg and the average blank sample value did not exceed this. Addition of progesterone to culture medium at a concentration of 10 ng/ml gave an assay mean ± SD of 10.3 ± 1.3 ng/ml (n = 28) and a coefficient of variation of 12.6% between assays.

17β-Oestradiol was measured by radioimmunoassay directly on the culture medium suitably diluted and incubated with antiserum (# 244) as in the assay of Korenman et al. (1974). The sensitivity of the standard curve was 2 pg and blank sample values were always less than this. Mean (± SD) assay value for 17β-oestradiol added to culture medium at a concentration of 0.5

ng/ml was 0.51 ± 0.03 ng/ml (n = 14). Interassay and intra-assay coefficients of variation were 6.6% (n = 110) and 4.5% (n = 20), respectively.

Results

a. *Hormone production and flow rate of perfusion fluid*

Increasing flow rates in the range 3-40 ml/hr gave increasing production of progesterone and 17β-oestradiol (Figs. 1 and 2). A plateau effect was evident above about 15-20 ml/hr in all tissues, but especially in those perfused with 5% calf serum.

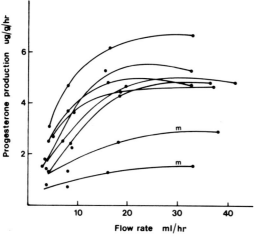

Fig. 1. Progesterone production with increasing flow rate of perfusing fluid – 5% calf serum or MEM (m).

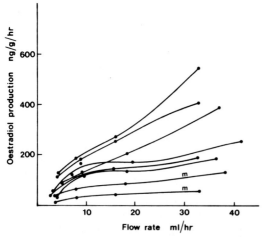

Fig. 2. 17β-Oestradiol production with increasing flow rate of perfusing fluid.

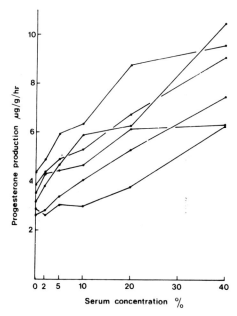

Fig. 3. Progesterone production with increasing concentration of calf serum in perfusing fluid.

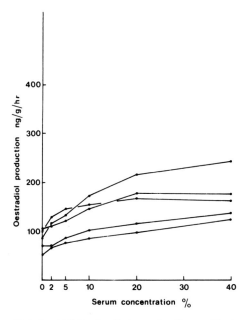

Fig. 4. 17β-Oestradiol production with increasing concentration of calf serum in perfusing fluid.

b. Hormone production and serum concentration

Increasing concentrations of newborn calf serum gave successive increases in progesterone and 17β-oestradiol production (Figs. 3 and 4).

Discussion

The advantages of a flow perfusion system for study of ovarian function were outlined by Anderson et al. (1973) and Watson and Leask (1975). Such an approach is necessary if individual functional elements of the gonad are to be studied and a dynamic method used. Division of the gland into small pieces and allocation of these into several groups assumes that the luteal tissue is homogeneous, while microscopy demonstrates that this is not the case. Anderson et al. (1973) stressed the problem of sample-to-sample variability in their studies of the rat ovary. In the present studies, replicate samples, while showing a moderate range of levels of steroidogenesis, have shown the same qualitative response to changes in the perfusion fluid. To the extent examined in these studies the tissue perfusion system can be said to be useful in providing information on the function of the human corpus luteum.

The rate of fluid flow is seen to have an important bearing on steroido-genesis of human corpus luteum tissue in vitro. This observation is of importance in specification of conditions of tissue perfusion experiments. It also has bearing on recent reports of the part played by flow rates of blood in determining the function of endocrine tissues. The effect of increase in perfusion fluid or blood flow may act through a greater supply of nutrients, substrates or gonadotrophins (Lee and Novy, 1978) or through a more rapid removal of the products of steroidogenesis, in this case, progesterone (Shinada et al., 1978; Caffrey et al., 1979).

There have also been studies on the importance of plasma proteins in the enhancement of steroidogenesis (Westphal, 1975; Ewing et al., 1976; Caffrey et al., 1979). In a similar way to that described for increased flow of blood or perfusion fluid, an increase in serum proteins is seen as increasing the removal of steroid products and reducing end production inhibition (Caffrey et al., 1979). The present studies provide evidence that these mechanisms operate in the human corpus luteum as in other tissues.

Acknowledgements

The technical assistance of Mrs. Christine Meikle and Miss Vicki Dolan is gratefully acknowledged.

References

Abraham, G.E., Manlimos, F.S., Solis, M., Garza, R. and Moroulis, G.B. (1975): *Clin. Biochem., 8,* 369.

Abraham, G.E., Swerdloff, R., Tulchinsky, D. and Odell, W.D. (1971): *J. Clin. Endocr., 32,* 619.

Anderson, L.M., Turnipseed, M.R. and Ungar, F. (1973): *Endocrinology, 92,* 265.

Biggs, J.S.G. and Baker, T.G. (1978): *J. Reprod. Fertil., 54,* 221.

Caffrey, J.L., Nett, T.M., Abel, J.H., Jr. and Niswender, G.D. (1979): *Biol. Reprod., 20,* 279.

Ewing, L.L., Chubb, C.E. and Robaire, B. (1976): *Nature (Lond.), 264,* 84.

Hammerstein, J., Rice, B.F. and Savard, K. (1964): *J. Clin. Endocr., 24,* 597.

Hashimoto, I., Asano, T. and Wiest, W.G. (1975): *Endocrinology, 96,* 421.

Korenman, S.G., Stevens, R.H., Carpenter, L.A., Robb, M., Niswender, G.D. and Sherman, B.M. (1974): *J. Clin. Endocr., 38,* 718.

L'Age, M., Gonzalez-Luque, A. and Yates, F.E. (1970): *Amer. J. Physiol., 219,* 281.

Lee, W. and Novy, M.J. (1978): *Biol. Reprod., 18,* 799.

Lowry, P.J. and McMartin, C. (1974): *Biochem. J., 142,* 287.

Marsh, J.M., Savard, K. and Lemaire, W.J. (1976): In: *The Endocrine Function of the Human Ovary,* p. 37. Editors: V.H.T. James, M. Serio and G. Giusti. Academic Press, London.

Shinada, T., Yokota, Y. and Igarashi, M. (1978): *Fertil. and Steril., 29,* 84.

Watson, J. and Leask, J.T.S. (1975): *J. Endocr., 64,* 163.

Westphal, U. (1975): In: *Normal and Abnormal Growth of the Prostate,* p. 616. Editor: M. Goland. Charles C. Thomas, Springfield, Illinois.

226

Follicle at the crossroads: hormonal determinants and biochemical correlates of incipient atresia*

RUTH H. BRAW, A. TSAFRIRI and H.R. LINDNER

Department of Hormone Research, Weizmann Institute of Science, Rehovot, Israel

Definition of problem and experimental approach

Of every thousand oocytes present in the human ovary at birth, only one is likely ever to be ovulated; and in the course of every oestrous cycle of the adult mouse, about 50 follicles are believed to undergo atresia (Byskov, 1978). Thus it is possible to view ovulation, the central theme of this symposium, in a somewhat perverted sense as an escape from atresia. We still do not fully understand the factors that regulate the numerical ratio between follicles that will reach maturity and those destined to undergo regression and degeneration. However, elegant work in the laboratory of G. Ross (Ross et al., 1979) suggests that the balance between androgenic and oestrogenic steroids within the follicle may be an important determinant of its subsequent fate.

One difficulty in investigating atresia is that it is usually recognized only in retrospect, after the follicle has developed extensive morphological signs of degeneration. We therefore looked for early functional correlates of follicular atresia. To this end we compared the steroidogenic pathways in normal preovulatory rat follicles with those in a synchronized follicle population destined to undergo atresia as a consequence of experimental manipulation of the animals. As an additional functional criterion of atresia we chose the loss of the ovulatory response to exogenous human chorionic gonadotrophin (hCG), using the same animal model, viz. rats in which the cyclic LH-surge is suppressed by repeated administration of pentobarbitone sodium.

The number of eggs shed at each cycle is normally maintained within narrowly defined limits characteristic of the species. Variations in this rate of ovulation may conceivably result either from changes in the number of oocytes recruited from the resting pool during the preceding cycle or from a change in the fraction of that cohort which will suffer atresia during its final

*These studies were supported by generous grants (to H.R.L.) of the Ford Foundation, The Rockefeller Foundation, and the Population Council, Inc., N.Y. H.R.L. is the Adlai E. Stevenson III Professor of Endocrinology and Reproduction Biology at the Weizmann Institute of Science. The contribution of R.B. was in partial fulfilment of the requirements for the Ph.D. degree of the Weizmann Institute's Graduate School.

growth spurt (Peters, 1979). To clarify the relative importance of these two factors, we examined the effects of a superovulatory dose of pregnant mare serum gonadotrophin (PMSG) on follicle kinetics in the prepubertal rat ovary.

FSH rescues antral follicles

Wistar-derived 26-day-old female rats were given a maximally effective dose of PMSG (Gestyl®, Organon, Oss, 15 I.U. in saline, subcutaneously), a preparation containing predominantly FSH-like activity. This dose of PMSG induces the release of 49 ± 11.6 (S.E.M.) ova/treated rat. Treated and vehicle-injected rats were sacrificed 6, 12, 24 or 48 hr after injection and the ovaries were subjected to histological examination. Follicles were classified by development stage (types 2-7; modified after Pedersen and Peters, 1968) and degree of atresia (stages I-III). Briefly, types 2-4 are preantral follicles with less than 200 granulosa cells in their largest cross-section (GC/S_m); the largest of these, type 4 (81-200 GC/S_m), are 120-170 μm in diameter, with a mean oocyte diameter of 49.9 μm, showing small, scattered pockets of follicular fluid accumulation. Types 5-6 have 201-600 and 601-1000 GC/S_m, respectively (follicle diameters 170-500 μm and oocyte mean diameter 56.3-58.0), while type 7 are mature preovulatory follicles. Stage I of atresia denotes follicles with 1-10% pyknotic nuclei in the membrana granulosa, with a mitotic index (1.8 ± 0.2 S.E.M.) significantly below that of normal follicles (3.0 ± 0.1). In Stage II atresia (Fig. 1), 10-30% of granulosa cell nuclei are pyknotic, the mitotic index is low (0.4 ± 0.1) and the oocyte showed meiosis-like changes such as condensed chromosomes in metaphase or polar bodies. In Stage III atretic follicles most of the granulosa cells are replaced by macrophages or debris, the antrum may have collapsed, the theca interna is hypertrophic and the oocyte is often fragmented or irregularly cleaved. The developmental stage from which the latter follicles are derived is usually difficult to determine.

Little of note happened in the preantral follicle population in response to the PMSG treatment, except for a transient rise in mitotic index 24 hr after injection: there was no significant change in total follicle number, the pyknotic index or the incidence of atresia. The salient finding was a sharp decline in the incidence of atresia in the antral follicle population (Fig. 2), and particularly in follicles of type 5. This change was evident within 12 hr of the hormone injection, at which time 7% ± 5 of type 5 follicles were classed as atretic in the ovaries from treated rats (pyknotic index 4.2 ± 0.9) compared with 66% ± 9 (p.i. = 14.8 ± 1.4) in those from untreated controls. Again, there was no increase in the total number of antral follicles (Fig. 2), except for a rise in type 6 follicles after 48 hr (Braw and Tsafriri, 1980a), probably attributable to the diminished rate of atresia of their type 5 precursors.

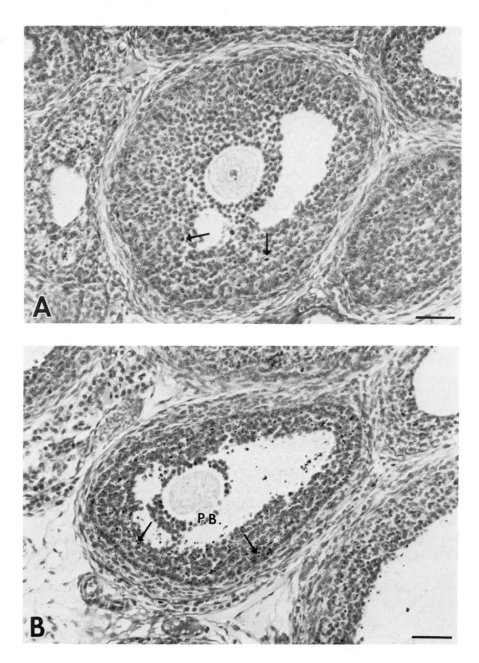

Fig. 1. (A) Non-atretic antral follicle. Note mitotic figures (arrows). (B) Follicle at stage II atresia. Note structure resembling polar body (P.B.) near oocyte and numerous pyknotic nuclei scattered throughout membrana granulosa (arrows). The follicular antrum contains much cell debris. Haematoxylin and eosin. Bar: 50 μm. (From Braw and Tsafriri, 1980a, *J. Reprod. Fertil.*, by permission).

It appears then, that PMSG induces superovulation in the rat not by recruiting preantral follicles smaller than type 4 into the pool of growing follicles, but rather by salvaging antral follicles from atresia, particularly at the type 5 stage. A similar conclusion has been reached with regard to the effect of PMSG on the immature mouse ovary (Peters, 1979). Likewise, Hirshfield and Midgley (1978) produced evidence that in the cyclic rat follicles of 200-400 μm diameter, corresponding roughly to our type 5 follicles, are in a labile stage of development and will perish unless supported by FSH. By contrast, the superovulatory effect of PMSG on the cyclic hamster ovary has been attributed chiefly to stimulation of the growth of small preantral follicles (Chirvas and Greenwald, 1978), though a sparing effect on larger follicles was also observed; aṅd in the sheep, it has been inferred that rescue of follicles from atresia does not play a significant role in the observed increase in the number of large follicles following administration of PMSG 'in vivo' (Dott et al., 1979).

The effect of PMSG is likely to be due to its FSH-like activity. FSH has a dual action on the follicle: it renders the granulosa cells responsive to LH, by inducing LH-receptors (Richards and Midgley, 1976; Lindner et al., 1977; Nimrod et al., 1977) and it stimulates oestrogen synthesis (Lamprecht et al., 1976), probably by inducing a granulosa cell aromatase (Dorrington et al., 1975; Fortune and Armstrong, 1977). It is possible that this oestrogen is responsible for the follicle-maintaining action of FSH, since oestrogen prevents follicular atresia in immature hypophysectomized rats (Harman et al., 1975). Besides, the increased aromatase activity by the FSH-stimulated follicle may prevent the accumulation of androgen, which has been implicated as a causative agent in follicular atresia (Louvet et al., 1975).

Loss of ovulability precedes atretic degeneration of mature follicles

The administration of pentobarbitone sodium during a critical period on the day of pro-oestrus – in our colony between 13.30 and 16.30 hr – prevents ovulation (Everett and Sawyer, 1950) by suppressing the cyclic surge of LH and FSH (Ayalon et al., 1972). Spontaneous ovulation will occur on the next day, but Everett and Sawyer (1950) observed that repetition of the barbiturate treatment for 3 days resulted in degeneration of the overmature crop of Graafian follicles. It appeared that this regimen could provide a useful model for studying early events in a cohort of follicles known to be doomed to atresia. The experimental design (Braw and Tsafriri, 1980b) is shown in Figure 3.

The capacity of the mature follicles to undergo ovulation was assessed by counting the number of tubal ova 16-18 hr after administration of hCG at a dose maximally effective in acutely barbiturate-blocked rats (Pregnyl®, Organon, Oss, 4 I.U./rat), given immediately after the last barbiturate injection. The results, summarized in Figure 4, show that ovulability of the follicles declined progressively with the duration of the blockade of the gonadotrophin surge, the effect attaining statistical significance on day 2 before any morphological evidence of atresia was evident. Inhibition of ovulation was about 50% on day 3, by which time most of the large follicles had reached stage I of atresia, and was maximal (69%) on day 4 after the

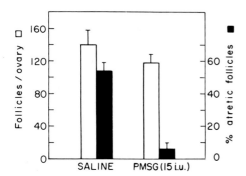

Fig. 2. Effect of Pregnant Mare Serum Gonadotrophin (PMSG) on the total number of type 5 + 6 follicles and the percentage of atretic follicles in this population 12 hr after injection of the hormone. Vertical brackets, S.E.M. for 4 animals.

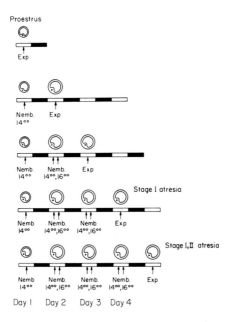

Fig. 3. Experimental design. Pentobarbitone sodium (30mg/kg body weight) was injected once on day of pro-oestrus between 13.30 hr and 14.00 hr (arrows) and twice on each subsequent day between 14.00 hr and 16.00 hr, as indicated. Follicles were explanted (Exp) between 8.00 and 12.00 hr on the day following the last barbiturate administration.

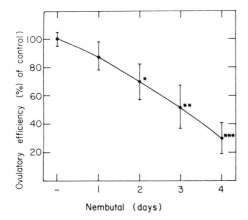

Fig. 4. Effect of duration of barbiturate treatment on ovulatory response to exogeneous hCG (4 I.U./rat). Ovulatory efficiency (% of control) is defined as

$$\frac{\text{No. of ova shed/rat treated} \times 100}{\text{No. of ova shed/control rats}}$$

For details of barbiturate treatment see Figure 3. Significant treatment effects (Student's t-test) are indicated by $*p < 0.05$, $**p < 0.01$, or $***p < 0.001$.

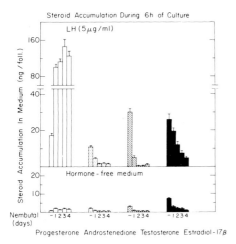

Fig. 5. Effect of continued suppression of cyclic gonadotrophin surge on accumulation of steroids in medium during 6 hr culture of Graafian follicles from pentobarbitone-treated rats in hormone-free or LH-containing (5 μg/ml) medium. Rats were treated with sodium pentobarbitone (Nembutal®; see Figure 3) for number of days indicated. Each bar represents the mean ± S.E.M. (vertical brackets) of 6-10 determinations. Androstene-dione, androst-4-ene-3,17-dione.

start of barbiturate injections when atresia had progressed to stage II in many of these follicles. Loss of the capacity to ovulate in response to a standardized dose of hCG therefore clearly precedes the gross morphological hallmarks of atresia, such as the appearance of pyknotic granulosa cell nuclei. The ovulatory response to hCG is lost even earlier after hypophysectomy, viz. 12 hr after the operation (Talbert et al., 1951, and own observations). It should be noted, however, that barbiturate treatment suppresses only the cyclic gonadotrophin surge while permitting tonic gonadotrophin secretion (Daane and Parlow, 1971; Ashiru and Blake, 1978); the latter component of the pituitary secretion may be adequate to delay the atretic degeneration of the mature follicles.

Altered pattern of steroidogenesis heralds atresia

Using the same experimental model (Braw and Tsafriri, 1980b), an even earlier indication of incipient atresia was obtained by studying the production of steroids in organ cultures of follicles explanted on the morning (8.00-12.00 hr) after the last barbiturate injection. Normal preovulatory follicles explanted before the gonadotrophin surge under these conditions accumulate predominantly oestrogen and very small amounts of progesterone and androgen, but the progesterone/oestrogen ratio is reversed within 4-6 hr after adding LH to the culture medium (Lindner et al., 1974 and present results, Figure 5). Upon repeated blockade of the gonadotrophic surge, both basal and LH-stimulated progesterone formation by the explanted follicles increased, but even more striking was the progressive decline in oestrogen formation and the lack of androgen accumulation even after LH-stimulation (Fig. 5). These changes, shown in Figure 5 for 6 hr cultures, were clearly recognizable even in follicles explanted on day 1 after barbiturate administration, and became quite pronounced on day 2. The increase in basal progesterone accumulation, i.e. without LH supplementation of the medium, was seen even more clearly in 24 hr incubations: the rate was doubled on day 1 and increased 4-fold by day 2 (data not shown). The unstimulated progesterone/oestradiol ratio increased about 25-fold from 0.2 in the control follicles to 5.0 on the 4th day of barbiturate block.

This marked stimulation of progesterone accumulation by LH even at an advanced stage of atresia (day 4) makes it clear that these follicles have not lost their responsiveness to LH, though a study by Carson et al. (1979) indicated a decline in LH-receptor density during atresia in ovine follicles.

Oestrogen production was restored to normal in follicles explanted on day 1 or 4 from barbiturate-treated rats by addition of testosterone to the culture medium (Fig. 6). This finding indicates that 17:20 sidechain splitting activity, rather than aromatase activity, limits oestrogen formation in this type of atretic follicle of the rat. Oestrogen formation is also impaired in atretic follicles of the sheep (Moor et al., 1978) and mare (Condon et al.,

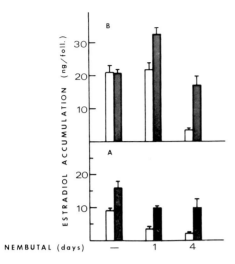

Fig. 6. Effect of continued suppression of cyclic gonadotrophin surge on aromatase activity in preovulatory Graafian follicles. The accumulation in the medium of 17β-oestradiol during 6 hr culture of the follicles with (hatched columns) or without (open columns) addition of testosterone (1 μg/ml) to the medium is shown. A, no added LH; B, LH (5 μg/ml) added to medium. Rats received pentobarbitone sodium (Nembutal; see Figure 3) for number of days indicated. Each bar represents mean ± S.E.M. of 3-10 incubations.

1979). However, Moor et al. (1978) found increased androgen accumulation in the atretic ovine follicle and concluded that aromatase activity was impaired. The discrepancy between the results obtained in the sheep and the present findings with rat follicles may represent an interspecific difference; alternatively the ovine follicles may have been examined at a more advanced stage of atresia.

When gonadotrophic support was withdrawn by hypophysectomy, rather than by barbiturate treatment, similar changes in steroidogenesis, viz. increased progesterone and diminished 17β-oestradiol accumulation, were observed in cultured follicles explanted as early as 6-12 hr after the operation (Braw and Tsafriri, unpublished). An altered pattern of follicular steroidogenesis, akin to that of the luteal cell, is thus the earliest concomitant of incipient follicular atresia identified to date. Since these studies have been confined to mature follicles, it remains to be established whether the conclusions reached also apply to follicles of stage 5, at which the incidence of atresia is highest.

It was recently observed that granulosa cells carry androgen receptors (Schreiber and Ross, 1976) and that androgen synergizes the stimulatory action of FSH on progestin formation (Armstrong and Dorrington, 1976; Nimrod and Lindner, 1976; Hillier et al., 1977). This positive androgen effect, the significance of which is still unclear, was somewhat surprising since androgens had been associated with follicular atresia (Louvet et al., 1975). In view of the present findings, is it possible that androgens promote atresia by inducing premature differentiation and quasi-luteinization of the granulosa cell, while abrogating the oestrogen-mediated proliferative response to FSH? And is such abortive luteinization a general feature of atretic follicles, including those that become atretic at earlier stages of development than examined in the present study? These questions invite further investigation.

Conclusions

The induction of superovulation by FSH or PMSG in the rat depends principally on the rescue of large antral follicles, that is type 5 and 6 follicles, from atresia, rather than on the recruitment of resting follicles smaller than type 4 into the actively growing pool. A similar situation prevails in the mouse, but in hamster both processes are believed to be operative, and in the sheep recruitment of small follicles, rather than the salvage of large ones from atresia, is said to determine the number of eggs reaching ovulation. Perhaps the relative importance of the two control mechanisms differs between habitually monotocous and polytocous mammals.

A model is described in which functional attributes of impending atresia can be defined in a synchronized follicle population. It is found that the capacity to ovulate in response to a standardized dose of hCG is lost before morphological signs of atresia become evident. Furthermore, at an even earlier stage, follicles destined for atresia are shown to be deficient in their ability to produce oestrogen, chiefly due to impaired 17,20-side-chain splitting activity. This conforms with the concept that oestrogens are capable of counteracting atresia, based on 'in vivo' results with hypophysectomized animals. On the other hand, the atretic follicles, even at a very early stage of the process, are characterized by a high rate of progesterone accumulation, which can be stimulated by LH.

Androgens, long suspected of causing follicular atresia, have been shown, paradoxically, to synergize FSH in stimulating progestin production by granulosa cells. We suggest, tentatively, that premature differentiation — i.e. quasi-luteinization — of granulosa cells may be the basis of the atresia-promoting action of androgen.

References

Armstrong, D.T. and Dorrington, J.H. (1976): *Endocrinology, 99,* 1411.
Ashiru, O.A. and Blake, C.A. (1978): *Life Sciences, 23,* 1507.
Ayalon, D., Tsafriri, A., Lindner, H.R., Cordova, T. and Harell, A. (1972): *J. Reprod. Fertil., 31,* 51.
Braw, R.H. and Tsafriri, A. (1980a): *J. Reprod. Fertil.,* in press.
Braw, R.H. and Tsafriri, A. (1980b): *J. Reprod. Fertil.,* in press.
Byskov, A.G. (1978): In: *The Vertebrate Ovary,* p. 533. Editor: R.E. Jones. Plenum Publishing Corp., New York.
Carson, R.S., Findlay, J.K., Burger, H.G. and Trounson, A.O. (1979): *Biol. Reprod., 21,* 75.
Chiras, D.D. and Greenwald, G.S. (1978): *Biol. Reprod., 19,* 895.
Condon, W.A., Ganjam, V.K., Kenney, R.M. and Channing, C.P. (1979): In: *Ovarian Follicular Development and Function,* p. 75. Editors: A.R. Midgley and W.A. Sadler. Raven Press, New York.
Daane, T.A. and Parlow, A.I. (1971): *Endocrinology, 88,* 653.
Dorrington, J.H., Moon, Y.S. and Armstrong, D.T. (1975): *Endocrinology, 97,* 1328.
Dott, H.M., Hay, M.F., Cran, D.G. and Moor, R.M. (1979): *J. Reprod. Fertil., 56,* 683.
Everett, J.W. and Sawyer, C.H. (1950): *Endocrinology, 47,* 198.
Fortune, J.E. and Armstrong, D.T. (1977): *Endocrinology, 100,* 1341.
Harman, S.M., Louvet, J.P. and Ross, G.T. (1975): *Endocrinology, 96,* 1145.
Hillier, S.C., Knazek, R.A. and Ross, G.T. (1977): *Endocrinology, 100,* 1539.
Hirshfield, A.N. and Midgley, A.R., Jr. (1978): *Biol. Reprod., 19,* 606.
Lamprecht, S.A., Kohen, F., Ausher, J., Zor, U. and Lindner, H.R. (1976): *J. Endocr., 68,* 343.
Lindner, H.R., Amsterdam, A., Salomon, Y., Tsafriri, A., Nimrod, A., Lamprecht, S.A., Zor, U. and Koch, Y. (1977): *J. Reprod. Fertil., 251,* 215.
Lindner, H.R., Tsafriri, A., Lieberman, M.E., Zor, U., Koch, Y., Bauminger, S. and Barnea, A. (1974): *Recent Progr. Hormone Res., 30,* 79.
Louvet, J.-P., Harman, S.M., Schreiber, J.R. and Ross, G.T. (1975): *Endocrinology, 97,* 366.
Moor, R.M., Hay, M.F., Dott, H.M. and Cran, D.G. (1978): *J. Endocr., 77,* 309.
Nimrod, A. and Lindner, H.R. (1976): *Mol. Cellular Endocr., 5,* 315.
Nimrod, A., Tsafriri, A. and Lindner, H.R. (1977): *Nature, 267,* 632.
Pedersen, T. and Peters, H. (1968): *J. Reprod. Fertil., 17,* 555.
Peters, H. (1979): In: *Ovarian Follicular Development and Function,* p. 1. Editors: A.R. Midgley and W.A. Sadler. Raven Press, New York.
Richards, J.S. and Midgley, A.R., Jr. (1976): *Biol. Reprod., 14,* 82.
Ross, G.T., Hillier, S.G., Telesnide, A.J. and Knazek, R.A. (1979): In: *Research on Steroids,* Vol. VIII, p. 185. Editors: A. Klopper, L. Lerner, H.J. van der Molen and F. Sciarra. Academic Press, London, New York.
Schreiber, J.R. and Ross, G.T. (1976): *Endocrinology, 99,* 590.
Talbert, G.B., Meyer, R.K. and McShan, W.H. (1951): *Endocrinology, 49,* 687.

Induction of ovulation in chronic anovulatory syndrome through a weak estrogen supplementation*

P.M. KICOVIC[1], C. MASSAFRA[2], G.D'AMBROGIO[2] and A.R. GENAZZANI[2]

[1] *Reproductive Medicine Programme, Medical Unit, Organon, Oss, The Netherlands; and* [2] *Department of Obstetrics and Gynecology, University of Siena, Siena, Italy*

Anovulation is a pathologic condition which may be related to both ovarian and/or hypothalamic-pituitary disturbances. Different clinical pictures such as anorexia nervosa, hyperprolactinemia, isolated deficiency of pituitary gonadotrophins, panhypopituitarism, primary or secondary ovarian failure with or without genetic disturbances are associated with the anovulatory syndrome. In addition, there are other conditions in which chronic anovulation is due to an inadequate regulation of the sensitivity and functioning of feedback mechanisms regulating the hypothalamic-pituitary-ovarian axis (Lasley and Judd, 1978). The latter conditions are characterized by impaired fertility with minor menstrual disorders. Chronic anovulatory syndrome (CAS) is the primary cause of prolonged, unopposed endometrial proliferation and stimulation of mammary glands, which is known to be a risk factor in the etiopathogenesis of corresponding malignancies.

HMG and HCG (Lunenfeld, 1963; Oelsner et al., 1978), antiestrogens — mainly clomiphene (Greenblatt and Barfield, 1961; Gorlitsky et al., 1978) and long-acting LHRH analogues (Schally et al., 1976), alone or in combination, have been used for the treatment of the CAS, primarily aimed at the restoration of fertility. Our recent data (Genazzani et al., 1978) showed that administration of epimestrol† induced (a) a rise in circulating gonadotrophins, and (b) an increase in LH response to LHRH in patients suffering from normogonadotrophic-normoprolactinemic secondary amenorrhea. When tested in a few patients with CAS (Genazzani et al., 1979) epimestrol proved to be an efficient means of restoring ovulation and an adequate luteal phase (ALP). The present study extends our previous knowledge on the validity of epimestrol in the treatment of CAS and supports weak estrogen supplementation as a new approach in the treatment of this syndrome.

*This study was partly supported by the Consiglio Nazionale delle Ricerche Project 'Biology of Reproduction'.

†(16α,17α)-3-methoxyestra-1,3,5(10)-triene-16,17-diol (Stimovul, Organon, Oss, The Netherlands).

TABLE 1.

Chronic anovulatory syndrome

No.	Patient	Age	Cl. diagnosis	Hormone levels (range)				
				LH (mU/ml)	FSH (mU/ml)	E$_2$ (pg/ml)	P (pg/ml)	PRL (ng/ml)
1	M.P.	28	Oligomenorrhea	14.8-20.3	9.8-17.5	165-205	391- 620	5-12
2	Z.M.T.	25	Sterility	9.5-12.3	5.2-8.3	138-175	540-1500	11-28
3	P.A.	28	Sterility	10.5-15.0	7.8-10.2	165-195	480- 910	6-15
4	P.M.	28	Sterility	3.3-12.8	3.5- 8.7	80-130	430- 710	5-10
5	L.A.M.	39	Sterility	11.1-27.0	3.4- 8.0	126-204	480- 610	3-14
6	M.D.	28	Sterility	9.7-19.7	5.5- 7.2	176-299	400-2900	8-19
7	P.M.	30	Sterility	5.0-53.0	8.0-11.3	69-170	850-1100	12-21
8	C.C.	31	Sterility PCT neg.*	12.4-32.2	4.3-10.3	117-219	755-1220	5-13
9	F.S.	30	Sterility OS**	8.0-13.5	4.0- 9.2	159-239	1450-2700	11-22
10	S.P.	31	Sterility PCT neg.*	20.0-40.0	5.8-12.9	103-137	740-2900	12-19
11	G.A.	23	Oligomenorrhea	2.0-18.5	4.0- 9.5	75-105	380- 524	5-14
12	G.M.	27	Oligomenorrhea	10.5-46.0	5.8-13.5	70-112	425-1508	8-13
13	F.N.	36	Oligomenorrhea	14.4-36.2	10.4-30.5	200-360	420- 900	5-11
14	D.M.P.	26	Polymenorrhea	7.8-27.6	4.3-14.0	210-247	380- 850	5-11
15	S.N.	26	Oligomenorrhea	8.9-31.8	5.5-10.9	121-182	350- 717	7-13

*PCT neg. = Post Coital Test Negative; **OS = Oligospermia.

Material and methods

Patients

Fifteen anovulatory patients (Table 1) aged 23-39 yrs, were selected for the study. In each patient diagnosis of chronic anovulation was made on the basis of both clinical symptoms such as oligomenorrhea and/or sterility without galactorrhea, hirsutism or ovarian enlargement, and an endocrinological follow-up for at least 1 cycle. After diagnosis patients were monitored for a further 2 cycles in order to verify the anovulatory condition. In each patient blood samples were drawn every 2-4 days, starting from day 6, 7 or 8 of the cycle to evaluate plasma levels of FSH, LH, estradiol (E$_2$) and progesterone (P). Furthermore, thyroid function and prolactin levels were investigated during control cycles. In sterile patients hysterosalpingography, postcoital test (PCT) and sperm analysis of the husband were also performed.

TABLE 2.

Effect of epimestrol treatment in chronic anovulatory syndrome

No.	Patient	Age	Treatment Type	Length (cycles)	Results	
1	M.P.	28	A	2	Adeq. L.P.	Pregnant
2	Z.M.T.	25	B	2	Adeq. L.P.	Pregnant
3	P.A.	28	A	1	Adeq. L.P.	Pregnant
4	P.M.	28	B	2	Short L.P.	
			C	2	Adeq. L.P.	Pregnant
5	L.A.M.	39	A	1	Short L.P.	
			A	4	Adeq. L.P.	
6	M.D.	28	A	2	Adeq. L.P.	Pregnant
7	P.M.	30	A	4	Adeq. L.P.	
8	C.C.	31	A	6	Adeq. L.P.	
9	F.S.	30	A	3	Adeq. L.P.	
10	S.P.	31	A	2	Anovulat.	
			B	2	Inadeq. L.P.	
			D	10	Adeq. L.P.	
11	G.A.	23	A	2	Adeq. L.P.	
12	G.M.	27	A	2	Short L.P.	
			A	5	Adeq. L.P.	
13	F.N.	36	A	2	Adeq. L.P.	
14	D.M.P.	26	A	1	Anovulat.	
			B	1	Short L.P.	
15	S.N.	26	A	3	Inadeq. L.P.	

A = 10 mg/day/10 days   C = 20 mg/day/10 days
B = 15 mg/day/10 days   D = 15 mg/day/15 days

Treatment

Epimestrol treatment was started in each patient on the 5th day of the cycle (Table 2). Standard treatment (2 x 5 mg/day for 10 days) was applied in 13 cases; the remaining 2 patients (nos. 2 and 4) started with 3 x 5 mg/day for 10 days. Depending on the individual response in 3 patients (nos. 4, 10 and 14) the daily dose was increased and, in 1 case (no. 10) the duration of treatment was also increased to 15 days (Table 2).

Assays

The plasma hormone levels were measured by radioimmunoassay. FSH, LH and prolactin were measured using Biodata Kits (Milano, Italy). After ether extraction of the plasma, E_2 and P were measured using antisera from Sorin

(Saluggia, Italy), tritiated molecules from NEN Chemicals GmbH and chromatographically pure E_2 and P standards. The radioimmunoassays involved overnight incubation at 4°C and a dextran-coated charcoal separation.

Results

Clinical evaluation

In 9 out of 15 cases ovulation with an ALP was obtained from the first treatment cycle onwards (Table 2). Of the other 6 patients, 2 remained anovulatory (nos. 10 and 14) and 4 ovulated but showed a short luteal phase (SLP) (nos. 4 and 12) or an inadequate luteal phase (ILP) (nos. 5 and 15). The 2 patients who failed to ovulate underwent treatment with a higher dose of epimestrol (15 mg/day for 10 days), one (no. 14) immediately and the other (no. 10) in a second cycle with the original treatment. As a result, both ovulated but showed either SLP (no. 14) or ILP (no. 10). In these patients the increase in the duration of treatment to 15 days for 10 consecutive cycles induced consistent ovulation and ALP. Of the 2 patients showing SLP after the first 2 cycles of treatment, one with 10 mg/day (no. 12) and the other with 15 mg/day (no. 4), the first showed ALP in 5 successive cycles without any change in the treatment schedule, and the second patient who received a dose of 20 mg/day for two cycles, showed ALP and became pregnant during the second cycle.

Concerning the 2 cases with ILP during the first cycle of treatment (10 mg/day for 10 days) one (no. 5) improved in the following cycles showing ALP, while the other (no. 15), monitored for further 2 cycles, constantly showed ILP.

The ovulation rate calculated from a total of 59 cycles was 95% and the ALP rate was 76%.

Concerning the number of pregnancies obtained in sterile couples with a normal sperm count and a positive PCT, 5 out of 7 became pregnant, one during the first, and the other 4 during the second, cycle of treatment displaying ALP (Table 2).

Endocrinological evaluation

The hormonal assays carried out before treatment showed more or less stable values in all cases for LH, FSH and E_2 associated with a very low concentration of P which did not vary throughout the cycle (Table 1, Figs. 1-6). During therapy, ovulation occurred either before (Fig. 1), just at the end (Fig. 2), or a few days after (Fig. 3), treatment. In each case the occurrence of an LH ovulatory peak corresponded to a rise in plasma E_2 levels indicative of follicular maturation. The E_2 rise varied from patient to

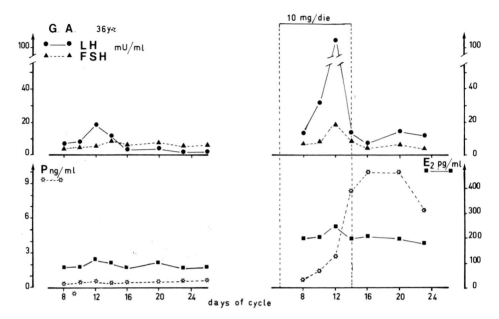

Fig. 1.   C.A.S. patient no. 11. LH, FSH, E$_2$ and P plasma levels in a control cycle (left) and during epimestrol treatment.

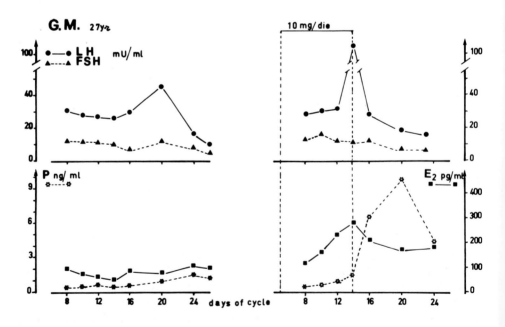

Fig. 2.   C.A.S. patient no. 12. As Figure 1.

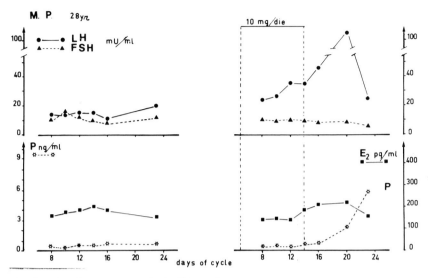

Fig. 3. C.A.S. patient no. 1. As Figure 1.

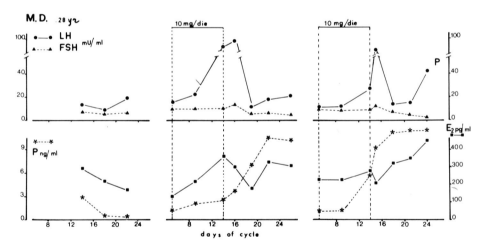

Fig. 4. C.A.S. patient no. 6. Effect of two consecutive cycles of epimestrol treatment on LH, FSH, E_2 and P plasma levels compared to control cycle (right).

patient. This biological situation may have occurred during treatment (Fig. 1), at the end of treatment (Fig. 2) or a few days later (Fig. 3). When ovulation and ALP were obtained, the same dose of epimestrol was constantly able to maintain its efficacy (Fig. 4) and in each cycle the occurrence of an LH ovulatory peak was always related to the endogenous E_2 pattern.

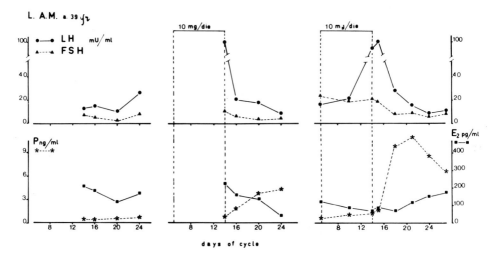

Fig. 5.   C.A.S. patient no. 5. As Figure 4.

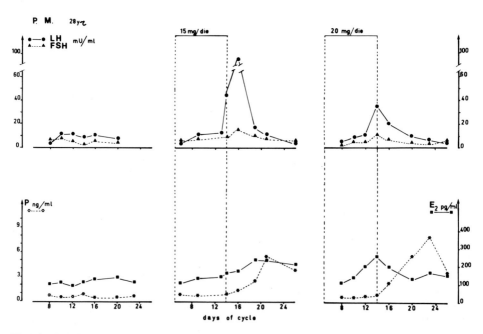

Fig. 6. C.A.S. patient no. 7. Effect of increasing the daily dose of epimestrol on LH, FSH, E$_2$ and P plasma levels compared to control cycle (right).

When ovulation and ILP were obtained during the first treatment cycle, the same regimen was able to induce ALP in subsequent cycles (Fig. 5) in patient no. 5, but not in patient no. 15.

When the treatment induced ovulation, followed by a SLP (Fig. 6), an increase in the daily dose of epimestrol resulted in a more rapid and a higher increase in E_2 followed by an ALP. With this treatment regimen the patient conceived during the second cycle.

Discussion

The efficacy of epimestrol in the treatment of CAS shown in previous studies (Schmidt-Elmendorff and Daemmerling, 1977; Genazzani et al., 1979) has been confirmed in the present study by the occurrence of a 95% ovulation rate in all cycles examined. As far as luteal function is concerned, ALP was present in 76% of the cycles and ILP or SLP in 19%. It is interesting to note that in 3 out of 5 patients, in whom anovulation or SLP occurred during the first treatment cycle, increasing the daily dose and/or the duration of treatment was always able to improve luteal function. Furthermore, in 2 cases showing SLP during the first or second treatment cycle, improved luteal function was seen without any change in the treatment schedule. The validity of epimestrol in restoring fertility is also shown by a high pregnancy rate in couples displaying a positive PCT. No side effects were observed in any of the 59 treatment cycles.

Concerning other drugs in current use for the treatment of anovulation, previous reports showed the ovulation rate for clomiphene citrate, with or without HCG, to be between 55 and 95%, with a pregnancy rate ranging from 22.5 to 73.3% (Drake et al., 1978; Gorlitsky et al., 1978; March et al., 1979). The incidence of mild ovarian hyperstimulation syndrome (OHSS) was reported to be 13.5% (Kistner, 1975) and may be increased when combined therapy with gonadotrophins is used (Hammerstein, 1967). Detailed studies on circulating pituitary and gonadal hormones in clomiphene-induced cycles indicate the hypothalamic effect of the drug, not counteracted by an endogenous E_2 rise (Ross et al., 1970; Yen et al., 1970; Dawood and Saxena, 1978) and show the existence of frequent occurrence of hyperprogesteronemia due to multiple luteinization (Dawood and Saxena, 1978). This last phenomenon is related to the incidence of side-effects (enlarged ovaries, hot flushes, etc.) in 11.5% patients (Gorlitsky et al., 1978). On the contrary, the pattern of endocrine indices during epimestrol treatment indicates that the rise of endogenous E_2 is the only factor responsible for the induction of an ovulatory LH peak. If this phenomenon occurs before the end of epimestrol treatment, neither LH pattern nor corpus luteum development and function are affected. This observation is in agreement with a complete absence of symptoms of OHSS and other minor side-effects in patients treated up to 14 consecutive cycles.

In conclusion, weak estrogen supplementation seems to be a physiological, efficient and safe method of inducing ovulation and ALP in patients suffering from CAS.

References

Crosignani, P.G. (Ed.) (1976): *Ovulation in the Human.* Academic Press, London.
Dawood, M.Y. and Saxena, B.B. (1978): *Obstet. and Gynec., 52/4,* 445.
Drake, T.S., Tredway, D.R. and Buchanan, G.C. (1978): *Fertil. and Steril., 30/3,* 274.
Genazzani, A.R., Facchinetti, F., De Leo, V., Picciolini, E., Franchi, F., Parrini, D. and Kicovic, P.M. (1978): *Fertil. and Steril., 30/6,* 654.
Genazzani, A.R., Massafra, C., D'Ambrogio, G. and Kicovic, P. (1979): In: *Psycho-neuroendocrinology in Reproduction,* p. 321. Editors: L. Zichela and P. Pancheri. Elsevier/North-Holland Biomedical Press, Amsterdam-New York-Oxford.
Gorlitsky, G.A., Kase, N.G. and Speroff, L. (1978): *Obstet. and Gynec., 51/3,* 265.
Greenblatt, R.B. and Barfield, W.E. (1961): *J. Amer. Med. Ass., 178,* 101.
Hammerstein, J. (1967): *Geburtsh. u. Frauenheilk., 27,* 1125.
Kistner, R.W. (1975): In: *Progress in Infertility,* p. 509. Editor: S.J. Behrman. Little, Brown and Co., Boston.
Lasley, B.L. and Judd, H.L. (1978): *Clin. Obstet. Gynaec., 21/1,* 87.
Lunenfeld, B. (1963): *J. Int. Fed. Gynaec. Obstet., 1,* 153.
March, C.M., Davajan, V. and Mishell, D.R., Jr. (1979): *Obstet. and Gynec., 53/1,* 8.
Oelsner, G., Serr, D.M., Mashiach, S., Blankstein, J., Snyder, M. and Lunenfeld, B. (1978): *Fertil. and Steril., 30/5,* 538.
Ross, G.T., Cargille, C.M. and Lipsett, M.B. (1970): *Rec. Progr. Hormone Res., 26,* 1.
Schally, A.V., Kastin, A.J. and Coy, D.H. (1976): *Int. J. Fertil., 21,* 1.
Schmidt-Elmendorff, H. and Daemmerling, R. (1977): *Geburtsh. u. Frauenheilk., 37,* 531.
Yen, S.S.C., Vela, P. and Ryan, K.J. (1970): *J. Clin. Endocr., 31,* 7.

Ovulation. A morphological analysis by scanning and transmission electron microscopy*

P.M. MOTTA and S. MAKABE

Istituto di Anatomia Umana Normale, Facoltà di Medicina, Università di Roma, Rome, Italy, and Department of Obstetrics and Gynecology, Toho University School of Medicine, Tokyo, Japan

In these last few years it has become evident that the ovary can be easily investigated using a combination of various high resolution microscopic techniques (Zuckerman and Weir, 1977).

Particularly, Scanning Electron Microscopy (SEM) seems to be a very suitable method for obtaining a more complete three-dimensional superficial view of the mammalian ovary and of the ovulatory process (Motta and Van Blerkom, 1975; Van Blerkom and Motta, 1979).

The purpose of this study is to analyse by SEM and transmission electron microscopy (TEM) the morphological changes occurring within the mature follicle and on the ovarian surface at the time of ovulation in various mammals and humans, with the aim of contributing to a better morphodynamic elucidation of the events leading to ovulation.

Material and methods

Ovaries were obtained from adult dogs, mice, rats, rabbits and cats. For mice and rats, the phase of the estrus cycle was determined by vaginal smears. Rabbits and cats, which are reflex ovulators, had their ovaries removed at intervals of hours after copulation.

Human ovaries were obtained from patients undergoing elective surgery. A few cases for control were selected in which the histological examination revealed a normal functioning ovary.

All the material, fixed by immersion and/or perfusion in a solution of 2.5% glutaraldehyde (0.18 M; pH 7.3), was critical point dried and prepared for SEM using procedures previously described in detail (Motta and Van Blerkom, 1975; Makabe and Hafez, 1979).

*Supported by grants of Toho University and Kanda 2nd Clinic, Tokyo and from C.N.R.: grant No. C.T. 76.01288.04.

Results and discussion

Granulosa cells of large Graafian follicles possess an irregularly spherical shape and their surface is populated by an increasing number of cellular projections as microvilli, blebs, cilia and other larger cytoplasmic evaginations (Figs. 1 to 4).

The changes on the granulosa cell surface in preovulatory follicles are probably dependent upon hormonal stimulation. They likely reflect an increase of cell surface which is, in these elements, an expanded site useful for binding an increased amount of gonadotropins (Amsterdam et al., 1975; Makabe and Hafez, 1979; Motta, 1979).

Furthermore, the development of large cellular expansions in granulosa cells is concomitant with the presence of large bundles of contractile filaments in the cortical areas of the cytoplasm of the same elements.

These findings suggest that the contractility of the granulosa cells 'in vivo' may contribute, just prior to ovulation, to a progressive detachment of the cumulus oophorus from the granulosa layer with a consequent liberation of the 'cumulus oophorus' within the large antrum filled with a very diluted 'liquor folliculi' (Motta and DiDio, 1974).

At the time of ovulation the oocyte is not always covered by a continuous layer of corona cells. The zona pellucida when evident shows an irregular surface provided with a number of pores, crypts and channels (Fig. 5). These fenestrations, corresponding to those regions where the granulosa cell processes traversed the zona (Motta and Van Blerkom, 1975; Dudkiewicz et al., 1976) clearly demonstrate that they are retracted at the time of ovulation (Motta and Van Blerkom, 1975).

Both companion cells and zona pellucida are covered with a fine granular material which can be interpreted as proof of a continuous secretory process of these cells even at the time of ovulation (Figs. 5 and 6).

Only rare and small desmosomes, zonulae adherentes and gap (communicating) junctions are present between oocyte and corona cells prior to ovulation (Motta et al., 1971). The gradual loss of such intercellular contacts, believed to promote a coordinate activity of the oocyte and granulosa cells within the developing follicle (Motta et al., 1971), in the hours preceding ovulation accounts for an independent role of these two cellular components.

The presumptive ovulatory areas are very obvious if viewed with SEM because they appear in the form of swellings on the surface of the ovary (Fig. 7). The ovarian epithelium covering these blister-like structures shows typical cellular changes which likely prelude to the dehiscence of the large preovulatory follicles (Figs. 7 and 8).

The superficial cells of the basal areas of these follicles are polyhedral and covered with numerous slender microvilli and occasional solitary cilia. Similar features are shown also from epithelial cells in other zones of the ovary not related to the ovulatory sites (Fig. 7). The superficial cells

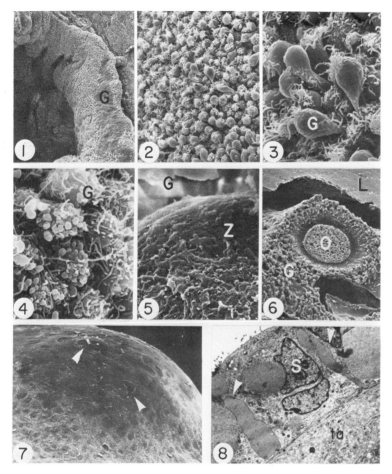

Figs. 1-4. Granulosa cells (G) of human Graafian follicles possess large cellular evaginations (Figs. 1, 2), long microvilli (Fig. 3), blebs and thin isolated cilia (Fig. 4). x150; x750; x3300; x3300: SEM.

Fig. 5. Zona pellucida (Z) with a few granulosa cells (G) in a mouse antral follicle. x3600:SEM

Fig. 6. Cumulus oophorus of a dog Graafian follicle. O = oocyte; G = granulosa cells; L = liquor folliculi. x560:SEM.

Fig. 7. Apex of a preovulatory follicle in the dog ovary. Note numerous exfoliating cells in necrosis (arrows). x260:SEM

Fig. 8. Superficial epithelium (S) of the apex of a rabbit preovulatory follicle. A fluid(*) accumulates into the tunica albuginea (ta) and distends (arrows) the spaces between apical cells in necrosis. x4300:SEM.

distributed on the lateral and periapical regions are elongated and possess a few short microvilli. On the apex the covering epithelium is made up of very flattened cells with very rare and distorted microvilli. In some cases the superficial cells, apparently in necrosis, degenerate and slough off. Several intercellular spaces may become evident and where the exfoliation of the surface epithelium occurs large areas of the underlying 'tunica albuginea' are evident. In other zones of the apex a fluid-like substance exudes in the form of small irregular droplets from intercellular spaces where superficial cells become uncoupled from each other (Figs. 7 and 8).

When sectioned and studied under TEM the same apical areas appear infiltrated by this fluid, which also dissociates the collagen tissue of the tunica albuginea and, accumulating under the basal lamina, penetrates and fills the intercellular spaces of the superficial epithelium until its final dissolution and rupture.

The tissue changes occurring prior to ovulation, as viewed by correlated SEM and TEM, suggest that an increase of fluids (edema) in the perifollicular stroma is the final and apparent cause of rupture of the weakened apical wall of the preovulatory follicle (Motta and Van Blerkom, 1975). These events are the partial morphological results of a more complex series of bio-chemical, functional and endocrine factors which can be appropriately followed by using different methods.

References

Amsterdam, A., Koch, Y., Liebermann, E. and Linder, H.R. (1975): *J. Cell Biol., 67,* 894.
Dudkiewicz, A.B., Shivers, C.A. and Williams, W.L. (1976): *Biol. Reprod., 14,* 175.
Makabe, S. and Hafez, E.S.E. (1979): In: *Human Ovulation,* Chapter 3, p. 39. Editor: E.S.E. Hafez. Elsevier/North-Holland, Amsterdam-New York.
Motta, P.M. (1979): In: *Psychoneuroendocrinology in Reproduction, Vol. V,* p. 145. Editors: L. Zichella and P. Pancheri. Elsevier/North-Holland, Amsterdam-New York.
Motta, P.M. and DiDio, L.J.A. (1974): *J. Submicrosc. Cytol., 6,* 15.
Motta, P.M., Takeva, Z. and Nesci, E. (1971): *Acta Anat. (Basel), 80,* 537.
Motta, P.M. and Van Blerkom, J. (1975): *Amer. J. Anat., 143,* 241.
Van Blerkom, J. and Motta, P.M. (1979): *Subcellular Basis of Mammalian Reproduction.* Urban and Schwarzenberg, Baltimore-Munich.
Zuckerman, S. and Weir, B.J. (Eds.) (1977): *The Ovary, 2nd Ed.* Academic Press, New York.

Disturbances of the menstrual cycle*

B. LUNENFELD[1] and A. ESHKOL

Institute of Endocrinology, The Chaim Sheba Medical Center, Tel-Hashomer, and [1]Department of Life Sciences, Bar-Ilan University, Ramat-Gan, Israel

The regulation of the menstrual cycle and ovulation are the result of balanced and coordinated effects of the hypothalamic gonadotrophin releasing hormone (GnRH), the pituitary gonadotrophins, and the ovarian responses (Fig. 1). The GnRH secreted by the hypothalamus in a specific quantity must be received and interpreted by the target cell of the pituitary, and these cells, in turn, must be capable of synthesizing and releasing gonadotrophins in adequate quantities and with a specific rhythm. The gonadotrophic hormones then act on the ovary and stimulate 3 balanced and appropriately coordinated processes, namely, growth of the follicle, differentiation of the follicular cells, and steroid production. The secretion of appropriate steroids at the proper time and in the correct amount, serves several purposes. These steroids serve in the messenger system of the feedback mechanism which regulates the secretion of the gonadotrophins, they modulate follicular responsiveness to gonadotrophins and act upon various functional compartments of the ovary, including the vascular apparatus; they stimulate changes in the genital organs in preparation for the transport of the ovum and the sperm cells, and prepare the endometrium for implantation of the fertilized eggs.

The above described events are reflected by characteristic hormonal patterns. In order to analyze the correlation between the various hormones which are changing at different rates, the ovulatory cycle has to be divided into several phases.

The *early follicular phase* is characterized by relatively elevated levels of FSH and low levels of LH, estrogens and progesterone. During this phase the growth of a number of follicles is set into motion. The number of FSH receptors in the follicles increases, and they acquire LH receptors. LH stimulates androgen production by the theca interna cells and FSH enhances aromatase activity of the granulosa cells and conversion of androgens to estrogens. The appearance of estrogens in the circulation marks the beginning of the *mid follicular phase.*

This phase is characterized by increasing levels of estrogens and relative low levels of FSH, LH and progesterone. The first significant rise of

*This work was supported in part by the Ford Foundation (Grant No. 67-470), and the World Health Organization.

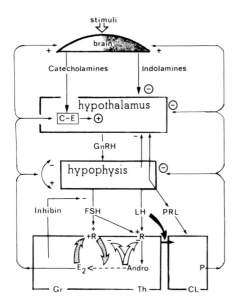

Fig. 1. Control and feedback mechanism regulating ovarian function. Control and co-ordination of ovarian (Gr = granulosa cells; Th = theca cells; CL = corpus luteum) function is accomplished through actions of 3 different types: (1) stimulation along the brain-hypothalamus-hypophysis-ovarian axis by catecholamines, indolamines, catechol-estrogens (C-E), gonadotrophin-releasing hormones (GnRH), follicle stimulating hormone (FSH), luteinizing hormone (LH) and prolactin (PRL); (2) intraovarian modulation of hormone receptors (R) by positive influence of FSH and estrogens (E_2) and negative effect of androgens (Andro); (3) feedback signals, positive (+) and negative (−), by ovarian steroids (E_2 and progesterone, P) and inhibin. (Reproduced from Lunenfeld and Eshkol, 1979).

estrogens occurs about 82 hr before ovulation (Boyers et al., 1980). When a proper (individually specific) level of estrogens is reached, positive feedback signals acting on the 'Cyclic center of the hypothalamus' will induce LH release. With the rise of LH, luteinization of the follicle(s) is induced, associated with cessation of granulosa cell proliferation. As luteinization of follicle(s) proceeds, progesterone rises and estrogen levels fall. The first rise of LH occurs approximately 32 hr before ovulation and marks the beginning of the *peri-ovulatory phase* of the cycle.

This phase is characterized by estrogens, LH and FSH rising to their peak values and their subsequent decrease. During this period the first significant rise in progesterone is observed. The temporal relationship of these events as correlated to ovulation is shown in Figure 2.

The major event of this phase is the rupture of a mature follicle, extrusion of the ovum (ovulation), and the differentiation of the follicular remnant into a corpus luteum; follicles which at the time of the rising LH did not attain their full maturity, will luteinize and the even less developed ones will undergo atresia.

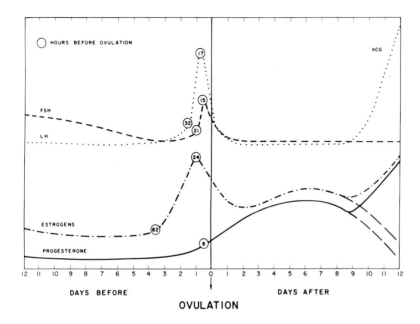

Fig. 2. Human menstrual cycle − schematic presentation of temporal relationships of hormonal profiles. (Data adapted from Boyers et al., 1980). The numbers in circles denote only approximately the time of the observed changes in the hormonal patterns in relation to ovulation.

The *post ovulatory phase* or *luteal phase* is characterized by a marked rise of progesterone which reaches a plateau level about 4 days after ovulation. The pattern of estrogen secretion in this phase parallels that of the progesterone. The association of estrogens and progesterone inhibits FSH and LH secretion via negative feedback control at the hypothalamic and pituitary levels. FSH and LH levels remain low during the luteal phase.

If ovulation is followed by fertilization and conception, then by the 9th post-ovulatory day hCG appears in the circulation. Its rapid rise stimulates corpus luteum function and estrogen and progesterone levels increase.

In the absence of conception, the corpus luteum regresses and estrogen and progesterone levels start to decline around the 10th day after ovulation. This marks the beginning of the *late luteal phase* or *premenstrual phase.*

Any disruption in the delicately coordinated interaction between the integrated components of the hypothalamic-pituitary-ovarian axis, which have to operate within precise quantitative limits and accurate temporal sequence, may lead to anovulation, cycle disturbances, or infertility.

The understanding of the basic mechanisms regulating reproductive processes, as summarized above, has enabled us to transform the approach to female infertility from an empirical to a scientifically more rational basis. Furthermore, it prompted the development or use of effective drugs and hormones, based on their specific actions, in modulating the function of the hypothalamic-pituitary-ovarian axis.

These can be classified into 3 main groups: (1) Human gonadotrophins. (2) Chlorotrianisene analogues. (3) Ergoline derivatives.

Each group of these agents acts through a different mechanism. Gonadotrophins stimulate the ovary directly, chlorotrianisene analogues stimulate the hypothalamic-pituitary system, and ergoline derivatives inhibit excessive prolactin secretion which interferes with the normal reproductive function.

Each of these agents may be used at various dosage levels and in different treatment schemes sometimes in combination, or in conjunction with estrogens or anti-gonadotrophins, and all of them carry risks of various complications.

Effective and optimal application of such drugs requires the recognition of the cause of the ovulatory failure. In this paper an attempt is made to classify anovulatory states into several entities and to suggest optimal management for each category.

Gonadotrophic insufficiency

Gonadotrophic insufficiency is due to either pituitary or hypothalamic insufficiency. In this situation pituitary secretion of gonadotrophins is absent or severely diminished. Follicular development does not reach the stage of estrogen secretion and cyclic ovarian function is not initiated. Patients pertaining to this etiological entity will be amenorrheic, without evidence of ovarian estrogen production, and low or unmeasurable gonadotrophin levels. The treatment of choice for this group of patients is human menopausal gonadotrophins (hMG) followed by human chorionic gonadotrophins (hCG). For a detailed description of the treatment scheme, the monitoring of gonadotrophic therapy, an assessment of its results and complications, see Lunenfeld and Insler (1978). This group does not include patients with hyperprolactinemia or with space-occupying lesions in the hypothalamic-pituitary region.

Impaired hypothalamic-pituitary responsiveness and/or function

The majority of anovulatory patients fall into this heterogenous category. The etiology leading to this type of dysfunction may be: (a) due to inappropriate sensitivity to negative or positive feedback signals at the hypothalamic-pituitary level; (b) induced by excessive prolactin secretion; (c) induced by inappropriate secretion of adrenal or ovarian steroids; (d) secondary to other endocrine dysfunction such as primary hypothyroidism; (e) iatrogenically induced.

Patients, belonging to any of the above subgroups, will be women with a variety of menstrual disturbances, luteal insufficiency, anovulatory cycles, or amenorrhea. They will all have distinct evidence of ovarian estrogen production.

Inappropriate sensitivity of the hypothalamic-pituitary system to feedback signals

Hypersensitivity to negative feedback signals will cause inappropriate gonado-trophin secretion during the early follicular phase of the cycle. This results in insufficient follicular maturation which is reflected by an absence of an estrogen rise capable of eliciting an appropriate midcycle LH surge. Under these circumstances, the follicles which developed will undergo atresia. For this group of patients the treatment of choice should be drugs which compete with estrogen receptors e.g. chlomiphene citrate, tamoxifen etc. The administration of these drugs to such patients results almost invariably in significant elevation of FSH and LH levels. This should result in a significant rise of estrogens and subsequent LH surge. A discrepancy between the ovulation rate and conception rate following clomiphene therapy has been shown (Table 1). This may be due to the antiestrogenic effect of the drug on the uterine cervix. In such cases combined clomiphene/estrogen treatment may significantly improve the results (Sharf et al., 1971; Insler et al., 1973; Skei et al., 1973). Furthermore, an inappropriate release of LH may lead to luteinization with a hormonal profile resembling ovulation.

Patients who do not respond to this drug or who do not become pregnant with the 'ovulatory' dose of clomiphene within 4 treatment cycles, would be considered for clomiphene plus hCG or hMG/hCG therapy.

TABLE 1.

Ovulation and pregnancy rates following clomiphene therapy as reported by different authors using Clomid

Authors		No. patients	Ovulation rate (%)	Pregnancy rate (%)
Greenblatt and Dala Pria	(1971)	257	77.0	
Kase et al.	(1967)	81	60.5	25.9
Kistner	(1965)	50	96.0	26.0
MacGregor et al.	(1968)	6714	70.0	32.7
Murray and Osmond-Clarck	(1971)	328	66.5	25.0
Pildes	(1965)	36	50.0	11.1
Seegar-Jones and Moraes-Ruehsen	(1967)	73	83.0	30.1
Spellacy and Cohen	(1967)	35	80.0	20.0
Whitelaw et al.	(1964)	37	72.9	45.9
MacLeod et al.	(1970)	118	77.0	31.0

(Reproduced from Lunenfeld and Insler, 1978).

Impaired pituitary responsiveness secondary to excessive prolactin secretion

Although it is well established that prolactin in rodents is the main stimulus of luteal function, its role during the menstrual cycle is not well understood. The recent development in prolactin radioimmunoassays and their massive introduction as a routine clinical investigation in infertile women has demonstrated that prolactin, if excreted in excess, may cause anovulation or luteal insufficiency. The mechanism(s) by which prolactin interferes in the hypothalamic-pituitary ovarian axis has not been completely elucidated. To date evidence has accumulated which indicates that prolactin may act on the hypothalamus, the pituitary (Bohnet et al., 1976; Boyar et al., 1976; Forsbach et al., 1977; Gudelsky et al., 1977) and on the ovary (McNatty et al., 1974; Faglia et al., 1977). Irrespective of the site(s) at which it acts, the end result will be similar i.e. anovulation or luteal insufficiency. Patients pertaining to this etiological entity will be women with a variety of menstrual cycle disturbances (luteal phase insufficiency, anovulatory cycle, and amenorrhea) with distinct evidence of ovarian estrogen production and with elevated prolactin levels.

For patients belonging to this group, ergoline derivatives (e.g. lisuride, metergoline, bromocriptine) should be the treatment of choice since they are capable of suppressing prolactin secretion. The ovulating dose of ergoline derivatives is maintained for up to 6 months and if no pregnancy occurs, combination therapies should be considered (e.g. adding clomiphene or human gonadotrophins).

Excessive prolactin secretion can also be due to prolactin secreting tumors. The interference will be similar to that outlined above, except that in these patients evidence of a space-occupying lesion in the hypothalamic pituitary region will be found (e.g. abnormality in pituitary tomography and/or visual fields). Some patients pertaining to this group have micro-adenomas (lesions less than 1 cm in diameter). These patients can also be treated with ergoline derivatives after consultation with neurosurgeons and/or neurologists, and after having been informed in detail of all the risks involved.

Impaired hypothalamic/pituitary responsiveness and/or function induced by inappropriate secretion of adrenal or ovarian steroids

In a situation where adrenal or ovarian steroids, especially androgens are secreted in excess, they may interfere in the complex feedback mechanism regulating the ovarian cycle. The severity of the cycle disturbances will be relative to the quality and amount of the steroids secreted and the responsiveness of the target cells. Patients pertaining to this etiological entity will be women with a variety of menstrual cycle disturbances and usually with some clinical signs of androgenization, virilization and a tendency to obesity. The origin of the steroids should be identified by evaluating them before and after selective suppression tests of ovarian function and of adrenal function. In the case where the origin is the ovary, estrogen/ progesterone combination is the choice of treatment, or preferentially, a combination of estrogen with an antiandrogen having a progestational activity e.g. cyproterone acetate. The latter will at the same time also have a beneficial effect on the clinical expression of androgenization.

This treatment should be continued for 6 months. If after this period ovulation is not restored, treatment with clomiphene or, if necessary, with hMG/hCG should be attempted. Treatment with corticosteroids or their analogues is indicated when the adrenal is the origin of the excessive androgen production. In addition to their suppressive effect on the pituitary-adrenal axis, they will serve as substitution therapy in cases of cortisol insufficiency (e.g. adrenogenital syndrome).

In cases where this therapy fails to induce ovulation, it has to be supplemented with chlorotrianisene analogues or if even this fails, with hMG/hCG therapy.

Impaired hypothalamic-pituitary responsiveness and/or function due to primary hypothyroidism

In cases where thyroid-stimulating hormone is excreted in excess (e.g. hypothyroidism) prolactin will also be elevated and some of the effects will be similar to those of the hyperprolactinemic hypothalamic pituitary dysfunction.

Treatment of the underlying cause by supplementation with thyroid hormones or their analogues will in most cases correct the metabolic disturbance, suppress the excessive TRH, and the consequent hyperprolactinemia.

Iatrogenically induced hypothalamic-pituitary responsiveness and/or function

Since the central nervous system (CNS) also participates in the regulation of hypothalamic function, drugs affecting this axis may interfere with neural signals to the hypothalamus.

Drugs with antidopaminergic properties which interfere in the regulation of prolactin secretion are a well known example.

However, other drugs acting on the level of neurotransmitters might also have similar effects on the ovulatory cycle. In a similar way, environmental and ecological factors can influence reproductive performance (e.g. college amenorrhea, anorexia nervosa etc.).

Furthermore, oral contraceptives may lead to transient or permanent dysfunction of the hypothalamic-pituitary-ovarian axis in predisposed women.

256   B. Lunenfeld and A. Eshkol

Therapy for this group of patients has to be considered for each case individually.

Ovarian failure

In this situation the ovary will be irresponsive to gonadotrophic stimulation and follicular development will be absent. Lack of ovarian estrogens will result in hypersecretion of FSH and LH. Patients pertaining to this etiological entity will be amenorrheic women with elevated FSH and LH levels and with no evidence of estrogen production. For patients of this group no fertility promotion therapy exists. Symptomatic therapy may be offered to patients with severe symptoms of estrogen deficiency.

We have tried to show in this short review that menstrual disorders have manyfold origins — each with their own characteristic hormonal and symptomatic patterns. Recognition of the underlying cause, and choice of the optimal therapy have revolutionized the treatment of anovulatory infertility and radically changed its prognosis. It seems justified to conclude that at present anovulation is a treatable symptom as far as infertility is concerned.

References

Bohnet, H.G., Dahlen, H., Wuttke, W. and Schneider, H.P.G. (1976): *J. Clin. Endocr., 42*, 132.
Boyar, R., Kapen, S., Weitzman, E.D. and Hellman, B. (1976): *New Engl. J. Med., 294*, 263.
Boyers, S.P., Carenza, C., Collins, W.P., Cheviakoff, S. et al. (1980): Submitted for publication.
Faglia, G., Beck-Pecoz, B., Travaglini, B., Ambrosi, M. et al. (1977): In: *Prolactin and Human Reproduction. Proceedings of Serono Symposia.* Editors: P.G. Crosignani and C. Robyn. Academic Press, London.
Forsbach, G., Soria, J., Canales, E.S., Guzman, V. et al. (1977): *Obstet. and Gynec., 50*, 139.
Gudelsky, G.A., Simpson, J., Mueller, G.P., Meites, J. et al. (1977): *Neuroendocrinology, 22*, 206.
Insler, V., Zakut, H. and Serr, D.M. (1973): *Obstet. and Gynec., 41*, 602.
Lunenfeld, B. and Insler, V. (1978): In: *Infertility: Diagnosis and Treatment of Functional Infertility*, p. 61. Grosse Verlag, Berlin.
Lunenfeld, B. and Eshkol, A. (1979): In: *Human Ovulation, Vol. III*, Chapter 12, p. 221. Editor: E.S.E. Hafez. North-Holland Publishing Company, Amsterdam-New York-Oxford.
McNatty, K.P., Sawers, R.S. and McNeilly, A.S. (1974): *Nature (Lond.), 250*, 653.
Sharf, M., Graff, G. and Kuminski, T. (1971): *Amer. J. Obstet. Gynec., 110*, 423.
Skei, M., Tayima, C., Maeda, H.R., Saki, K. and Yoshihara, T. (1973): *Amer. J. Obstet. Gynec., 116*, 388.

Effect of epimestrol treatment on endocrine and clinical features of the short and inadequate luteal phase*

A.R. GENAZZANI[1], G. D'AMBROGIO[1], C. MASSAFRA[1] and
P.M. KICOVIC[2]

[1] Clinica di Ostetricia e Ginecologia, Università di Siena, Siena, Italy, and
[2] Reproductive Medicine Programme, Medical Unit, Organon, Oss, The
Netherlands

The luteal phase defect represents, according to Jones (1976), the factor responsible for infertility in 3.5% of all cases. This syndrome may be divided into short luteal phase (SLP) and inadequate luteal phase (ILP), the former being characterized by a prompt rise of plasma progesterone (P) levels following LH peak, rapidly declining after a few days (Strott et al., 1970). ILP, originally described by Sherman and Korenman (1974), is characterized by a rise of circulating P after ovulation to levels less than half of those expected; the length of the luteal phase is, however, more or less normal. The etiology of these syndromes has been related either to ovarian or central factors (Jones, 1976). Since corpus luteum development depends on follicular maturation, it has been shown that factors involved in follicular maturation are responsible for luteal function. FSH induces the appearance of specific LH-receptors in granulosa cells (Richards and Midgley, 1976) and as a consequence, the number of LH binding sites per cell rises 40-fold during the development of the secondary follicle (Kammerman and Ross, 1975). This leads to the development of high affinity and avidity receptors for LH, typical of the preovulatory follicle (YoungLai, 1975). Impaired development of granulosa cells has been shown to be related to deficient FSH secretion during the follicular phase or to the induction of an insufficient midcycle LH surge (Jones and Madrigal-Castro, 1970; Strott et al., 1970), or to the presence of higher than normal prolactin levels (Seppala et al., 1976). The latter is responsible for reduced P secretion from the granulosa cells, both 'in vitro' (McNatty et al., 1974) and 'in vivo' (Del Pozo et al., 1979).

It has become evident that the treatment of the luteal phase defect should induce adequate follicular growth and a sufficient LH peak. The observation that in chronic anovulatory patients epimestrol° (E) treatment induced adequate follicular maturation, as shown by a progressive rise in plasma

*This study was partly supported by the Consiglio Nazionale delle Ricerche Project 'Biology of Reproduction'.

°(16α,17α)-3-methoxyestra-1,3,5(10)-triene-16,17-diol (Stimovul, Organon, Oss, The Netherlands).

estradiol (E_2) levels (Genazzani et al., 1979) and in cases of normoprolactinemic secondary amenorrhea (Genazzani et al., 1978) stimulated both synthesis and secretion of LH, suggests that this compound may provide a useful means of treating the luteal phase defect in normoprolactinemic subjects.

Material and methods

Patients. Nine patients with ILP and 7 with SLP, aged 26-43 yrs were studied (Table 1). Thirteen were sterile and 5 had oligomenorrhea. Three were not married and complained of oligomenorrhea. Dysmenorrhea was also present in most of the patients. SLP or ILP diagnosis was made on the basis of serial endocrinological examinations during a whole cycle, confirmed in the following 2 cycles by 3-4 plasma P measurements during the luteal period. In the sterile cases, hysterosalpingography, post coital test (PCT) and sperm analysis of the husband were also performed. In 4 cases oligospermia was

TABLE 1.

Hormone levels in ILP and SLP patients

No.	Age (yrs)	Clin. diagnosis	Hormone levels (range)				
			LH (mU/ml)	FSH (mU/ml)	E_2 (pg/ml)	P (pg/ml)	PRL (ng/ml)
ILP							
1	38	Sterility	12.3-22.5	5.8- 7.4	185-215	950-2250	7-22
2	33	Sterility	3.3-28.5	3.5- 8.8	55-116	320-3060	8-14
3	26	Sterility	14.0-50.0	7.6-14.5	94-204	257-3961	7-23
4	38	Sterility	14.5-100	8.5-22.5	66-240	400-1880	7-15
5	30	Oligomenorrhea	8.6-82.0	9.3-11.6	82-116	450-3465	7-12
6	34	Sterility*	3.1-100	4.9-15.2	72-276	430-3000	15-23
7	33	Oligomenorrhea	3.6-62.0	2.8-15.0	119-340	630-4750	9-15
8	38	Oligomenorrhea	14.1-36.1	5.2-11.6	128-208	435-2085	8-13
9	43	Oligomenorrhea	10.5-13.5	4.8- 7.0	120-230	800-1600	5-10
SLP							
10	27	Sterility*°	23.3-68.5	5.9-13.8	104-396	750-6550	6-13
11	26	Sterility	2.9-23.8	5.7- 7.3	135-150	1450-4080	5-15
12	35	Sterility	10.4-100	3.7-20.9	30-120	544-12500	6-14
13	29	Sterility	16.1-70.0	5.8-12.6	98-300	920-13400	8-10
14	30	Sterility	25.0-100	8.3-19.0	95-233	480-6748	13-16
15	28	Sterility*	10.0-100	9.5-35.0	121-277	608-7500	12-27
16	31	Infertility°	12.0-17.0	7.0- 9.5	145-180	720-5080	10-19

°Post Coital Test Negative; *Oligospermia

TABLE 2.

Effect of epimestrol treatment in ILP and SLP

No.	Age (yrs)	Treatment Type	Length (cycles)	Results (luteal phase)
ILP				
1	38	A	1	ILP
		B	2	ALP
2	33	A	3	ALP
3	26	A	2	ILP
		F	2	ILP
		D	5	ALP
4	38	A	3	ALP
5	30	A	4	ALP
6	34	A	4	ALP
7	33	A	1	SLP
		B	1	ALP
8	38	A	2	SLP
9	43	A	2	SLP
		C	2	ALP
SLP				
10	27	A	3	ALP
11	26	A	1	ALP Pregnant
12	35	A	5	ALP Pregnant
13	29	A	5	ALP Pregnant
14	30	A	2	ILP
		B	2	ILP
		E	3	ALP
15	28	A	2	ILP
		C	2	ALP
16	31	A	4	ALP

A	= 10 mg/day/10 days	D	= 15 mg/day/20 days
B	= 15 mg/day/10 days	E	= 15 mg/day/15 days
C	= 10 mg/day/20 days	F	= 20 mg/day/10 days

found, 2 cases had a negative PCT (Table 1). In each patient blood samples were taken every 2-4 days from the 6th, 7th or 8th day of cycle until the end of the cycle. Blood sampling was done in the control cycle and during the first month of each different type of treatment in all subjects to measure LH, FSH, E_2 and P. Thyroid function and prolactin levels were also investigated during the control cycles. The occurrence of an adequate luteal phase (ALP) was checked with 3-4 blood samples collected in the luteal period in successive therapy cycles.

Treatment. E treatment was started on the 5th day of the cycle (Table 2). All subjects began with a standard treatment (5 mg x 2/day x 10 days). Depending on the individual response, the daily dose was increased to 15 mg (nos. 1, 7, 14) or 20 mg (no. 3) for 2 cycles. In 2 of the above the treatment was also prolonged to 15 (no. 14) and 20 (no. 3) days. In 2 patients (nos. 9, 15) the standard treatment was prolonged to 20 days after the first 2 cycles (Table 2).

Assays. Plasma hormone levels were measured by radioimmunoassay (RIA). FSH, LH and prolactin were measured using Biodata kits (Milan, Italy). After ether extraction of the plasma, E_2 and P were measured using antisera from Sorin (Saluggia, Italy), tritiated molecules from NEN (Dreieichenhain, FRG) and chromatographically pure E_2 and P standards. The RIAs involved overnight incubation at $4°C$ and a dextran-coated charcoal separation.

Results

Clinical evaluation (Table 2)

ILP. In 4 cases the standard treatment induced an ALP while 3 patients (nos. 7, 8, 9) showed SLP and in 2 (nos. 1, 3) the luteal phase was not modified. Increasing the daily dose to 15 mg (no. 7) or prolonging the treatment from 15-20 days corrected SLP, inducing constant ALP. In 2 patients (nos. 1, 3) the standard treatment did not significantly modify the clinical picture but an increased dose induced an ALP (case 1, 15 mg; case 3, 20 mg). None of the 5 sterile patients became pregnant during the observation period of 3-9 months.

SLP. Five out of 7 cases of SLP responded to the standard treatment with an ALP. The other 2 cases required longer treatment (15-20 days) with the same (no. 15) or increased (no. 14) doses of E (Table 2). Three out of 4 patients with SLP and sterility became pregnant in the first 5 cycles of ALP.

Endocrinological evaluation

ILP. During the control period different patients (nos. 1, 2, 3, 5, 8, 9) were found to have low E_2 levels during follicular maturation (Fig. 1) or values suggesting adequate follicular maturation (Fig. 2) (nos. 4, 6, 7) on the basis of patterns and absolute concentrations. The FSH plasma levels were at the lower limit of the normal range or even lower in most patients (Figs. 1-3). The LH pattern showed reduced (nos. 1, 2, 7-9) (Fig. 1) or normal (nos. 3, 4, 5, 6) (Figs. 2, 3) mid-cycle values, always followed by a markedly deficient P rise. In cases with E_2 levels in the follicular phase, suggesting impaired follicular maturation, the treatment succeeded in increasing E_2 levels (Fig. 1) to concentrations suggesting a better development and maturation of the

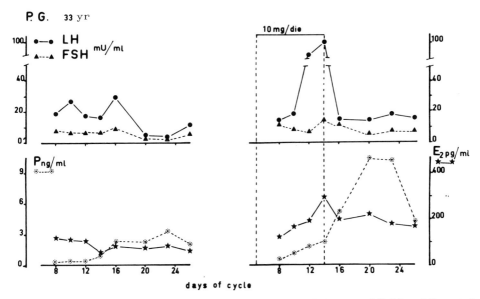

Fig. 1. *ILP case no. 2:* Plasma levels of LH, FSH, E$_2$ and P in control (left) and E treated cycle (right).

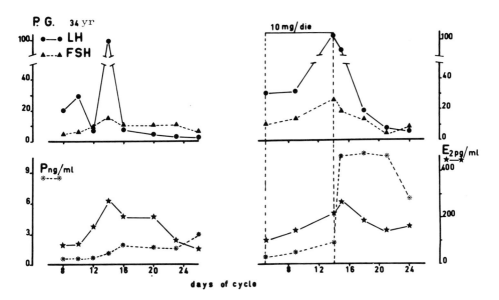

Fig. 2. ILP case no. 6: As in Figure 1.

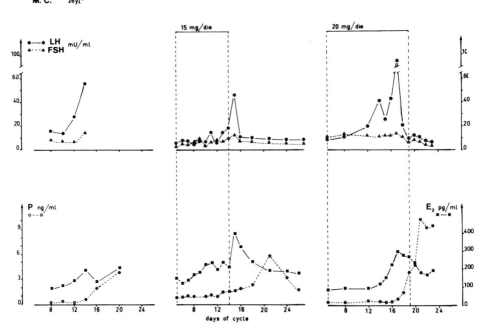

Fig. 3. ILP case no. 3: Effect of increasing daily dose of E and length of treatment on LH, FSH, E$_2$ and P plasma levels compared to control cycle (left).

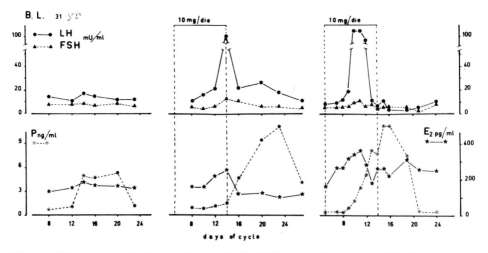

Fig. 4. SLP case no. 16: Plasma levels of LH, FSH, E$_2$ and P in control (left) and in two consecutive cycles under the same E treatment.

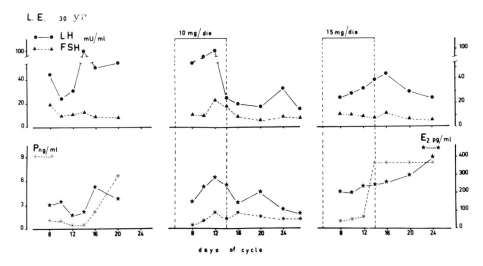

Fig. 5. SLP case no. 14: Effect of increasing dose of E on LH, FSH, E$_2$ and P plasma levels in 2 different cycles compared to control cycle.

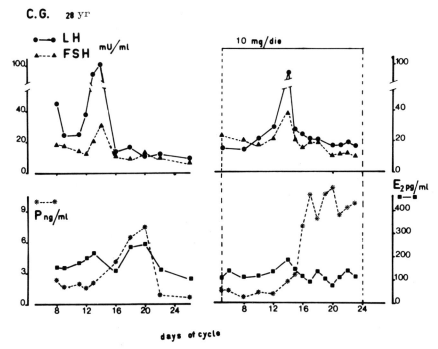

Fig. 6. SLP case no. 15: Effect of a 20-day E treatment on LH, FSH, E$_2$ and P plasma levels compared to a control cycle (left).

follicle followed by a greater LH discharge from the pituitary. The luteal phase was characterized by adequate P concentrations. A similar picture was also found during luteal phase in those cases (Fig. 2) in whom a clear defect of follicular development was apparent before treatment. Patient no. 3(Fig. 3) who was unresponsive to doses of 10 and 15 mg/day x 10 days responded with an ALP to longer treatment, the LH peak and early luteal development occurring during treatment.

SLP. The endocrinological features of patients with SLP suggested impaired follicular development in some cases (nos. 11, 12, 14, 16) (Figs. 4, 5). FSH plasma levels were found to be lower than normal in most patients; the LH mid-cycle peak was depressed in patients 11 and 16, and normal in the others. The early luteal phase showed mean P values (days +1, +2 from the LH peak: $3,540 \pm 1,434$ pg/ml; days +3, +4: $5,377 \pm 2,147$ pg/ml, M $\pm$ SD), similar to those reported in normal subjects (Genazzani et al., 1977) but from 5th-7th day after LH peak. P concentrations declined rapidly showing the typical feature of SLP. During treatment, the cases which responded positively to 10 mg/day x 10 days during the first cycle showed similar responses in subsequent cycles (Fig. 4); the LH peak was found either at the end of, or during treatment. Patient no. 14 who responded with ILP to the standard treatment showing E_2 values suggesting improved follicular maturation and a normal LH ovulatory peak, responded to an increased dose with sustained E_2 concentrations and an adequate luteal P rise. Similarly patient no. 15 who did not respond to standard treatment (Fig. 6) gave ALP with increased length of treatment (20 days).

Discussion

In 11 cases, E treatment with 10 mg/day x 10 days succeeded in inducing an ALP; similar results were obtained in the other 5 patients after increasing the daily dose or the length of treatment.

A significant finding was that in all cases the occurrence of the LH ovulatory peak either during, or at the end, or after the end of treatment was always related to the endogenous E_2 peak. This suggests that it is not E itself, but ovarian E_2 which activates the positive feedback on LH secretion responsible for ovulation. From the present findings it appears evident that E therapy during the luteal phase does not affect corpus luteum development or function and that it is without luteolytic activity.

The lack of pregnancies in patients who had an ILP (cases 1-5) despite the attainment of an ALP is in agreement with other findings reporting a lack of pregnancies despite adequate substitution therapy (Ruehsen et al., 1969) and may suggest the existence of primitive ovarian factors responsible for ILP and impaired pituitary secretion of gonadotropins. The findings of Jones et al. (1969) on the existence of chromosomal anomalies and/or reduced numbers of ovarian follicles in such patients agrees with the above conclusion.

On the other hand, the cases with SLP showed a high pregnancy rate (3/4), and the corpus luteum function markedly improved during treatment. In these cases, the depressed FSH secretion during follicular maturation and the occurrence of a lower LH mid-cycle peak than in controls, with significantly lower E_2 levels (control cycles in 15 fertile ALP patients: E_2 = 328 ± 72 pg/ml, SLP (present cases): E_2 = 175 ± 89 pg/ml (p < 0.001) all point to a central defect in gonadotropin regulation as the major cause of SLP. The presence of insufficient amounts of FSH and E_2 may be responsible for impaired maturation and development of granulosa cells (Erikson et al., 1974; Richards et al., 1976) and a reduction of the number of LH receptors on these cells (Richards and Midgley, 1976). This is probably the biological situation responsible for a SLP.

The effectiveness of E in inducing ALP in cases of ILP and SLP and its absence of side effects, or of ovarian hyperstimulation, sustain the validity of follicular phase treatment with a weak estrogen in correcting luteal phase defects.

References

Del Pozo, E., Wyss, H., Tolis, G., Alcaniz, J., Campana, A. and Naftolin, F. (1979): *Obstet. and Gynec., 53/3,* 282.

Erickson, G., Challis, J. and Ryan, K. (1974): *Develop. Biol., 40,* 208.

Genazzani, A.R., Facchinetti, F., De Leo, V., Picciolini, E., Franchi, F., Parrini, D. and Kicovic, P. (1978): *Fertil. and Steril., 30/6,* 654.

Genazzani, A.R., Magrini, G., Facchinetti, E., Romagnino, S., Pintor, C., Felber, J.P. and Fioretti, P. (1977): In: *Androgens and Antiandrogens,* p. 247. Editors: L. Martini and P.M. Motta. Raven Press, New York.

Genazzani, A.R., Massafra, C., D'Ambrogio, G. and Kicovic, P. (1979): In: *Psychoneuro-endocrinology in Reproduction,* p. 321. Editors: L. Zichella and P. Pancheri. Elsevier/North-Holland Biomedical Press, Amsterdam-New York-Oxford.

Jones, G.S. (1976): *Fertil. and Steril., 27/4,* 351.

Jones, G.S. and Madrigal-Castro, V. (1970): *Fertil. and Steril., 21,* 1.

Jones, G.S., Ruehsen, M., Johanson, A., Raiti, S. and Blizzard, R. (1969): *Fertil. and Steril., 20,* 14.

Kammerman, S. and Ross, J. (1975): *J. Clin. Endocr., 41,* 546.

McNatty, K.P., Sawers, R.S. and McNeilly, A.S. (1974): *Nature (Lond.), 250,* 653.

Richards, J.S., Ireland, J., Rao, M.C., Bernath, G., Midgley, A. and Reichert, L. (1976): *Endocrinology, 99,* 1562.

Richards, J.S. and Midgley, A. (1976): *Biol. Reprod., 14,* 82.

Ruehsen, M.D., Jones, G., Burnett, L. and Baramki, T. (1969): *Amer. J. Obstet. Gynec., 103,* 1059.

Seppala, M., Hirvonen, E. and Ranta, T. (1976): *Lancet, 1,* 229.

Sherman, B. and Korenman, S. (1974): *J. Clin. Endocr., 39,* 145.

Strott, C., Cargille, C., Ross, G. and Lipsett, M. (1970): *J. Clin. Endocr., 30,* 246.

YoungLai, E. (1975): *J. Endocr., 67,* 289.

Plasma steroid response of pubertal girls to human menopausal gonadotropin*

M. ZACHMANN[1], B. MANELLA[1], L. SANTAMARIA[1], W. ANDLER[2] and A. PRADER[1]

[1] *Department of Pediatrics, University of Zurich, Kinderspital, Zurich, Switzerland, and* [2] *Department of Pediatrics, Universitätsklinikum, Essen, F.R.G.*

The plasma or urinary testosterone (T) response to human chorionic gonadotropin (hCG) is widely used to evaluate gonadal function or to diagnose anorchia in prepubertal or pubertal boys and the response of T-precursors is helpful to differentiate defects of the T-biosynthesis in male pseudohermaphroditism. In contrast surprisingly little information is available concerning similar stimulation tests of the ovaries in girls.

Theoretically and from the experience of treatment of infertility in adult women, an estrogen response can be obtained in females after stimulation with hCG, human menopausal gonadotropins (hMG), or both. Generally, a more marked estrogen response is to be expected after hMG-stimulation, while hCG is more effective in inducing ovulation (Keller, 1975).

In adults and possibly even more so in prepubertal or pubertal children, the sex hormone secretion of the ovaries seems to respond less and more slowly to stimuli than that of the testes. We and many others have shown that a single dose of hCG (e.g. 5000 IU/m² i.m.) is sufficient to induce significant T- and precursor increments in prepubertal boys (Zachmann, 1972). By contrast, in females including adult women, a single dose of hCG, or of hMG, or a combined dose appears to be insufficient for a diagnostically useful estrogen response. The present investigation was performed to evaluate the plasma steroid response to hMG in pubertal girls.

Material and methods

The following test was carried out to evaluate the plasma steroid response to hMG in pubertal girls. Blood was drawn for estimation of 17β-estradiol (E_2), estrone (E_1), and − in some cases − other steroids. Five daily i.m. injections of hMG (150 IU of LH and FSH activity, Pergonal 50, Serono, Italy) were then given and blood was again drawn on the 6th day. The test was performed in 32 girls aged 8 to 19 yrs (Table 1). Eight of them can be

*Supported by the Swiss National Science Foundation (Grant No. 3.883.077).

TABLE 1.

Plasma steroid response to hMG. Number of subjects

Diagnosis	Age (yrs) mean (range)	n	No. of estimations					
			E_2	E_1	T	△4A	17-OHP	DHA
Normal girls	13.9 (13-18)	8	8	5	3	3	3	–
XO Turner syndrome	11.8 (8-16)	11	11	9	2	2	2	2
XO/XX Turner mosaicism	13.3 (12-14)	4	4	4	–	–	–	–
Various disorders	16.0 (13-19)	9	9	7	4	2	3	5
Total	13.7	32	32	25	9	7	8	7

E_2 = estradiol, E_1 = estrone, T = testosterone, △4A = androstenedione, 17-OHP = 17-OH-progesterone, DHA = dehydroepiandrosterone.

considered as endocrinologically normal. They were premenarchic girls with tall stature, whose gonadal function was to be evaluated before estrogen treatment in high doses (Zachmann et al., 1975). All of them had appropriate pubertal development for bone age, normal LHRH test results, and spontaneous subsequent menstruations after discontinuation of estrogen treatment. For ethical reasons, completely normal girls could not be studied. Eleven girls had XO Turner syndrome and 4 XO/XX Turner mosaicism. Nine additional girls suffered from various disorders: one had bilateral adrenal hyperplasia with hirsutism and high plasma dehydroepiandrosterone (DHA); one had the syndrome of acanthosis nigricans, diabetes mellitus, and virilization. Two girls had congenital adrenal hyperplasia (CAH); one, mild untreated 21-hydroxylase-, and one, severe treated 3β-hydroxysteroid dehydrogenase deficiency. In addition, studies were performed on one girl with gonadotropin deficiency and anosmia, one with testicular feminization (gonadectomized), and one with hypergonadotropic hypogonadism of unknown cause. Finally, 2 girls with malignant disease (1 sarcoma, 1 Hodgkin's disease) were studied under treatment with cytostatic drugs.

Plasma E_2 and E_1 were determined radioimmunologically according to Bidlingmaier et al. (1973), using antibodies from NEN Chemicals, Dreieichenhain (E_2) and from Biodata-Hypolab (E_1). DHA, 17-OH-progesterone, T, and △4-androstenedione were determined by unpublished radioimmunoassays using antibodies from Biodata-Hypolab, Dr. F. Bidling-

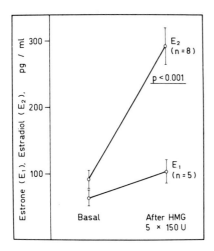

Fig. 1. Plasma 17β-estradiol and estrone response to hMG in endocrinologically normal girls.

maier (Dept. of Pediatrics, University of Munich, FRG), Dr. U. Goebelsmann (Dept. of Obstetrics and Gynecology, University of Southern California, Los Angeles), and from Miles laboratories, respectively.

Results and Discussion

In the normal girls, mean plasma E_2 increased from 91 to 292 pg/ml (Fig. 1). This increment is highly significant ($p < 0.001$). E_1 increased only slightly from 64 to 104 pg/ml (not significant). The other steroids, determined in 3 girls only, showed no change (Table 2).

In the girls with XO Turner syndrome, neither E_2, nor E_1 changed significantly, mean values being 47 and 55 pg/ml (E_2) and 67 and 63 pg/ml (E_1) before and after hMG, respectively (Fig. 2). The other steroids also showed no change. In XO/XX Turner mosaicism, there was a slight E_2-response from 55 to 77 pg/ml (not significant), and no E_1-response (73 and 81 pg/ml, Fig. 3).

TABLE 2.

Plasma steroid response to hMG. Normal girls (ng/dl, n = 3, Mean ± SEM)

	Basal	After hMG
Testosterone	93 ± 13	78 ± 13
△4-androstenedione	167 ± 27	177 ± 44
17-OH-progesterone	273 ± 52	222 ± 46

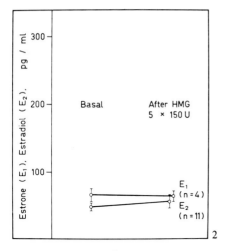
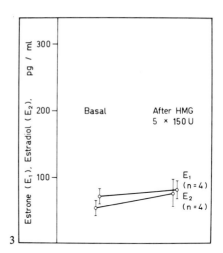

Fig. 2. Plasma 17β-estradiol and estrone response to hMG in girls with XO Turner syndrome.

Fig. 3. Plasma 17β-estradiol and estrone response to hMG in girls with XO/XX mosaicism.

In the individual cases, the following results were obtained: In acquired adrenal hyperplasia, a normal response was found. In acanthosis nigricans, diabetes mellitus and virilization, E_2 did not increase (43 and 38 pg/ml), but surprisingly and unlike in any of the other patients, T increased markedly (214 to 678 ng/dl), suggesting defective steroid aromatization. The other steroids including DHA, remained unchanged. In CAH due to 21-hydroxylase deficiency, E_2 did not respond (92 and 52 pg/ml), but basal E_1 and 17-OH-progesterone were high as expected (279 pg/ml and 992 ng/dl, respectively). In 3β-hydroxysteroid dehydrogenase deficiency (tested under adrenal suppression with hydrocortisone 40 mg daily), E_2 (48 and 43 pg/ml) and E_1 (35 and 32 pg/ml) did not respond, but DHA increased from 312 to 450 ng/dl, indicating that the enzyme defect is probably also present in the ovaries. In hypergonadotropic hypogonadism, there was no E_2-response (25 and 22 pg/ml), while in hypogonadotropic hypogonadism, there was a slight response (25 to 49 pg/ml). There was also no response in the gonadectomized patient with testicular feminization as well as in the 2 patients with malignancies. Although the number of patients studied is small, this preliminary investigation suggests the following conclusions:
1. Five injections of hMG are sufficient to significantly increase plasma E_2 in premenarchic, pubertal normal girls. Whether the mixture of gonadotropins contained in the hMG-preparation acts mainly on the steroidogenesis in the follicles, the corpora lutea, or the ovarian stroma (Marsh et al., 1976) is unknown before a menstrual cycle has been established.

2. There is no or an insignificant response if ovarian tissue is absent (as in XO Turner syndrome) or deficient (as in XO/XX mosaicism).
3. Estrogen precursor estimations are useful in certain conditions such as congenital defects of steroid biosynthesis.

References

Bidlingmaier, F., Wagner-Barnack, M., Butenandt, O. and Knorr, D. (1973): *Pediat. Res.,* *7*, 901.

Keller, P.J. (1975): In: *Ovulation und Ovulationsauslösung.* Editors: W. Obolensky and O. Käser. Huber, Bern-Stuttgart-Wien.

Marsh, J.M., Savard, K. and Lemaire, W.J. (1976): In: *The Endocrine Function of the Human Ovary,* p. 37. Editors: V.H.T. James, M. Serio and G. Giusti. Academic Press, London-New York-San Francisco.

Zachmann, M. (1972): *Acta Endocr. (Kbh.), 70, Suppl.,* 164.

Zachmann, M., Ferrandez, A., Mürset, G. and Prader, A. (1975): *Helv. Paediat. Acta, 30,* 11.

Hormonal changes at female surgical castration*

D.H. BARLOW, R. FLEMING, M.C. MACNAUGHTON and J.R.T. COUTTS

Department of Obstetrics and Gynaecology, Glasgow University, Royal Maternity Hospital, Glasgow, U.K.

Female surgical castration by bilateral oophorectomy causes an acute transition to a postmenopausal state in which any ovarian contribution to hormone production is absent.

Studies of the acute endocrine changes at bilateral oophorectomy were initiated by Bulbrook et al. (1958) who demonstrated a significant fall in oestrogen excretion in premenopausal subjects but not in postmenopausal subjects. Subsequent workers have reported on aspects of the transition, usually in small groups of subjects. The gonadotrophin changes alone were examined by Ostergard et al. (1970), Wallach et al. (1970), Yen and Tsai (1971) and Monroe et al. (1972). Daw (1974) studied oestradiol and luteinizing hormone changes and recently Utian et al. (1978) observed oestradiol and gonadotrophin changes. All workers agree that there is a rapid decline in circulating oestradiol levels and a slower, but substantial, rise in gonadotrophin levels. The purpose of the present study was to define closely the endocrine changes in a spectrum of relevant hormones in a larger group of patients.

Material and methods

Patients

Women undergoing gynaecological surgery were studied by daily sequential peripheral blood sampling. Ten women undergoing surgery without oophorectomy were examined to demonstrate any hormone changes caused by surgery and anaesthesia. Twenty-three women undergoing bilateral oophorectomy, usually at hysterectomy, were studied to demonstrate the hormonal changes secondary to surgical castration.

Blood sampling

Plasma samples were obtained pre-operatively, at 1, 3, 6, 12 and 24 hr post-operatively and then at daily intervals until discharge from hospital.

*This work was supported by the Medical Research Council (UK) during Dr. Barlow's tenure of an M.R.C. Training Fellowship.

Routine follow-up was achieved at 6-8 weeks and longer term follow-up has been maintained. Plasma samples were stored at $-20°C$ until assay.

Hormone assay

The hormones studied included the principal postmenopausal oestrogen — oestrone (OE_1), its precursor, androstenedione ($\triangle_4 A$) and its major metabolite, oestrone sulphate ($OE_1 S$) as well as 17β-oestradiol (OE_2), luteinizing hormone (LH) and follicle stimulating hormone (FSH). The assays were standard specific radioimmunoassay techniques with the exception of the $OE_1 S$ method. Following the extraction of OE_1 from the plasma sample, the $OE_1 S$ in the aqueous phase was hydrolysed to OE_1 which was then extracted and assayed by the OE_1 method.

Results and discussion

Pre-operative hormone profiles confirmed a premenopausal pattern in all subjects examined. The two subject groups were not matched groups, therefore absolute hormone levels could not be compared between the groups. No cases involved hormonally active tumours.

Non-oophorectomy 'control' group

The only significant change detected was a transient peak of $\triangle_4 A$ in the first hours after surgery (Fig. 1a). This outpouring of $\triangle_4 A$ is part of the adrenal stress response mediated by adrenocorticotrophin as observed by Charters et al. (1969) in patients undergoing surgery. There was no significant alteration in the other hormone profiles (Fig. 1b-f).

Oophorectomy group

The most marked effect of bilateral oophorectomy was a fall in the mean level of OE_2 to 25 pg/ml by 3 hr post-operation (Fig. 1d). After 3 hr the OE_2 level remained at this basal level throughout the period of observation. Utian et al. (1978) observed similar basal levels on their first post-operation sample at 24 hr.

The nature of hypothalamo-pituitary feedback mechanisms determines that withdrawal of OE_2 mediated feedback inhibition should evoke a maximal gonadotrophin response. Although circulating OE_2 levels were basal by 3 hr after oophorectomy a gonadotrophin response was not detectable for several days. The earlier and more marked response was in FSH (Fig. 1f), the levels of which were detectably rising by 2 days and had risen into the post-menopausal range by 8 days. LH levels rose more slowly from day 4 and had doubled by 8 days (Fig. 1e). These findings are consistent with those

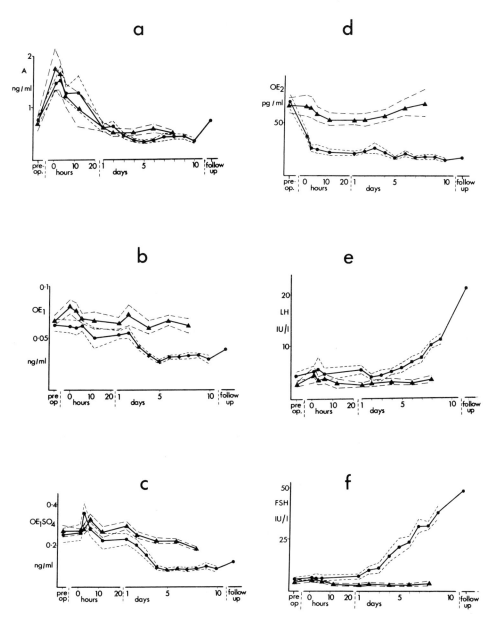

Fig. 1. Hormone levels in women post-oophorectomy (●——●) compared with those in women subjected to abdominal surgery with conservation of the ovaries (▲——▲) during the pre- and immediately post-operative period: a = Androstenedione; b = Oestrone; c = Oestrone sulphate; d = Oestradiol; e = LH; f = FSH.

TABLE 1.

Androstenedione levels (mean ± SEM) in symptomatic and asymptomatic post-oophorectomy patients

	Androstenedione (ng/ml)	
	Symptomatic patients	Asymptomatic patients
Pre-operation	0.64 ± 0.14	0.84 ± 0.14
8 days post-operation	0.37 ± 0.09	0.50 ± 0.08
Follow-up (6 weeks)	0.48 ± 0.06*	0.94 ± 0.10*

*Significant difference p = < 0.01.

reported by Utian et al. (1978). Monroe et al. (1972) observed a transient depression in gonadotrophin levels in the first few days which was not confirmed in this study. The more marked FSH response is consistent with the pattern of gonadotrophin levels observed by Sherman and Korenman (1975) in perimenopausal women and attributed by Van Look et al. (1977) to either an alteration in feedback sensitivity or the withdrawal of a specific FSH-inhibiting substance of ovarian origin, an 'inhibin-like' substance.

The 'stress' mediated peak of $\triangle_4$ A was observed after oophorectomy and was followed by a significant depression of $\triangle_4$ A levels (p < 0.01) compared with the pre-operative state (Fig. 1a). This depression may be due to the loss of the 25% ovarian contribution to circulating $\triangle_4$ A levels detected by Horton et al. (1966). By 6 to 8 weeks the mean $\triangle_4$ A level had returned to pre-operative levels, possibly by adrenal compensation.

Circulating OE_1 levels were maintained for 2 days following oophorectomy then fell to a baseline which was maintained throughout follow-up (Fig. 1b). In the premenopausal woman, OE_1 is derived from ovarian OE_2 by interconversion and by aromatisation in peripheral tissues of circulating $\triangle_4$ A. After the menopause the principal source of OE_1 is well established to be circulating $\triangle_4$ A (Grodin et al., 1973). The more gradual fall in OE_1 compared to OE_2 may reflect the more complex nature of OE_1 production.

Circulating OE_1 S levels were found to parallel the pattern observed with OE_1 (Fig. 1c). It is likely that the substantial circulating pool of OE_1 S is a further source of OE_1 by hydrolysis. This route of interconversion is exploited in some forms of 'natural oestrogen' replacement therapy (Jacobs et al., 1977).

Follow-up at 6-8 weeks was achieved in 21 oophorectomy subjects and 7 (33%) experienced distressing vasomotor symptoms at this time. There was no correlation between circulating oestrogen or gonadotrophin levels and the occurrence of these symptoms. The symptomatic patients were found at follow-up to have significantly lower (p < 0.01) $\triangle_4$ A levels than in the asymptomatic subjects (Table 1). The mechanism for this difference and any possible role of the reduced $\triangle_4$ A in the symptomatology of these patients is not clear at present. There was no such difference in $\triangle_4$ A levels during the peri-operative period.

References

Bulbrook, R.D., Greenwood, F.C., Hadfield, G.J. and Scowen, E.F. (1958): *Brit. Med. J.*, 2, 7.

Charters, A.C., Odell, W.D. and Thompson, J.C. (1969): *J. Clin. Endocr.*, 29, 63.

Daw, E. (1974): *Curr. Med. Res. Opinion, 2*, 256.

Grodin, J.M., Siiteri, P.K. and MacDonald, P.C. (1973): *J. Clin. Endocr.*, 36, 207.

Horton, R., Romanoff, E. and Walker, J. (1966); *J. Clin. Endocr.*, 26, 1267.

Jacobs, H.S., Hutton, J.D., Murray, M.A.F. and James, V.H.T. (1977): *Curr. Med. Res. Opinion, 4, Suppl. 3*, 58.

Monroe, S.E., Jaffe, R.B. and Midgley, A.R. (1972): *J. Clin. Endocr., 34*, 420.

Ostergard, D.R., Parlow, A.F. and Townsend, D.E. (1970): *J. Clin. Endocr., 31*, 43.

Sherman, B.M. and Korenman, S.G. (1975): *J. Clin. Invest., 55*, 699.

Utian, W.H., Katz, M., Davey, D.A. and Carr, P.G. (1978): *Amer. J. Obstet. Gynec., 132*, 297.

Van Look, P.F.A., Lothian, H., Hunter, W.M., Michie, E.A. and Baird, D.T. (1977): *Clin. Endocr., 7*, 13.

Wallach, E.E., Root, A.W. and Garcia, C. (1970): *J. Clin. Endocr., 31*, 376.

Yen, S.C.C. and Tsai, C.C. (1971): *J. Clin. Invest., 50*, 1149.

Oestrogen provocation test amplification of GnRH test in secondary amenorrhoea

E. MAININI and C. MAZZI

Divisione di Endocrinologia, Ospedale S. Antonio, Gallarate (VA), Italy

It is known that oestrogens exert both negative and positive influences on gonadotrophin secretion (Labrie et al., 1977; Yen, 1978). The positive effect has been used to assess the functional state of the hypothalamus-pituitary axis in cases of secondary amenorrhoea.

Material and methods

The present study was carried out in 41 female patients, aged 20 to 38 yrs, 19 (Group A) hospitalized for amenorrhoea existing for at least 3 months (average, 77 days), 22 (Group B) hospitalized for amenorrhoea of more than 9 months duration (average, 13 months). Gonadotrophins LH, FSH, prolactin (PRL) and 17β-oestradiol (E_2) levels were measured in all patients at 7.30-8.00 a.m. GnRH test ($100\,\mu g$ i.v.) was performed 2 hr before and 72 hr after the administration of oestradiol benzoate (5 mg i.m.) (OPT: Oestrogen Provocation Test). LH and FSH were measured immediately before and 20, 30, 40, 60, 120 min after the injection of 'Relisorm L' (Serono, Rome). LH, FSH, PRL, E_2 were measured immediately before and 8, 16, 24, 32, 40, 48, 56, 72 hr after the injection of 'Progynon B Oleoso' (Schering, Berlin) (oestradiol benzoate 5 mg). The hormone values were determined with radioimmunological methods: LH, FSH, PRL using materials supplied by Biodata (Rome), E_2 using material supplied by CEA Sorin (Saluggia). Serum was separated and stored at $-20^{\circ}C$ until assayed. Since we were dealing with data on patients which were in themselves controls, the F test for significance was used instead of Student's t test for the comparison of mean values.

Results and discussion

All the patients showed basal hormone levels similar to values found in normal women during the early follicular phase of the cycle. All showed a normal response of LH and FSH to GnRH stimulus carried out before OPT (Table 1).

The OPT was considered to show a positive feedback effect if the peak values of LH, between 48 and 72 hr were significantly elevated ($p < 0.001$)

TABLE 1.

Basal hormone levels and gonadotrophin responses (mean ± SE) to GnRH test

	No. patients	E_2 (ng/100 ml)	PRL (ng/ml)	LH (mIU/ml) Baseline	Peak	FSH (mIU/ml) Baseline	Peak
Group A	19	8.6 ± 1.3	7 ± 2	5.5 ± 0.9	30.5 ± 3.3*	9.7 ± 1.1	21.8 ± 3.7*
Group B	22	6.0 ± 1.9	7 ± 3	3.9 ± 1.0	27.7 ± 3.6*	7.6 ± 1.2	21.6 ± 3.1*

* $p < 0.01$ with respect to baseline values.

TABLE 2.

Pituitary response (mean ± SE) to oestradiol benzoate administration

	No. patients	LH (mIU/ml) Baseline	Peak	FSH (mIU/ml) Baseline	Peak	PRL (ng/ml) Baseline	Peak
Group A	10	6.6 ± 0.9	27.2 ± 3.2*	11.8 ± 1.1	14.6 ± 2.4	7 ± 3	35 ± 3*
	9	4.5 ± 0.6	5.4 ± 0.8	5.9 ± 0.7	8.2 ± 1.5	8 ± 2	40 ± 4*
Group B	8	4.4 ± 1.8	18.9 ± 3.3*	7.9 ± 1.7	9.5 ± 1.8	5 ± 3	25 ± 2*
	14	3.0 ± 0.7	4.6 ± 0.4	6.5 ± 0.8	8.0 ± 0.7	9 ± 3	45 ± 4*

* $p < 0.01$ with respect to baseline values.

TABLE 3.
Oestradiol levels following oestradiol benzoate administration and its effects on release of gonadotrophins in response to second GnRH test (mean ± SE)

	No. patients	E_2 (ng/100 ml)	LH (mIU/ml) Baseline	LH (mIU/ml) Peak	FSH (mIU/ml) Baseline	FSH (mIU/ml) Peak
Group A	10	81.3 ± 6.1	21.6 ± 4.0 (1)**	44.4 ± 2.4 (1)**(2)**	12.6 ± 2.0	32.4 ± 4.5 (2)**
	9	98.6 ± 8.0	8.2 ± 1.6	35.9 ± 2.7 (2)**	4.0 ± 0.6	24.7 ± 4.6 (2)*
Group B	8	68.1 ± 5.3	15.1 ± 3.5 (1)*	47.0 ± 3.6 (1)*(2)**	8.1 ± 2.0	28.9 ± 4.3 (2)**
	14	95.9 ± 7.1	3.7 ± 0.4	22.7 ± 3.5 (2)**	4.4 ± 0.6	17.4 ± 3.1 (2)**

* $p < 0.05$; ** $p < 0.01$
(1) With respect to pre-administration levels. (2) With respect to baseline values.

above baseline (Shaw et al., 1975). Ten patients from Group A (52.6%) and 8 from Group B (36.3%) showed an increase in circulating LH levels as an indication of positive feedback release (Table 2).

The second GnRH test, carried out 72 hr after the injection of oestradiol benzoate, caused a further significant increase in the LH response in the 18 patients (Table 3). We conclude that the test described gives more detailed information regarding the relationships between oestrogens and basal secretion of LH and its release induced by GnRH, as a guide to diagnosis and indications regarding the results of subsequent treatment. On the contrary OPT did not modify the FSH secretion and so we must suppose that, in the cases examined, the negative feedback has not been efficacious. The OPT, moreover, caused increased PRL secretion, in accordance with other studies which used pharmacological doses of oestrogens (Kandeel et al., 1979) but without interfering with the gonadotrophin release.

References

Labrie, F., Lagacé, L., Dronin, J., De Léan, A., Kelly, P.A., Ferland, L., Beaulieu, M., Raymond, V., Dupont, A. and Cusan, L. (1977): In: *Les Oestrogènes. Rapports présentés à la XIV Réunion des Endocrinologistes de Langue Francaise (Paris),* p. 3. Masson, Paris.

Kandeel, F.R., Butt, W.R., Rudd, B.T., Lynch, S.S., London, D.R. and Logan Edwards, R. (1979): *Clin. Endocr., 10,* 619.

Shaw, R.W., Butt, W.R., London, D.R. and Marshall, J.C. (1975): *Clin. Endocr., 4,* 267.

Yen, S.S.C. (1978): In: *Reproductive Endocrinology. Physiology, Pathophysiology and Clinical Management,* p. 126. W.B. Saunders Company, Philadelphia.

Hyperprolactinaemia syndrome

C. ROBYN

Human Reproduction Research Unit, Université Libre de Bruxelles, Hôpital Saint-Pierre, Brussels, Belgium

Since the first measurement of prolactin in serum by radioimmunoassay (RIA), it is increasingly recognized that hyperprolactinaemia is an extremely frequent condition. That hyperprolactinaemia is associated not only with major alterations of the menstrual cycle (amenorrhoea, anovulatory bleeding) but also with minor modifications (short luteal phase, reduced progesterone secretion) is also well documented. All these alterations in the menstrual cycle result in infertility or at least in sub-fertility.

Three types of hyperprolactinaemia have been identified: a physiological hyperprolactinaemia (long-lasting lactation), a pathological hyperprolactinaemia and a pharmacological hyperprolactinaemia (use of dopamine-antagonists).

In order to understand the mechanisms by which hyperprolactinaemia can induce alterations of the menstrual cycle, it is essential to briefly describe the physiological control of prolactin secretion.

Control of prolactin secretion

Prolactin secretion is under a permanent inhibitory influence exerted by the hypothalamus. For a rather long time isolation of prolactin inhibiting factor (PIF) from the hypothalamus was disappointing. However, it was known that, in vitro, prolactin release is inhibited by low concentrations of dopamine; such inhibition disappears as soon as dopamine is removed from the incubation medium (McLeod and Lehmeyer, 1972). Dopamine has been found in an hypothalamic extract exhibiting high PIF activity (Takahara et al., 1974). Actually, the amount of dopamine present was enough to explain all PIF activity of the extract. After unsuccessful attempts due to rapid denaturation of dopamine (Kamberi et al., 1971), it was found that injection of this amine in a portal vessel induces prolactin inhibition (Takahara et al., 1974). The amount of dopamine found in the hypothalamus and portal blood accounts for the extent of physiological inhibition of prolactin secretion (Shaar and Clemens, 1974; Ben Jonathan et al., 1977). Thus, dopamine appears to be a major PIF, if not the only PIF, in physiological conditions. In teleost fish, dopaminergic terminals establish synaptic contacts with the lactotrophs in the pituitary gland (Ingleton et al., 1977).

Such connections have been lost through evolution. In mammals, dopamine reaches the anterior pituitary through the portal vessels and controls prolactin secretion via specific postsynaptic receptor sites on the lactotrophs (Caron et al., 1978; McLeod and Lamberts, 1978a, b; Shin, 1978). The ability of a wide variety of dopamine agonists and antagonists to interact with dopamine binding sites on pituitary membranes correlates well with the relative potency of their in vitro action on prolactin secretion (Caron et al., 1978). However, such correlation is not obvious for all substances, especially not for some dopamine antagonists. Similar discrepancies were described between clinical potencies of anti-schizophrenic drugs and their ability to compete for dopamine receptors in the brain. It seems, that in the brain, separate agonist and antagonist states of dopamine receptor exist (Creese et al., 1976a, b). Clinical potencies of anti-schizophrenic drugs correlate more closely with their ability to inhibit tritiated haloperidol (dopamine antagonist) binding than with their ability to inhibit dopamine binding (Creese et al., 1976a, b). A similar situation exists at the level of the pituitary gland. Some drugs, such as haloperidol and pimozide are dopamine antagonists at low concentrations. At higher concentrations, these agents have, alone, a powerful action to inhibit prolactin secretion (McLeod and Lamberts, 1978a, b). Apparently, haloperidol and pimozide preferentially bind, in low concentration, to the dopamine antagonist site: thus they do not block the binding of the dopamine to the agonist site but they suppress its physiological action. At higher concentrations, haloperidol and pimozide bind to the agonist site, eventually blocking the binding of dopamine, and inhibiting prolactin secretion (McLeod and Lamberts, 1978b).

There are several factors other than dopamine involved in the regulation of prolactin secretion. It is known that oestrogens stimulate the release and the synthesis of prolactin by a direct effect on the lactotrophs (Apfelbaum and Taleisnik, 1977; Jacobi et al., 1977). Oestrogens exert also a mitogenic effect on these pituitary cells (Jacobi et al., 1977). Hyperplasia of the lactotrophs during pregnancy in women is the consequence of such oestrogenic stimulation. In experimental animals, chronic treatment with oestrogens results in the development of pituitary tumours (El Etreby et al., 1973, 1977). Oestrogens influence prolactin secretion during the menstrual cycle: serum prolactin levels are higher at mid-cycle (Vekemans et al., 1977) and at the same time prolactin release induced by thyrotrophin releasing hormone (TRH) is increased (Reymond and Lemarchand-Béraud, 1976).

Several recent reports indicate an inhibitory effect of progesterone on prolactin secretion. This effect seems to be more apparent when prolactin secretion is enhanced by oestrogens (Libertum et al., 1979). Cramer et al. (1979) have recently shown that large doses of progesterone injected into rats enhances dopamine concentration in portal blood.

TRH releases not only thyrotrophin but also prolactin. This tripeptide acts via specific receptors located on the TSH cells and on the lactotrophs (Robyn, 1976). TRH enters these hypophysial cells (Tixier-Vidal et al.,

1978). There is indirect evidence that TRH has no major physiological significance in the control of prolactin secretion (Robyn, 1976; Frantz, 1978). Even, in most cases of hypothyroidism, it appears that deficiency in thyroid hormones is enough to explain the hyperprolactinaemia, and the excessive prolactin response to various stimuli such as TRH and dopamine antagonists. In hyperthyroidism, prolactin secretion is less sensitive to such releasers than in normal subjects (Robyn, 1976).

The serotoninergic control of prolactin secretion appears to be mediated by the dopaminergic neurones of the hypothalamus. Serotonin is a prolactin releaser but it has no direct effect in vitro on prolactin secretion by the lactotrophs (McLeod and Lamberts, 1978a, b).

Enkephalins and endorphins also enhance prolactin secretion in vivo, (Cusan et al., 1977; Grandison and Guidotti, 1977; Shaar et al., 1977). However, none of these drugs influence in vitro prolactin secretion by anterior pituitary tissue (Rivier et al., 1977). Therefore their influence is likely also mediated by the dopaminergic pathway.

Gamma aminobutyric acid (GABA) inhibits prolactin secretion in some experimental conditions (Grandison and Guidotti, 1979). Specific GABA receptors are found in the rat anterior pituitary (Grandison and Guidotti, 1979). It is not yet clear whether GABA exerts any physiological role in the regulation of prolactin secretion.

An important control of prolactin secretion is that exerted by prolactin itself. Indeed, it is well established that prolactin inhibits its own secretion, likely by increasing dopamine turn-over at the level of tuberoinfundibular dopaminergic neurones (Fuxe et al., 1978). In the median eminence, there are very close relationships between the dopaminergic terminals and the terminals of the LHRH neurones. However, it is obvious that dopamine and LHRH are in different neurones (Kizer et al., 1975). Such close relationships between dopaminergic and LHRH terminals give a rather easy basis for the inhibitory effect of dopamine on LHRH release, and thus on LH secretion. Actually, dopamine seems to influence more the pulsatile character of LHRH release than the tonic secretion of this hypothalamic hormone. Intravenous injection of a large dose of haloperidol, a potent dopamine antagonist, in the rhesus monkey abolishes the pulsatile release of LH (Knobil, 1979).

There is good evidence that a prolactin releasing factor other than TRH exists (Valverde et al., 1972): its nature and mechanism of action are not yet elucidated. Such prolactin-releasing factor-like activity has been found in plasma of hyperprolactinaemic patients in direct relationship to the serum prolactin concentration (Garthwaite and Hagen, 1978).

Types of hyperprolactinaemia

Hyperprolactinaemia occurs under the influence of physiological, pathological and pharmacological factors.

Physiological hyperprolactinaemia

Major hyperprolactinaemia occurs during pregnancy. This is only seen in man and in primates in whom large amounts of oestrogens are produced by the feto-placental unit. In all mammals, delivery is followed by a period of hyperprolactinaemia associated with lactation (Robyn, 1979). The duration of such hyperprolactinaemia is directly influenced by the duration of lactation. During this period, fertility is suppressed or completely abolished (Short, 1976).

In man, it took rather a long time before the significance of this endocrine mechanism was recognized (Robyn, 1979). In industrialized countries, lactation is usually of very short duration, ranging from a few days to 1 or 2 months, and the number of feedings per day rarely exceeds six. In these conditions, lactational hyperprolactinaemia is of short duration too, no more than a few weeks. In non industrialized countries, especially in rural areas, the situation is quite different. Mothers give the breast for 2 years or more. In addition, since the infant is always with the mother, day and night (he sleeps beside the mother), he can reach the breast each time he wants to: he has not to cry to get the breast. In such conditions, the average number of feedings is often around 13 (Vis and Hennart, 1978). Delvoye et al. (1976, 1977a) reported that in these populations of nursing mothers, hyperprolactinaemia persists for 18 months.

Nipple stimulation during suckling induces prolactin release by a neuro-endocrine reflex (Robyn, 1979). However, such prolactin release following suckling is no longer significant after the first 3 postpartum months. This is also true during long-lasting lactation (Delvoye et al., 1976). However, in mothers nursing for at least 2 yrs, basal levels of serum prolactin remain high for more than 1 yr when the number of feedings exceeds 6 per day (Delvoye et al., 1977b). Thus, if after the third postpartum month, each suckling episode is not followed by a significant rise in serum prolactin, repeated nipple stimulations are required to maintain a permanent hyperprolactinaemia.

As reported by Delvoye et al. (1978a, b, 1980) such lactational hyper-prolactinaemia is associated with alterations of the menstrual cycle (amenor-rhoea, anovulatory cycles or inadequate corpus luteum) and thus with infertility or sub-fertility.

In nursing rats, exteroceptive stimuli, such as sounds from the young in distress, also stimulate prolactin release (Terkel et al., 1978). So far, the influence of such stimuli has not been established in nursing women (Robyn, 1979).

In rural areas of developing countries oral administration of infusions prepared with various parts of plants is often used to stimulate lactation. Whether such plant extracts act by enhancing prolactin release, is not yet known. This should be investigated in the view of the contraceptive effects associated with hyperprolactinaemia and with the dopaminergic control of prolactin secretion.

Pathological hyperprolactinaemia

Pathological hyperprolactinaemia was originally described as the amenor-rhoea-galactorrhoea syndrome. It is, however, fallacious to keep such a restrictive denomination for this syndrome and to make distinctions between Chiari-Frommel, Argonz-del Castillo and Forbes-Albright syndromes. Indeed, boundaries between these categories are very often unclear.

In almost half of the cases of non puerperal galactorrhoea, there is no hyperprolactinaemia (Kleinberg et al., 1977). In a variable proportion of cases (10-50%) non puerperal hyperprolactinaemia is not associated with galactorrhoea.

The most common alteration of the menstrual cycle associated with hyperprolactinaemia is amenorrhoea. But other alterations of the menstrual cycle are also seen in hyperprolactinaemic patients: anovulatory bleeding, inadequate corpus luteum (Robyn et al., 1976, 1977).

Thus, the hyperprolactinaemia-infertility syndrome is a more realistic denomination than the amenorrhoea-galactorrhoea syndrome (Crosignani and Robyn, 1977). There are many underlying causes to this syndrome: hypothyroidism, hypothalamic dysfunction, hyperplasia of the lactotrophs, pituitary adenoma secreting prolactin (prolactinoma), interruption of vascular connections between the hypothalamus and the pituitary gland (extension of large pituitary tumours, pituitary stalk section).

It is not yet established whether a prolactinoma is a primitive disease of the pituitary gland or whether it is the consequence of a hypothalamic dysfunction. In some cases, however, it is well documented that complete removal of a micro-adenoma can be followed by complete recovery of a normal hypothalamic control of prolactin secretion, including restoration of the circadian variation of circulating prolactin concentration (Jacquet et al., 1978). This suggests that at least some prolactinomas may have a pituitary origin.

Chronic administration of oestrogens to laboratory animals induces the development of prolactinomas. Would oral contraceptives have the same effect in women? There is no clearcut answer to this question. In most women, combined contraceptive pills do not induce clearcut hyperprolactinaemia. Galactorrhoea, hyperprolactinaemia and pituitary tumours were found to be more frequent in post-pill amenorrhoea than in non pill-related amenorrhoea (March et al., 1977). However, among women with amenorrhoea-galactorrhoea syndrome, the incidence of pituitary tumours was reported to be almost the same following discontinuation of oral contraceptives and in cases unrelated to the pill (Van Campenhout et al., 1977). It seems reasonable to avoid the use of oral contraceptives in hyperprolactinaemic women.

The incidence of hyperprolactinaemia among amenorrhoeic women varies between 15 and 30% (Crosignani and Robyn, 1977). In about one third of hyperprolactinaemic women, alterations of the sella turcica are found by careful radiological tomography examination (L'Hermite et al., 1978a, b). However, micro-adenomas were found in hyperprolactinaemic patients even though no alterations of the sella turcica were detected (Vezina and Sutton, 1974). Such high incidence of pathological hyperprolactinaemia was ignored until 1971, when RIA of human prolactin became available. Previously, visual field defects revealed the existence of a large pituitary tumour. The treatment was only surgical. The disease that we see today is quite different: it is revealed by alteration of the menstrual cycle and confirmed by the measurement of prolactin in serum. Often, it is a non-tumoural condition and the treatment is medical using prolactin inhibitors. Even when there is good radiological evidence for the presence of an adenoma in the sella turcica, it is of small dimensions (micro-adenoma) and thus only potentially dangerous: reports indicate that rapid expansion of a prolactinoma during pregnancy induced in amenorrhoeic women can cause dramatic visual field defects.

Of particular interest is the high incidence of hyperplasia of the lactotrophs as revealed by systematic examination of the pituitary gland at autopsy (McKeel et al., 1978). Adenomatous hyperplasia was found in 5.6% of the glands. So far, very little is known about the natural history of the hyperprolactinaemia-infertility syndrome. Such history includes the aetiology, the patho-physiological mechanisms and the progression (reversible or not) of the disease.

Pharmacological hyperprolactinaemia

Most drugs producing hyperprolactinaemia are psychotropic drugs. They are phenothiazines, substituted benzamides and butyrophenones. The mechanism of action common to all these drugs appears to be a blockade of dopaminergic transmission. As shown in vitro (Caron et al., 1978; McLeod and Lamberts, 1978a, b) such interference by these dopamine antagonists occurs at the level of all accessible dopamine receptors not only in the brain but also at the level of the lactotrophs. Actually, hyperprolactinaemia induced by neuroleptics or related drugs appears to be primarily due to disinhibition of prolactin secretion by a direct effect at the pituitary level (McLeod and Robyn, 1977). The blood-brain barrier is not very permeable to some of these drugs. Among others, this is the case for sulpiride, a substituted benzamide. Still this substance is a very potent prolactin releaser (McLeod and Robyn, 1977; L'Hermite et al., 1978a, b).

Endocrine profile of the hyperprolactinaemia syndrome

The endocrine profile is very similar whatever the cause of the hyperprolactinaemia might be.

Basal levels

Serum *prolactin* levels are increased. It should be emphasized that hyper-prolactinaemia is not easy to establish. The 95% upper limit of the normal distribution is hazy: 30 ng/ml or 650 μU/ml is a common limit in non amenorrhoeic women. But when serum prolactin is repeatedly at that level, or even slightly below, it may be associated with minor alterations of the menstrual cycle (short luteal phase) and infertility. Even intermittent hyperprolactinaemia, particularly during the follicular phase, can be associated with alterations of the menstrual cycle (Robyn, 1979). Serum prolactin levels above 5400 μU/ml (300 ng/ml) are seen in the case of prolactin secreting adenomas (Frantz, 1978). In most instances, values repeatedly above 900 μU/ml (50 ng/ml) are associated with amenorrhoea. There are at least 3 populations of prolactin molecules in serum: they do not equally influence the available radioimmunoassays. More should be known about the physio-pathological significance of such molecular heterogeneity. It is more realistic to consider prolactin as a complex of molecules rather than as a single and unique peptide molecule. Prolactin secretion is extremely labile. It is enhanced by 'stress' of all kinds. There is a circadian periodicity in serum prolactin levels with peak values at night. However, the values often remain high in the early morning hours, at a time when blood samples are collected for most laboratory testings. The half-life of prolactin is short, some 15 min: surprisingly little is known about the metabolism of this hormone. Serum *oestradiol* levels are low in hyperprolactinaemic women. In most cases they are equal to or even below the levels seen in the early stages of the follicular phase of ovulatory cycles (Crosignani and Robyn, 1977). Circulating DHEA-S and urinary DHEA are clearly increased in women affected by amenorrhoea with hyperprolactinaemia. This is the consequence of direct or indirect effects of prolactin on the adrenal cortex (Carter et al., 1977; Giusti et al., 1977; Parker et al., 1978).

Serum *LH* and *FSH* levels are within the range of values found during the early follicular phase of ovulatory cycles. In hyperprolactinaemic lactating mothers basal serum FSH levels tend to be somewhat more elevated. In amenorrhoeic women with hyperprolactinaemia, the pulsatile release of LH is suppressed (Bohnet and Schneider, 1977).

Dynamic tests

Prolactin secretion. Testing of prolactin secretion with TRH has been proposed for the selection of patients with pituitary tumours from the group of women with non-tumoural hyperprolactinaemia. Actually, prolactin response to TRH is commonly suppressed, at least in relative terms, not only in patients with radiological evidence of a prolactinoma (Robyn, 1976), but also in cases of major non-tumoural hyperprolactinaemia (last trimester of pregnancy, first year of long-lasting lactation).

For the same purpose of differential diagnosis, the use of dopamine antagonists for testing prolactin release has been suggested by several authors. Some of them reported that a clearcut prolactin response indicates a non-tumoural hyperprolactinaemia (Boyd et al., 1977; Cowden et al., 1979). Actually, as for TRH, the relative increase of serum prolactin levels is more related to the degree of hyperprolactinaemia than to the presence of a pituitary adenoma: when the basal levels are high, the response is relatively small (Crosignani and Robyn, 1977).

Disappearance of the circadian variation in serum prolactin levels seems to be an early indication of the presence of a prolactinoma (L'Hermite et al., 1978; Cowden et al., 1979).

Similarily the use of prolactin inhibitors was found to be inadequate in differentiating patients with prolactinomas. This is valid for L-dopa, CB 154 and apparently also for nomifensine, although testing with this last substance was considered to be promising (Müller et al., 1978). Fine and Frohman (1978) reported that in patients with pituitary tumours, L-dopa alone led to prolactin suppression comparable with that in normal subjects. However, they showed that L-dopa plus carbidopa, which produces peripheral dopa-decarboxylase inhibition, resulted in much less suppression of plasma prolactin in patients with pituitary tumours than in normal controls.

Gonadotrophin secretion. In most hyperprolactinaemic women (Crosignani and Robyn, 1977; Bergh et al., 1977; Lachelin et al., 1977; Delvoye et al., 1978; L'Hermite et al., 1978a, b), the FSH response to LHRH is of increased amplitude as compared to that seen in normoprolactinaemic subjects (early follicular or luteal phase). The LH response to LHRH is more variable depending on the period of the menstrual cycle when control tests were performed. Decreased gonadotrophin reactivity to LHRH has been reported in patients with tumours and during bromocriptine treatment. In amenor-rhoeic women with hyperprolactinaemia, the pulsatile release of LHRH and thus also that of LH is abolished; it reappears during treatment with bromocriptine (Bohnet and Schneider, 1977). In these women with no pulsatile LH release the positive feedback of oestrogens on LH secretion is abolished (Glass et al., 1975; Delvoye et al., 1978; L'Hermite et al., 1978).

Mechanism of infertility

When in hyperprolactinaemic women, the endocrine changes related to ovulation are abolished, amenorrhoea prevails. When such changes still occur, corpus luteum deficiency is the rule. Prolactin affects the mechanisms controlling ovulation both at the hypothalamic and at the ovarian level.

Hypothalamus

There is good evidence that prolactin is involved in hypothalamic functions.

Some hypothalamic neurones contain prolactin in their cell bodies and in their terminals (Fuxe et al., 1978): there are even extra-hypothalamic localizations of prolactin. These localizations of prolactin in the brain persist after hypophysectomy (Toubeau et al., 1979). Some hypothalamic neurones in the preoptic area are responsive to prolactin: microiontophoretic administration of prolactin changes the rate of firing of these neurons (Barry et al., 1978). Specific binding sites for prolactin were found on ependyma of the rat choroid plexus (Walsh et al., 1978). The pituitary secretes to the brain: the neurohypophyseal capillary bed not only receives trophic hormones produced in the adenohypophysis but, under certain physiological circumstances, delivers those hormones directly to the brain. Thus, increased prolactin concentrations were found in blood samples taken from intracranial vessels (Bergland et al., 1977).

As already mentioned, prolactin stimulates dopamine turn-over in the median eminence (Advis et al., 1977). This is likely responsible for the mechanism of the short feedback loop by which prolactin influences LH secretion (Fuxe et al., 1978). Indeed, dopamine influences LH secretion (Leebaw et al., 1978). There are very close relationships in the median eminence between LHRH nerve terminals and dopaminergic nerve terminals (Kizer et al., 1975). Dopamine antagonists exert direct effects on LHRH neurones in hypophysectomized rats: pimozide markedly increases the LHRH content in the median eminence (Corbin et al., 1975). Injection of large amounts of haloperidol in the rhesus monkey abolishes the pulsatile release of LH (Knobil, 1979).

In cases of hyperprolactinaemic amenorrhoea consecutive to pituitary stalk section in the rhesus monkey (Knobil, 1979) and in hyperprolactinaemic patients with amenorrhoea (Leyendecker et al., 1979), a pulsatile release of LH can be restored by i.v. administration of small doses of synthetic LHRH at frequent and regular intervals. This is enough to restore ovulations with normal luteal function.

In conclusion, hypothalamic factors are very likely decisive in the suppression of ovulation as it often occurs in hyperprolactinaemic women; prolactin appears to regulate the pulsatile release of LHRH via a dopaminergic pathway.

Ovary

Besser and Thorner (1975) reported a resistance to the effect of exogenous gonadotrophins on ovarian steroidogenesis in hyperprolactinaemic patients; the resistance disappears after lowering prolactin levels by bromocriptine. However, it is not fully adequate to establish ovarian resistance on that basis. Indeed, follicular growth starts quite soon after initiation of bromocriptine therapy in hyperprolactinaemic women. It is obvious that growing follicles are more sensitive in producing oestrogens in response to exogenous gonadotrophins than non-growing follicles. Thus, an adequate comparison of the effects of gonadotrophins should involve ovaries at exactly the same stage of follicular growth. This is not the case in the study by Besser and Thorner (1975).

To support the contention of ovarian resistance in hyperprolactinaemia, the work of McNatty et al. (1974, 1977) has often been quoted. These authors reported that 'in vitro' progesterone synthesis by human granulosa cells from graafian follicles was impaired when prolactin concentration in the medium was increased above physiological levels. Such results, however, cannot be extrapolated to the effect of prolactin on oestrogen production by the growing follicles.

Sulpiride hyperprolactinaemia in normal women does not appear to induce ovarian refractoriness to exogenous gonadotrophins (Aono et al., 1978). In cases of anovulation, Kemmann et al. (1977) reported that normo- and hyperprolactinaemic patients showed no significant difference in the required dosage and duration of exogenous gonadotrophin treatment, plasma 17β-oestradiol response and ovulatory and pregnancy outcome. Archer and Josimovitch (1976) indicate also an absence of ovarian resistance to exogenous gonadotrophin in hyperprolactinaemic patients with amenorrhoea. When during sulpiride hyperprolactinaemia, ovulation is not abolished, serum oestradiol levels during the pre-ovulatory period are very similar to those seen in the same women during the same period of control cycles. However, the development of the granulosa cells seems to be grossly impaired (Robyn et al., 1976, 1977; L'Hermite et al., 1978a, b). Indeed, such cycles under sulpiride hyperprolactinaemia are characterized by very poor luteal phase (4-5 days) and with low serum progesterone levels (2-5 ng/ml). McNatty (1979, personal communication), recently reported for follicles of equivalent size a reduced number of granulosa cells in hyperprolactinaemic women as compared to normoprolactinaemic women.

When sulpiride hyperprolactinaemia is induced only from mid-cycle, i.e. after ovulation, the effects on the corpus luteum are much less apparent. The luteal phase is shorter but only by 1 or 4 days and serum progesterone levels are reduced but only by some 25% (Delvoye et al., 1974; Robyn et al., 1977).

Thus, prolactin exerts a direct ovarian effect only on the granulosa cells: excess of prolactin suppresses progesterone secretion by these cells. When during hyperprolactinaemia, the endocrine changes related to ovulation still occur, oestradiol production, as reflected by the circulating levels of this steroid, is normal. However, the development of granulosa cells is impaired. Whether this is due to a local effect of prolactin or to an impaired hypothalamic control on gonadotrophins secretion, remains to be elucidated.

References

Advis, J.P., Hall, T.R., Hodson, C.A., Mueller, G.P. and Meites, J. (1977): *Proc. Soc. Exp. Biol. (N.Y.), 155,* 567.

Aono, T., Yasuda, M., Shioji, T., Kondo, K. and Kurachi, K. (1978): *Acta Endocr. (Kbh.), 89*, 142.

Apfelbaum, M.E. and Taleisnik, S. (1977): *Acta Endocr. (Kbh.), 86*, 714.

Archer, D.F. and Josimovitch, J.B. (1976): *Obstet. and Gynec., 48*, 155.

Barry, J., Croix, D. and Poulain, P. (1977): In: *Progress in Prolactin Physiology and Pathology*, p. 253. Editors: C. Robyn and M. Harter. Elsevier/North-Holland Biomedical Press, Amsterdam.

Ben Jonathan, N., Oliver, C., Weiner, H.J., Mical, R.S. and Porter, J.C. (1977): *Endocrinology, 100*, 452.

Bergh, T., Nillius, S.J. and Wide, L. (1977): *Acta Endocr. (Kbh.), 86*, 683.

Bergland, R.M., Davis, S.L. and Page, R.B. (1977): *Lancet, 2*, 276.

Besser, G.M. and Thorner, M.O. (1975): *Path. et Biol. 23*, 779.

Bohnet, H.G. and Schneider, H.P.G. (1977): In: *Prolactin and Human Reproduction*, p. 153. Editors: P.G. Crosignani and C. Robyn. Academic Press, London.

Boyd, A.E., Reichlin, S. and Turksoy, N. (1977): *Ann. Intern. Med., 87*, 165.

Caron, M.G., Beaulieu, M., Raymond, V., Gagne, B., Drouin, J., Lefkowitz, R.J. and Labrie, F. (1978): *J. Biol. Chem., 253*, 2244.

Carter, J.N., Tyson, J.E., Warne, G.L., McNeilly, A.S., Faiman, C. and Friesen, H.G. (1977): *J. Clin. Endocr., 45*, 973.

Corbin, A., Beattie, C.W. and Upton, G.V. (1975): *Experientia (Basel), 31*, 613.

Cowden, E.A., Thomson, J.A., Doyle, D., Ratcliffe, J.G., MacPherson, P. and Teasdale, G.M. (1979): *Lancet, 1*, 1155.

Cramer, E.A., Parker, C.R. and Porter, J.C. (1979): *Endocrinology, 105*, 929.

Creese, I., Burt, D.R. and Snyder, S.H. (1976a): *Life Sci., 17*, 993.

Creese, I., Burt, D.R. and Snyder, S.H. (1976b): *Science, 192*, 481.

Crosignani, P.G. and Robyn, C. (1977): *Prolactin and Human Reproduction*, p. 305. Academic Press, New York-London.

Cusan, L., Dupont, A., Kledzik, G.C. and Labrie, F. (1977): *Nature (Lond.), 268*, 5644.

Delvoye, P., Badawi, M., Demaegd, M. and Robyn, C. (1978a): In: *Progress in Prolactin Physiology and Pathology*, p. 213. Editors: C. Robyn and M. Harter. Elsevier/North-Holland Biomedical Press, Amsterdam.

Delvoye, P., Delogne-Desnoeck, J. and Robyn, C. (1976): *Lancet, 7*, 288.

Delvoye, P., Delogne-Desnoeck, J. and Robyn, C. (1980): *Clin. Endocr., 3*, 243.

Delvoye, P., Delogne-Desnoeck, J., Uwayitu-Nyampeta and Robyn, C. (1977a): *Clin. Endocr., 7*, 257.

Delvoye, P., Demaegd, M., Delogne-Desnoeck, J. and Robyn, C. (1977b): *J. Biosoc. Sci., 9*, 447.

Delvoye, P., Demaegd, M., Uwayitu-Nyampeta and Robyn, C. (1978b): *Amer. J. Obstet. Gynec., 130*, 635.

Delvoye, P., Taubert, H.D., Jürgensen, O., L'Hermite, M., Delogne, J. and Robyn, C. (1974): *C.R. Acad. Sci. (Paris), 279*, 1463.

El Etreby, M.F., Richter, K.-D. and Günzel, P. (1973): In: *Human Prolactin*, p. 65. Editors: J.L. Pasteels and C. Robyn. Excerpta Medica, Amsterdam.

El Etreby, M.F., Schilk, B., Soulioti, G., Tushaus, U., Wiemann, H. and Günzel, P. (1977): *Endokirinologie, 69*, 202.

Fine, S.A. and Frohman, L.A. (1978): *J. Clin. Invest., 21*, 973.

Frantz, A.G. (1978): *New Engl. J. Med., 298*, 201.

Fuxe, K., Andersson, K., Hökfelt, T., Agnati, L.F., Ogren, S.O., Eneroth, P., Gustafsson, J.A. and Skett, P. (1978): In: *Progress in Prolactin Physiology and Pathology*, p. 95. Editors: C. Robyn and M. Harter. Elsevier/North-Holland Biomedical Press, Amsterdam.

Garthwaite, T.L. and Hagen, T.C. (1978): *J. Clin. Endocr., 47*, 885.

Giusti, G., Bassi, F., Borsi, L., Cattaneo, S., Giannotti, P., Lanza, L., Pazzagli, M., Vigiani,

C. and Serio, M. (1977): In: *Prolactin and Human Reproduction,* p. 239. Editors: P.G. Crosignani and C. Robyn. Academic Press, London.

Glass, M.R., Shaw, R.W., Butt, W.R., Logan Edwards, R. and London, D.R. (1975): *Brit. Med. J., 2,* 274.

Grandison, L. and Guidotti, A. (1977): *Nature (Lond.), 270,* 357.

Grandison, L. and Guidotti, A. (1979): *Endocrinology, 105,* 754.

Ingleton, P.M., Batten, T.F.C. and Ball, J.N. (1977): *J. Endocr., 73,* 9P.

Jacobi, J., Lloyd, H.M. and Meares, J.D. (1977): *J. Endocr., 72,* 35.

Jacquet, P., Grisoli, F., Guibot, M., Lissitsky, J.C. and Carayon, P. (1978): *J. Clin. Endocr., 46,* 459.

Kamberi, I.A., Mical, R.S. and Porter, J.C. (1971): *Endocrinology, 88,* 1012.

Kemmann, E., Gemzell, C.A., Beinert, W.C., Beling, C.B. and Jones, J.R. (1977): *Amer. J. Obstet. Gynec., 129,* 145.

Kizer, J.S., Arimura, A., Schally, A.V. and Brownstein, M.J. (1975): *Endocrinology, 96,* 523.

Kleinberg, D.L., Noel, G.L. and Frantz, A.G. (1977): *New Engl. J. Med., 296,* 589.

Knobil, E. (1979): *Rec. Progr. Hormone Res.,* in press.

Lachelin, G.C.L., Abu-Fadil, S. and Yen, S.S.C. (1977): *J. Clin. Endocr., 44,* 1163.

Leebaw, W.F., Lee, L.A. and Woolf, P.D. (1978): *J. Clin. Endocr., 47,* 480.

Leyendecker, G., Struve, T. and Plotz, E.J. (1979): In: *The Endocrine Society Meeting, 61st Annual Meeting,* Abstr. 926.

L'Hermite, M., Caufriez, A., Badawi, M., Sugar, J., Schwers, J., Robyn, C., Cordova, T., Ayalon, D., Legros, J.J. and Stevenaert, A. (1978): In: *Progress in Prolactin Physiology and Pathology,* p. 397. Editors: C. Robyn and M. Harter. Elsevier/North-Holland Biomedical Press, Amsterdam.

L'Hermite, M., Delogne-Desnoeck, J., Michaux-Duchene, A. and Robyn, C. (1978a): *J. Clin. Endocr., 47,* 1132.

L'Hermite, M., Denaycr, P., Golstein, J., Virasoro, E., Vanhaelst, L., Copinschi, G. and Robyn, C. (1978b): *Clin. Endocr., 9,* 195.

Libertum, C., Kaplan, S.E. and De Nicola, A.F. (1979): *Neuroendocrinology, 28,* 64.

March, C.M., Kletzky, O.A., Israel, R., Davajan, V. and Mishell, D.R. (1977): *Fertil. and Steril., 28,* 346.

McKeel, D.W., Fowler, M. and Jacobs, L.S. (1978): In: *The Endocrine Society Meeting, 60th Annual Meeting,* Abstr. 557.

McLeod, R.M. and Lamberts, S.W.J. (1978a): In: *Progress in Prolactin Physiology and Pathology,* p. 111. Editors: C. Robyn and M. Harter. Elsevier/North-Holland Biomedical press, Amsterdam.

McLeod, R.M. and Lamberts, S.W.J. (1978b): *Endocrinology, 103,* 200.

McLeod, R.M. and Lehmeyer, J.E. (1972): In: *Lactogenic Hormones,* p. 53. Editors: G.E.W. Wolstenholme and J. Knight. Churchill Livingstone, Edinburgh-London.

McLeod, R.M. and Robyn, C. (1977): *J. Endocr., 72,* 273.

McNatty, K.P., McNeilly, A.S. and Sawers, R.S. (1977): In: *Prolactin and Human Reproduction,* p. 109. Editors: P.G. Crosignani and C. Robyn. Academic Press, New York-London.

McNatty, K.P., Sawers, R.S. and McNeilly, A.S. (1974): *Nature (Lond.) 250,* 653.

Müller, E.E., Genazzani, A.R. and Murru, S. (1978): *J. Clin. Endocr., 47,* 1352.

Parker, L.N., Chang, S. and Odell, W.D. (1978): *Clin. Endocr., 8,* 1.

Reymond, M. and Lemarchand-Beraud, T. (1976): *Clin. Endocr., 5,* 429.

Rivier, C., Vale, W., Ling, N., Brown, M. and Guillemin, R. (1977): *Endocrinology, 100,* 238.

Robyn, C. (1976): In: *Proceedings of the First International Symposium on Basic Applications and Clinical Uses of Hypothalamic Hormones,* p. 319. Editors: A.L.

Charro-Salgado, R. Fernandez Durango and J.G. Lopez del Campo. Excerpta Medica, Amsterdam.

Robyn, C. (1979): In: *Human Placenta: Proteins and Hormones (Serono Symposia, Siena).* Editors: A. Klopper, A.R. Genazzani and P.G. Crosignani. Academic Press, London.

Robyn, C., Delvoye, P., Van Exter, C., Vekemans, M., Caufriez, A., Denayer, P., Delogne-Desnoeck, J. and L'Hermite, M. (1977): In: *Prolactin and Human Reproduction,* p. 71. Editors: P.G. Crosignani and C. Robyn. Academic Press, New York-London.

Robyn, C., Vekemans, M., Caufriez, A. and L'Hermite, M. (1976): *IRCS Med. Sci., 4,* 14.

Robyn, C., Delvoye, P., Vekemans, M., Aidara, D., Caufriez, A., Badawi, M. and L'Hermite, M. (1977a): In: *Actualités Gynécologiques,* p. 157. Editors: A. Netter and A. Gorins. Masson, Paris.

Robyn, C., Delvoye, P., Vekemans, M., Caufriez, A., Delogne-Desnoeck, J. and L'Hermite, M. (1978): In: *Functional Morphology of the Human Ovary,* p. 1. Editor: J.R.T. Coutts. MTP Press Limited, International Medical Publishers, Lancaster.

Shaar, C.J. and Clemens, J.A. (1974): *Endocrinology, 95,* 1202.

Shaar, C.J., Frederickson, R.C.A., Dininger, N.B. and Jackson, L. (1977): *Life Sci., 21,* 853.

Shin, S.H. (1978): *Life Sci., 22,* 67.

Short, R.V. (1976): In: *Breast-Feeding and the Mother (Ciba Symposium),* p. 73. Elsevier/North-Holland, Amsterdam.

Takahara, J., Arimura, A. and Schally, A.V. (1974): *Endocrinology, 95,* 462.

Terkel, J., Damassa, D.A. and Sawyer, C.H. (1978): In: *The Endocrine Society Meeting, 60th Annual Meeting,* Abstr. 232.

Tixier-Vidal, A., Brunet, N. and Gourdji, D. (1978): In: *Progress in Prolactin physiology and Pathology,* p. 29. Editors: C. Robyn and M. Harter. Elsevier/North-Holland Biomedical Press, Amsterdam.

Toubeau, G., Desclin, J., Parmentier, M. and Pasteels, J.L. (1979): *J. Endocr., 83,* 261.

Valverde, R., Chieffo, C.V. and Reichlin, S. (1972): *Endocrinology, 91,* 982.

Van Campenhout, J., Blanchet, P., Beauregard, M. and Papas, S. (1977): *Fertil. and Steril., 28,* 728.

Vekemans, M., Delvoye, P., L'Hermite, M. and Robyn, C. (1977): *J. Clin. Endocr., 44,* 989.

Vezina, J.L. and Sutton, T.J. (1974): *Amer. J. Roentgenol., 120,* 46.

Vis, H.L. and Hennart, Ph. (1978): *Acta Paediat. Belg., 31,* 195.

Walsh, R., Posner, B.I., Kopriwa, B.W. and Brawer, J.R. (1978): *Science, 201,* 1041.

Infertility with normal menstrual rhythm: hormone patterns before and during treatment with bromocriptine (CB 154)*

A. CRAIG[1], R. FLEMING[2], W.P. BLACK[2], M.C. MACNAUGHTON[2], P. ENGLAND[3] and J.R.T. COUTTS[2]

[1] *Clinpath Services Limited, High Wycombe, Bucks;* [2] *Department of Obstetrics and Gynaecology, Glasgow University, Royal Maternity Hospital, Rottenrow, Glasgow;* [3] *Department of Pathological Biochemistry, Glasgow Royal Infirmary, Glasgow, U.K.*

Elevated prolactin levels have been shown in the hyperprolactinaemia amenorrhoea syndrome to be responsible for anovulation. Reduction of these levels using the dopamine agonist bromocriptine (Sandoz Ltd., CB 154) results in a return of normal menstruation and in many cases a return of fertility (Thorner et al., 1974). The situation in women with unexplained infertility is much less clear. Lenton et al. (1977) reported a significantly increased pregnancy rate when women with unexplained infertility were treated empirically with bromocriptine. However, Wright et al. (1979), in a double blind trial, observed no significant difference between the pregnancy rates in infertile patients treated with either bromocriptine or a placebo. This paper reports the results of empirical treatment with bromocriptine of 17 patients with unexplained infertility.

Material and methods

Patients

Seventeen patients with a history of unexplained infertility were included in this study. All of these patients had apparently normal cycles of regular length, had husbands with potent sperm counts and had no ovarian anatomical abnormality on laparoscopic examination. Their only complaint was a lack of conception although they had been attempting to do so for a minimum of 3 yrs.

*Supported by a grant from the Higher Medicine Committee of the Greater Glasgow Area Health Board.

Blood samples

Each patient provided serial daily blood samples throughout 2 menstrual cycles. The first cycle was an investigation cycle and during the second cycle each patient was treated with 2.5 mg of bromocriptine daily. The plasma was separated from each blood sample and stored at −20°C until subjected to hormone assay.

Hormone assays

Using sensitive, specific, precise, radioimmunoassays (RIA) each plasma sample was assayed for the levels of prolactin (PRL), follicle stimulating hormone (FSH), luteinising hormone (LH), oestradiol (OE₂) and progesterone (P). The RIA were standard assays without chromatography; dextran coated charcoal was used to separate free and antibody bound fractions for the steroid assays while second antibody methods were employed for the protein hormones.

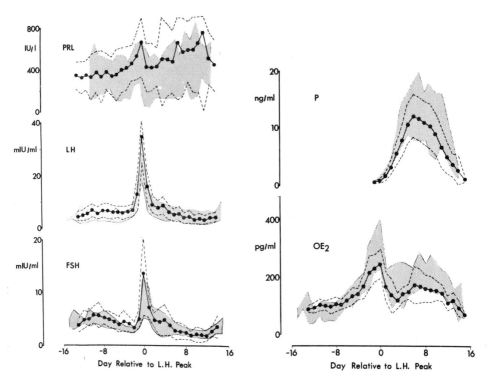

Fig. 1a and b. Hormone profiles (mean ± SD; ●———●) in investigation cycles from 17 patients with unexplained infertility compared with the 95% confidence limits of the normal ranges (hatched background).

Results

Thirteen of the patients in this study showed transient hyperprolactinaemia (T↑PRL) (Coutts et al., 1978), whilst the other 4 patients were normo-prolactinaemic. Figures 1a and b show the mean levels of the protein and steroid hormones respectively in the 17 investigation cycles compared with the 95% confidence limits of our laboratory normal cycle range. All levels are plotted relative to the day of the mid-cycle LH peak which is designated day 0. As a result of the T↑PRL the mean levels of PRL were in the high normal range in the patients; the levels of FSH and LH were generally normal although there was a slight elevation of LH in the follicular phase which was a function of elevated levels in 4 patients which will be discussed later; P and OE_2 levels in the luteal phase were at the lower end of the normal range whilst several patients also had lowered pre-ovulatory OE_2. Figures 2a and b show the protein and steroid hormone levels compared with our normal ranges for all 17 bromocriptine treatment cycles. The PRL levels

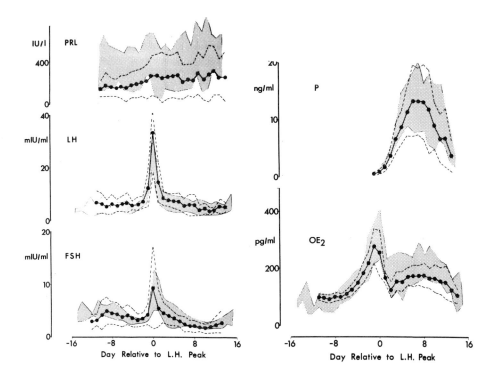

Fig. 2a and b. Hormone profiles (mean ± SD; ●——●) from bromocriptine treated cycles of 17 patients with unexplained infertility compared with the 95% confidence limits of the normal ranges (hatched background).

were reduced significantly, but there were no significant reductions in any of the other hormones on any day in the whole group. Although it was not significant, the overall profiles of the steroid hormones (OE_2 and P) appeared to be improved on bromocriptine therapy (Fig. 1b and 2b). One patient became pregnant on this treatment regime. A number of abnormalities were detected in the investigation cycles: (1) *poor follicular growth* – where the concentrations of OE_2 remained within the early follicular phase range prior to day –3 of the cycle (n = 7); (2) *poor P surge* – where levels of P between days +1 and +5 were below the normal range in at least 3 samples (n = 6); (3) *elevated follicular phase LH* – where LH levels were elevated above baseline in > 50% of samples up to day –3 (n = 4). Figure 3 shows the mean levels of OE_2 and P in the patients with poor follicular growth in both investigational and treatment cycles compared with the normal ranges. Bromocriptine improved the pre-ovulatory oestradiol levels although not significantly on any single day. This improved follicular maturation was further evidenced by the fact that the length of the follicular phase on bromocriptine (11.2 ± 2.4 days) was significantly shorter than it was in the investigation cycles (12.8 ± 2.3 days) for the whole group of treated patients (n = 17; p < 0.01 paired data). The patients with poor P surge showed no significant changes in hormone levels, apart from lowered

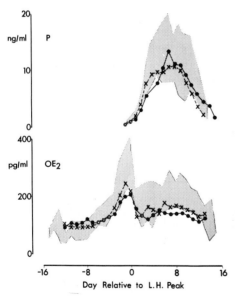

Fig. 3. Mean OE_2 and P levels from 7 patients with poor follicular growth in investigation (●——●) and bromocriptine treatment (X –– X) cycles compared with the 95% confidence limits of our normal ranges (hatched background).

PRL levels, on bromocriptine therapy. The mean levels of the hormones, in the group with elevated follicular LH levels, for both investigation and treatment cycles are shown in Figures 4a and b compared with the normal cycle range. Bromocriptine as well as lowering PRL levels, also caused a significant fall ($p < 0.01$ paired data) in the follicular phase LH levels (Fig. 4a) resulting in normalisation of this hormone. Within this group of patients, bromocriptine also apparently reduced the FSH levels (Fig. 4a) but this reduction was not statistically significant. The steroid hormone levels were not significantly changed by the treatment (Fig. 4b).

Discussion

On the group data from the 17 patients in this study our results confirm the observations of Wright et al. (1979) that bromocriptine is of little value in patients with unexplained infertility. Only one of these patients became pregnant. However, a number of interesting points were observed when the patients were sub-divided into categories on the basis of their investigation

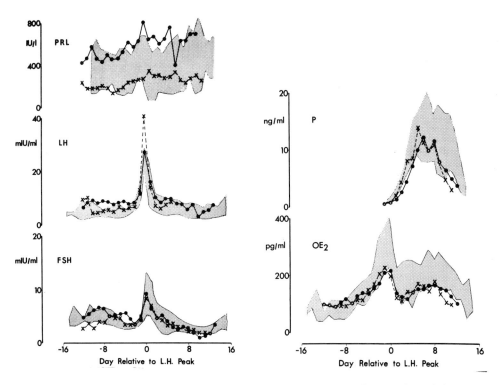

Fig. 4a and b. Mean hormone profiles in investigation cycles (●——●) and bromo-criptine treatment cycles (X —— X), from 4 patients with elevated follicular LH, compared with the 95% confidence limits of the normal cycle (hatched background).

cycles. Bromocriptine appeared to improve follicular growth and development as manifested by improved pre-ovulatory levels of OE_2 in a group of women with poor follicular growth and shortened follicular phases in the total group of treated women. Bromocriptine also normalised LH levels in a group of women with elevated follicular phase LH. Since the levels of LH observed in these women were similar to those observed by our group in women with polycystic ovarian disease (McConway et al., 1979) this may explain reports of successful bromocriptine therapy in patients with polycystic ovarian disease and normal PRL levels.

References

Coutts, J.R.T., Fleming, R., Carswell, W., Black, W.P., England, P., Craig, A. and Macnaughton, M.C. (1978): In: *Advances in Gynaecological Endocrinology*, p. 65, Editors: H. Jacobs. R.C.O.G., London.
Lenton, E.A., Sobonale, O.S. and Cooke, I.D. (1977): *Brit. Med. J., 2,* 1179.
McConway, M.G., England, P., Black, W.P., Macnaughton, M.C., Govan, A.D.T. and Coutts, J.R.T. (1979): In: *Research on Steroids, Vol. VIII,* p. 247. Editors: A. Klopper, L. Lerner, H.J. van der Molen and F. Sciarra. Academic Press, London.
Thorner, M.O., McNeilly, A.S., Hagen, C. and Besser, G.M. (1974): *Brit. Med. J., 2,* 419.
Wright, C.S., Steele, S.J. and Jacobs, H.S. (1979): *Brit. Med. J., 1,* 1037.

Prolactin response to nomifensine and deprenyl in hyperprolactinaemic polycystic ovary syndrome: further evidence for an oestrogen effect

P. FALASCHI, A. ROCCO, P. POMPEI, F. SCIARRA and G. FRAJESE

Clinica Medica V, Università di Roma, Italy

It is well known that prolactin (PRL) secreting pituitary adenoma is the most common cause of non-pharmacologically induced hyperprolactinaemia. However in about 27% of patients with the polycystic ovary (PCO) syndrome we found high basal plasma PRL levels (Falaschi et al., 1979). In most cases of hyperprolactinaemic PCO syndrome bromocriptine therapy was able to restore normal ovarian function and to improve peripheral hyperandrogenic symptoms together with the normalization of plasma PRL levels and a significant reduction of testosterone (T) and oestrone (E_1) levels (Rocco et al., 1979, 1980). Hyperprolactinaemic PCO patients show an exaggerated PRL response to TRH and dopamine (DA) blockade with haloperidol, strongly suggesting that elevated circulating oestrogen levels

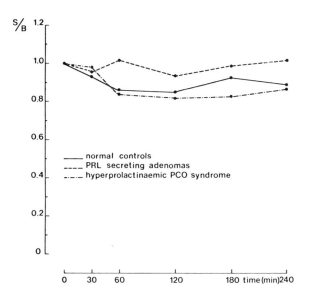

Fig. 1. Plasma PRL response to deprenyl (10 mg per os) in 10 women with hyperprolactinaemic PCO syndrome, in 10 female patients with PRL secreting adenomas and in 10 normal female controls (in terms of S/B ratio, mean).

sensitize the pituitary galactotrophs to oversecrete PRL (Falaschi et al., 1980). This excessive PRL response, in fact, is commonly observed in association with elevated circulating oestrogen levels (Buckman et al., 1976; Reymond and Lemarchand-Beraud, 1976; Guitelman et al., 1978).

Several pharmacological tests have been proposed to discriminate the so-called functional and tumoural hyperprolactinaemia (Barbarino et al., 1978; Fine and Frohman, 1978; Müller et al., 1978), most of which are based on the postulate that in PRL secreting pituitary adenomas a lack of presynaptic dopaminergic activity at hypothalamic level is present.

Nomifensine, for example, a DA reuptake inhibitor, which causes an increase of the DA concentration at the synaptic level, has been shown to reduce PRL levels in so-called functional and in puerperal hyperprolactinaemia, but not in PRL secreting adenomas (Müller et al., 1978).

In order to provide further information as to the mechanism involved in hyperprolactinaemia in PCO and to test our hypothesis on the oestrogen effect we studied the PRL response pattern to nomifensine and deprenyl in these patients. The latter drug is a MAO inhibitor (Yang and Neff, 1973), which blocks DA catabolism and increases the DA concentration at the synaptic level but via a different mechanism from nomifensine.

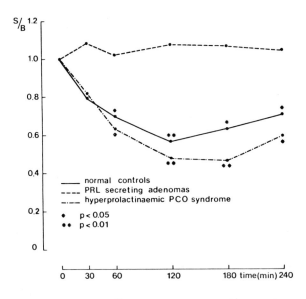

Fig. 2. Plasma PRL response to nomifensine (200 mg per os) in 10 women with hyperprolactinaemic PCO syndrome, in 10 female patients with PRL secreting adenomas and in 10 normal female controls (in terms of S/B ratio, mean).

Material and methods

Ten female patients with PRL secreting pituitary adenomas, aged 22-41 yrs, and 10 with hyperprolactinaemic PCO syndrome, aged 18-38 yrs, were studied. Ten normal female volunteers of comparable age were studied as controls in the follicular phase of the menstrual cycle. Diagnosis of pituitary adenoma was based on skull X-rays, CT scan and in 6 cases on surgical findings. Plasma PRL levels ranged between 25-3600 ng/ml. The patients with hyperprolactinaemic PCO syndromes were selected on the basis of the following parameters: hirsutism; oligo-amenorrhoea; enlarged ovaries (on laparotomy, laparoscopy, pelvigraphy or echography); high pulsatile LH levels with no midcycle peak; normal or low FSH levels; raised levels of T, androstenedione, dehydroepiandrosterone sulphate and E_1; normal or low levels of oestradiol; normal sella turcica. Blood for basal hormonal determinations (2 samples on different days) was drawn through a heparinized cannula inserted in an antecubital vein between 09.00 and 09.30 in rest conditions and after an overnight fast. Blood samples were collected between the 4th and 9th day of the menstrual cycle in normal subjects and in those presenting dysfunctional uterine bleeding. Blood samples were centrifuged at 3000 r.p.m. for 10 min and plasma obtained stored at $-20°C$. Plasma PRL, LH and FSH levels were determined by a double antibody radio-immunoassay (RIA) method using Biodata (Milan) reagents; plasma T levels were evaluated according to Sciarra et al. (1976) by a RIA method; plasma oestradiol levels were determined using Biodata kits and plasma E_1 levels were determined using Biodata antiserum antioestrone 3BSA. All blood samples of the same subject were evaluated in the same assay series.

All subjects, after basal hormonal assessment, were tested with nomifensine (Hoechst, Milan) at a dose of 200 mg per os and deprenyl (Chinion) at a dose of 10 mg per os. Vein blood was drawn through a cannula inserted into a forearm at time -45, -30, -15, 0 (drug administration), 30, 60, 120, 180 and 240 min. No relevant side effects were observed during the tests.

The results are expressed as the ratio between plasma PRL levels at each time period (S) and baseline (B) levels. The normal female range in our laboratory is up to 15 ng/ml.

Results and conclusions

The administration of deprenyl induced a slight, but not significant decrease in PRL in controls and in hyperprolactinaemic PCO. No change was observed in the group of patients with PRL secreting adenoma (Fig. 1).

Nomifensine significantly decreased PRL levels, in terms of S/B ratio, in the control subjects and in the PCO patients. Most patients with PRL secreting adenomas did not respond to the drug; only 2 cases showed a decrease in PRL levels.

TABLE 1.

Plasma PRL response (ng/ml) to nomifensine (NFS) (200 mg per os) and deprenyl (DEP) (10 mg per os) in 10 patients with hyperprolactinaemic PCO syndrome

Case	Drugs	Time (min)								
		−45	−30	−15	0	30	60	120	180	240
1	NFS	−	−	28.9	28.1	32.8	19.3	16.0	14.5	24.5
	DEP	−	−	40.0	36.1	36.9	32.0	30.0	28.7	30.6
2	NFS	−	−	32.7	29.0	29.7	26.5	26.8	28.3	29.1
	DEP	−	−	35.0	31.0	33.4	29.5	25.6	28.1	28.9
3	NFS	−	−	42.5	23.7	20.7	18.9	8.6	11.7	13.4
	DEP	−	−	30.3	26.0	26.8	24.7	22.1	19.1	23.3
4	NFS	−	−	17.4	18.8	13.4	10.7	10.7	5.0	21.4
	DEP	−	−	28.6	27.0	23.4	20.3	19.4	16.4	16.4
5	NFS	32.1	25.8	27.2	29.5	18.5	15.1	10.3	15.2	15.3
	DEP	33.0	26.9	29.0	25.2	26.5	20.0	20.8	22.6	27.9
6	NFS	23.5	17.9	21.9	19.3	20.1	12.2	9.0	9.3	8.1
	DEP	28.0	23.8	19.5	17.8	15.6	16.2	15.7	13.0	18.8
7	NFS	27.3	22.2	19.0	20.0	13.0	12.2	10.9	8.7	10.2
	DEP	19.0	24.3	23.3	20.7	18.7	14.7	16.5	16.6	20.5
8	NFS	15.9	18.8	16.3	17.4	8.4	8.7	8.4	7.4	8.8
	DEP	30.0	28.8	25.1	25.6	21.2	19.1	20.5	21.0	19.0
9	NFS	37.4	30.7	31.8	24.7	17.8	14.3	9.2	8.8	7.6
	DEP	33.0	24.2	21.8	20.7	24.3	16.3	15.0	17.8	15.6
10	NFS	29.1	32.4	41.0	26.0	23.5	16.5	6.8	8.2	7.5
	DEP	18.0	20.8	17.0	21.5	16.4	19.2	18.0	22.2	17.7

Table 1 shows the plasma PRL response, in terms of ng/ml, to nomifensine and deprenyl in individual subjects with hyperprolactinaemic PCO syndrome.

Evidence has been reported in the literature (Fine and Frohman, 1978; Müller et al., 1978; Van Loon et al., 1979), indicating that patients with PRL secreting adenomas show a decreased presynaptic DA activity at hypothalamic level. This appears to be supported by the lack of effect of nomifensine in PRL tumours. It is not possible to exclude, however, that some PRL adenomas may be due to pathogenetic events at the pituitary level, such as, for example, microinfarctions of portal capillaries, in the presence of normal dopaminergic activity at hypothalamic level. This hypothesis could possibly explain the PRL suppressive effect of nomifensine in some cases of prolactinomas as reported by other groups (Crosignani et al., 1979; Faglia et al., 1979).

The PRL response to nomifensine in the individual PCO patients, showed in 9 out 10 subjects studied a significant PRL suppression similar to that observed in physiological puerperal hyperprolactinaemia (Müller et al., 1978).

In conclusion, in our series of hyperprolactinaemic PCO patients the normal sella turcica, the elevated circulating E_1 levels, the excessive PRL response to TRH and haloperidol (Lusofarmaco, Milan), the PRL suppression with nomifensine, in fact strongly suggest that in this syndrome the hyperprolactinaemia is the functional consequence of an oestrogen effect, since the PRL response to pharmacological stimuli is very similar to that observed in subjects with elevated circulating oestrogen levels.

References

Barbarino, A., De Marinis, L., Maira, G., Menini, E. and Anile, L. (1978): *J. Clin. Endocr.,* *47,* 1148.
Buckman, M.T., Peake, G.T. and Srivastava, L.S. (1976): *J. Clin. Endocr., 43,* 901.
Crosignani, P.G., Ferrari, C., Mattei, A. and Picciotti, M.C. (1980): In: *Central and Peripheral Regulation of Prolactin Function,* p. 287. Editors: R.M. MacLeod and V. Seapagnini. Raven Press, New York.
Faglia, G., Moriondo, P., Nissim, M., Beck-Peccoz, P., Travaglini, P. and Ambrosi, B. (1979): In: *First International Symposium on Neuractive Drugs in Endocrinology, Milan.*
Falaschi, P., Del Pozo, E., Rocco, A., Toscano, V., Petrangeli, E., Pompei, P. and Frajese, G. (1980): *Obstet. Gynec., 55,* 579.
Falaschi, P., Rocco, A., Sciarra, F., Toscano, V. and Frajese, G. (1979): In: *Research on Steroids, Vol. VIII. Serono Symposia Vol. 21,* p. 241. Editors: A. Klopper, L. Lerner, H. Van der Molen and F. Sciarra. Academic Press, London.
Fine, S.A. and Frohman, L.A. (1978): *J. Clin. Invest., 61,* 973.
Guitelman, A., Aparicio, N.C., Mancini, A. and Debeljuk, L. (1978): *Fertil. and Steril., 30,* 42.
Müller, E.E., Genazzani, A.R. and Murru, S. (1978): *J. Clin. Endocr., 47,* 1352.
Reymond, M. and Lemarchand-Beraud, T. (1976): *Clin. Endocr., 5,* 429.
Rocco, A., Falaschi, P., Pompei, P., Del Pozo, E. and Frajese, G. (1979): In: *Psychoneuroendocrinology in Reproduction, Developments in Endocrinology, Vol. 5,* p. 387. Editors: L. Zichella and P. Pancheri. Elsevier/North-Holland Biomedical Press, Amsterdam.
Rocco, A., Falaschi, P., Toscano, V., Petrangeli, E., Sciarra, F. and Frajese, G. (1980): In: *Proceedings of International Symposium on Paediatric and Adolescent Gynaecology. Serono Symposia.* In press.
Sciarra, F., Toscano, V., Concolino, G., Sorcini, G., Marocchi, A. and Conti, C. (1976): *Hormone Res., 7,* 16.
Van Loon, G.R., Appel, N., Kim, C. and Ho, D. (1979): In: *First International Symposium on Neuractive Drugs in Endocrinology, Milan.* Abstr. 30.
Yang, H.Y.T. and Neff, N.H. (1973): *J. Pharmacol. Exp. Ther., 187,* 365.

Discontinuous therapy with bromocriptine in hyper-prolactinemic patients with amenorrhea

D. FONZO, G. GALLONE, M. MANENTI, R. SIVIERI and F. CERESA

Istituto di Medicina Interna, Clinica Medica B, Università di Torino, Italy

The incidence of hyperprolactinemia in secondary amenorrhea ranges from 15 to 25% (Canales et al., 1976; Bergh et al., 1977) and galactorrhea is present in the majority of hyperprolactinemic patients (Bohnet et al., 1976; Sèppala et al., 1977; Shearman and Fraser, 1977; Vekemans et al., 1977; Thorner and Besser, 1978).

Hyperprolactinemia may occur in association with pituitary tumors, although these tumors are often small and difficult to diagnose. Other causes of hyperprolactinemia include hypothalamic disease, disease or disruption of the hypothalamic/hypophyseal stalk, primary hypothyroidism and intake of certain drugs which block dopamine receptors at pituitary level (e.g. phenothiazines, butyrophenones, benzamides (metoclopramide and sulpiride), and pimozide), or deplete the stores of dopamine (e.g. reserpine and α-methyldopa) or act through non-dopamine mechanisms at the pituitary level (e.g. estrogens and thyrotrophin releasing hormone). In a previous study, 66 consecutive cases with menstrual disturbances and galactorrhea, alone or associated, were divided according to plasma prolactin (PRL) and all hyperprolactinemic patients were treated with bromocriptine (2.5 mg three times daily) (Table 1). All patients menstruated within 74 days: in 22 patients (84%), the first menstrual flow initiated between the

TABLE 1.

Normo- or hyperprolactinemia in 66 consecutive cases of menstrual disturbances and/or galactorrhea

	PRL < 25 ng/ml	PRL > 25 ng/ml	Total
Hypo-oligomenorrhea	18	4	22
Amenorrhea	14	4	18
Galactorrhea	2	6	8
Hypo-oligomenorrhea and galactorrhea	0	8	8
Amenorrhea and galactorrhea	0	10	10
Total	34	32	66

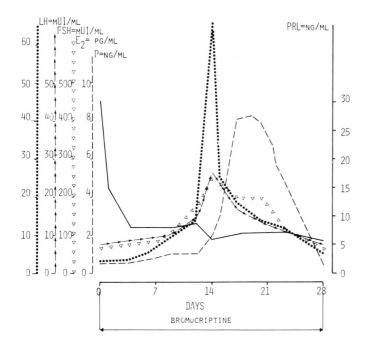

Fig. 1. Hyperprolactinemic patients: continuous treatment with bromocriptine (2.5 mg three times daily).

TABLE 2.

Hyperprolactinemic patients treated with bromocriptine (2.5 mg 3 times daily): interval between start of treatment and first menstruation

Patients menstruating between 24th and 31st day	22 (84%)
Patients menstruating after 31st day	4 (16%)
Total no. patients	26

24th and the 31st day of bromocriptine therapy, an interval which is the average duration of a normal menstrual cycle (Table 2).

Normalization of plasma PRL in these patients was followed by cyclic hormonal changes that closely mimicked a spontaneous ovulatory cycle, which apparently initiated with the beginning of bromocriptine therapy (Fig. 1).

Material and methods

In an attempt to elucidate the temporal relationships between hyperprolac-

tinemia and the neuroendocrine events leading to ovulation and to menstruation, we have studied the hormonal profile of 6 hyperprolactinemic patients
with secondary amenorrhea of at least 12 months duration. All patients had
been off therapy for at least 3 months, had a normal sellar profile and
menstruated within 31 days of continuous bromocriptine therapy (2.5 mg
three times daily) (Table 3).

After a few months of continuous therapy, bromocriptine was limited to
the first 10 days of the cycle and all endocrine parameters were measured.

Results and discussion

Table 4 shows that following bromocriptine withdrawal plasma PRL increased in all patients, but nevertheless normal menstrual flows occurred in
all subjects within 31 days.

All cycles were apparently ovulatory, since one patient was pregnant by

TABLE 3.

*Amenorrhea-galactorrhea patients treated with bromocriptine (2.5 mg 3 times daily con-
tinuous)*

Case	No.	PRL (ng/ml) basal	PRL (ng/ml) during therapy	First menses (day)
I.T.	1	34	8	31
B.F.	2	27	7	28
O.S.	3	31	6	27
C.T.	4	28	4	26
D.E.	5	47	5	30
M.G.	6	30	6	29

TABLE 4.

*Amenorrhea-galactorrhea patients: discontinuous bromocriptine treatment (2.5 mg 3
times daily for 10 days)*

Case	No.	PRL (ng/ml) during therapy (7th day)	PRL (ng/ml) following withdrawal of treatment (21st day)	Menses (day)
I.T.	1	4	32	pregnancy
B.F.	2	3	27	29
O.S.	3	6	35	31
C.T.	4	2	26	27
D.E.	5	6	42	28
M.G.	6	4	28	29

TABLE 5.

Clinical and hormonal findings in one patient with secondary amenorrhea

| Name: B.F. | Age: 30 | kg 71 | cm 166 |
| Married | Parity index: 0 | 0   0 | 0 |

Menstrual disturbances:	Secondary amenorrhea
	2 yrs 2 mths duration
Galactorrhea:	Present for 2 yrs 2 mths
Previous therapy:	None
Gynecological Ex.:	Normal
Sella X-ray:	Normal
Libido:	Decreased
Basal body temperature:	Monophasic

Basal hormonal profile

| | Weeks | | | |
	1	2	3	4
PRL (ng/ml)	32	25	34	27
FSH (mIU/ml)	5	7	4	3
LH (mIU/ml)	5	8	10	9
E_2 (pg/ml)	60	70	85	70
P (pg/ml)	570	390	460	380
Cortisol (μg/100 ml)	9	–	–	–
HGH (ng/ml)	3	–	–	–
TSH (μIU/ml)	4	–	–	–
T_4 (μg/100 ml)	11	–	–	–
Testosterone (ng/ml)	0.5	–	–	–

TABLE 6.

Continuous bromocriptine treatment (2.5 mg 3 times daily)

| B.F. age 30 yrs | Weeks | | | | | | | | |
| | | Bromocriptine | | | | | | | |
	4	5	6	7	8	9	10	11	12
PRL (ng/ml)	27	5	–	7	–	9	–	5	–
FSH (mIU/ml)	3	19	–	15	–	14	–	16	–
LH (mIU/ml)	9	15	–	12	–	16	–	9	–
E_2 (pg/ml)	70	70	–	205	–	80	–	170	–
P (pg/ml)	380	390	–	8500	6200	320	330	7400	6200
Galactorrhea	++	++	+	–	–	–	–	–	–

                                     ↑   ↑

                             Menses   Menses

the end of the cycle and the others showed a rise in progesterone in the second phase indicating the presence of a functioning corpus luteum. The hormonal profiles in one of these patients are reported as an example under basal conditions (Table 5), during continuous bromocriptine therapy (Table 6) and during discontinuous bromocriptine therapy (Table 7). Following bromocriptine withdrawal plasma PRL values increased and galactorrhea reappeared, but ovulation occurred in two consecutive cycles as is shown by the progesterone rise in the luteal phase.

These findings seemed to indicate that hyperprolactinemia inhibits ovulation and consequently menstruation, only when it is present in the first days of the cycle, as if the cyclic neuro-endocrine events, leading to follicle maturation and to ovulation, once started, can proceed automatically and independently from the surrounding endocrine situation.

TABLE 7.

Discontinuous bromocriptine treatment (2.5 mg 3 times daily) first 10 days of cycle

| B.F. age 30 yrs | Weeks | | | | | | | | |
| | Bromocriptine | | | | | Bromocriptine | | | |
	12	13	14	15	16	17	18	19	20
PRL (ng/ml)	–	3	2	27	32	6	4	28	35
FSH (mIU/ml)	–	6	–	7	–	5	–	6	–
LH (mIU/ml)	–	10	–	11	–	12	–	8	–
E$_2$ (pg/ml)	–	85	–	125	–	80	–	160	–
P (pg/ml)	6200	260	280	7400	6600	290	330	8200	7100
Galactorrhea	–	–	–	–	+	–	–	–	+
		↑ Menses				↑ Menses			↑ Menses

TABLE 8.

Amenorrhea-galactorrhea patients: discontinuous bromocriptine treatment (2.5 mg 3 times daily x 5 days)

| Case | No. | PRL (ng/ml) | | | | Menses (day) |
| | | During therapy (7th day) | Following withdrawal of treatment | | | |
			(14th day)	(21st day)	(28th day)	
C.T.	4	5	24	31	34	27
D.E.	5	8	31	40	46	28
M.G.	6	6	25	32	36	28

TABLE 9.

Clinical and hormonal findings in one patient with secondary amenorrhea

Name: C.T.	Age: 33	kg 62	cm 170
Married	Parity index: 2	0 0	2

Menstrual disturbances:	Secondary amenorrhea
	6 yrs duration
Galactorrhea:	Present for 6 yrs
Previous treatment:	hCG unsuccessful results
Discontinued:	For 2 yrs
Gynecological Ex.:	Normal
Sella X-ray:	Normal
Basal body temperature:	Monophasic

Basal hormonal profile

	Weeks			
	1	2	3	4
PRL (ng/ml)	27	25	28	26
FSH (mIU/ml)	3	11	5	8
LH (mIU/ml)	5	16	13	9
E_2 (pg/ml)	65	75	95	85
P (pg/ml)	250	330	480	840
Cortisol (μg/100 ml)	9	–	–	–
HGH (ng/ml)	2	–	–	–
TSH (μIU/ml)	6	–	–	–
T_4 (μg/100 ml)	8	–	–	–
Testosterone (ng/ml)	0.2	–	–	–

TABLE 10.

Continuous bromocriptine treatment (2.5 mg 3 times daily)

C.T.	Weeks									
		Bromocriptine								
age 33 yrs	4	5	6	7	8	9	10	11	12	13
PRL (ng/ml)	26	8	–	5	–	4	–	5	–	6
FSH (mIU/ml)	8	8	–	10	–	12	–	10	–	11
LH (mIU/ml)	9	10	–	8	–	12	–	7	–	11
E_2 (pg/ml)	135	95	–	130	–	150	–	130	–	150
P (pg/ml)	840	610	590	6500	8200	310	590	2200	6900	1500
Galactorrhea	+	+	–	–	–	–	–	–	–	–

                 ↑   ↑

         Menses   Menses

To further investigate this hypothesis bromocriptine treatment was reduced in 3 of the patients and limited to the first 5 days of the cycle. As shown in Table 8 plasma PRL levels, which were normal during bromocriptine treatment, increased following withdrawal, from the second week of the cycle. Nevertheless all patients menstruated in due time, even if in some instances low progesterone levels indicated impaired luteal function.

Since the basal temperature diagrams did not show a biphasic profile in all cycles studied, the question might be raised whether ovulatory cycles were always present in every patient.

The hormonal profile of one of these patients is reported as an example

TABLE 11.

Bromocriptine treatment (2.5 mg 3 times daily) first 10 days of cycle

C.T. age 33 yrs	Weeks								
	Bromocriptine					Bromocriptine			
	14	15	16	17	18	19	20	21	22
PRL (ng/ml)	6	3	2	20	26	5	7	22	30
FSH (mIU/ml)	11	8	–	7	–	12	–	9	–
LH (mIU/ml)	11	7	–	9	–	10	–	9	–
E$_2$ (pg/ml)	150	90	–	160	–	60	–	140	–
P (pg/ml)	1500	380	320	8400	6200	510	480	5100	6200
Galactorrhea	–	–	–	–	–	–	–	–	–
		↑ Menses				↑ Menses			↑ Menses

TABLE 12.

Bromocriptine treatment (2.5 mg 3 times daily) first 5 days of cycle

C.T. age 33	Weeks								
	Bromocriptine					Bromocriptine			
	22	23	24	25	26	27	28	29	30
PRL (ng/ml)	30	5	24	31	34	6	18	28	32
FSH (mIU/ml)	–	7	–	11	–	8	–	9	–
LH (mIU/ml)	–	9	–	10	–	8	–	8	–
E$_2$ (pg/ml)	–	80	–	200	–	100	–	140	–
P (pg/ml)	6200	420	510	2700	3200	400	310	3100	2000
Galactorrhea	–	–	–	–	–	–	–	–	–
		↑ Menses				↑ Menses			↑ Menses

prior to therapy (Table 9), during continuous bromocriptine treatment (Table 10), during the 10 days- (Table 11) and, finally, during the 5 day-schedule (Table 12).

PRL levels promptly increased every time bromocriptine was discontinued, but, even if progesterone levels in the luteal phase were slightly lower than normal, menstrual flows occurred in due time for two consecutive months.

A tentative explanation for our findings can be based on the observation that 17β-estradiol levels were low in our hyperprolactinemic patients, and did not show any consistent rise during the basal period of observation. In this condition the estrogenic impregnation of the hypothalamus might be insufficient for the local synthesis of catecholestrogens in the concentration needed to prevent norepinephrine catabolism, in order to stimulate gonadotropin release (Yen et al., 1974; Fishman and Norton, 1975; Wang and Yen, 1975; Paul and Axelrod, 1977).

The lowering of PRL in the first days of the cycle could allow the physiological rise of 17β-estradiol with hypothalamic estrogenic impregnation, leading to the cascade mechanism which, through the amplification of a cyclic neuroendocrine signal, exerts automatically the peak release of LH and ovulation (Fuxe and Eueroth, 1977; Müller and Nistico, 1978). Once started, the cascade of neuroendocrine events cannot be altered by a new PRL rise. In our experience the rise in PRL which follows bromocriptine withdrawal may only limit the corpus luteum secretion of progesterone.

References

Bergh, T., Nillius, S.J. and Wide, L. (1977): *Acta Endocr. (Kbh.), 86.*

Bohnet, H.G., Dahleu, H.G., Wuttke, W. and Schneider, H.P.G. (1976): *J. Clin. Endocr., 42,* 132.

Canales, E.S., Forsbach, G., Soria, J. and Zarate, A. (1976): *Fertil. and Steril., 27,* 1335

Fishman, J. and Norton, B. (1975): *Endocrinology, 96,* 1054.

Fuxe, K. and Eueroth, P. (1977): *Brain Res., 122,* 177.

Müller, E.E. and Nistico, G. (1978): *Neurotransmitters and Anterior Pituitary Function.* Academic Press, New York.

Paul, S.M. and Axelrod, J. (1977): *Science, 197,* 657.

Seppala, M., Lehtovita, P. and Rauta, T. (1977): *Acta Endocr. (Kbh.), 86,* 457.

Shearman, R.P. and Fraser, I.S. (1977): *Lancet, 1,* 1195.

Thorner, M.O. and Besser, G.M. (1978): *Acta Endocr. (Kbh.), Suppl. 216, 88,* 131.

Vekemans, M., Delvoye, P., L'Hermite, M. and Robyn, C. (1977): *J. Clin. Endocr., 44,* 989.

Wang, C.F. and Yen, S.S.C. (1975): *J. Clin. Invest., 55,* 201.

Yen, S.S.C., Vanden Berg, G. and Siler, T.M. (1974): *J. Clin. Endocr., 39,* 170.

Failure of progesterone to enhance prolactin response to TRH in estrogen-treated oophorectomized women*

P.M. KICOVIC[1] , F. FRANCHI[2] and M. LUISI[2]

[1] *Reproductive Medicine Programme, Medical Research Unit, Organon, Oss, The Netherlands;* [2] *Scuola di Perfezionamento in Endocrinologia ed Unità Endocrinologica del Consiglio Nazionale delle Ricerche, Università di Pisa, Pisa, Italy*

Estrogens play an important role in regulating prolactin (PRL) secretion at pituitary (Ajika et al., 1972) and hypothalamic (Meites, 1970) levels. However, changes in both basal levels of PRL (Friesen et al., 1972; L'Hermite et al., 1972; Franchimont et al., 1976) and the TRH-stimulated PRL release (Tyson and Friesen, 1973; McNeily and Hagan, 1974; Lemarchand-Béraud et al., 1977; Boyd and Sanchez-Franco, 1977) at different times of the menstrual cycle remain controversial. The reason for the discrepancies is not clear. In a recent study, Boyd and Sanchez-Franco (1977) found a significantly greater TRH-stimulated PRL response on day 21-22 than on day 7-8 of the menstrual cycle, but two very recent studies (Rutlin et al., 1977; Lachelin and Yen, 1978) have shown that estrogen treatment of post-menopausal women has no significant effect on the PRL response to TRH administration (though a sharp rise in basal PRL levels did occur). We therefore thought it pertinent to investigate whether progesterone (P) might play a role in the augmentation of PRL release observed in the luteal phase. The present study was undertaken because no information is available on the effect of P on PRL in humans.

Material and methods

Six oophorectomized women aged 39-45 yrs volunteered for this study. All had been shown previously to be healthy on physical examination and detailed endocrine evaluation. They were free of any steroid treatment for at least 6 months prior to the present study and had low circulating baseline PRL (3.3-7.0 ng/ml).

The subjects were given 25 μg/day of ethinylestradiol (EE) orally for 8 days. During the last 48 hr of EE treatment P was administered by continuous i.v. infusion at a rate of 20 mg/24 hr. P was dissolved in

*Supported by the Consiglio Nazionale delle Ricerche (Rome). Grant No. 78.02319.04/115.1130.

propylene glycol, sterilized by filtration and dissolved in human serum albumin and normal saline.

TRH (200 μg) was given as a rapid i.v. injection 3 times, i.e. before EE (day 0), and on days 6 (EE) and 8 (EE + P). Plasma samples were obtained before and 20, 40, 60 and 120 min after the injection. During the P-infusion plasma samples were obtained at 2 hr intervals.

PRL was measured daily at 10.00 hr prior to, and during, treatment, and also following TRH. P was measured during P-infusion. PRL and P were measured by radioimmunoassay (RIA) using Biodata (Milan, Italy) test-kits (codes 1803 and 1884, respectively). Plasma samples were frozen until assayed. All assays were carried out in duplicate, at the same time and with the same batches of reagents. The intra-assay coefficient of variation for PRL was 3.8% and for P was 4.9%. Results were evaluated by means of Student's t-test.

Results

Table 1 shows the changes in mean basal levels of PRL on days 6 and 8. The basal PRL level increased significantly ($p < 0.01$) from 4.4 ± 1.7 (mean ± SD) to 9.0 ± 2.4 (on day 6) and 9.4 ± 1.7 (on day 8).

The PRL response to TRH on days 0 and 6 is illustrated in Figure 1. No significant difference was found in the mean $max_\triangle PRL$ (34.8 vs 39.5 ng/ml, both at 20 min) or in the cumulative response (1816.0 ± 385.5 vs 2180.8 ± 529.5 ng/ml/2 hr).

Intravenous infusion of P at a rate of 20 mg/24 hr over a period of 48 hr induced a sharp rise in mean plasma P, which was maintained at levels of between 16.3 ± 1.8 and 20.6 ± 3.0 ng/ml (Fig. 2).

Figure 3 shows TRH-stimulated PRL release on days 6 and 8. As can be seen, neither the mean $max_\triangle PRL$ (39.5 vs 38.8 ng/ml, both at 20 min) nor the cumulative response (2180.8 ± 529.5 vs 2225.7 ± 402.5 ng/ml/2 hr) was influenced by P-infusion.

TABLE 1.

Mean (±SD) plasma PRL levels (ng/ml) prior to (day 0) and during EE (day 6) and EE + P (day 8) administration

	Day 0	Day 6	Day 8
Mean	4.4	9.0*	9.4*
SD	1.7	2.4	1.7

*0.001 > p < 0.01.

Discussion

In the present experiment, the use of i.v. infusion of P, in an attempt to
simulate the P pattern seen during the luteal phase of normal menstrual
cycle, has disclosed that the high P levels of between 16 and 20 ng/ml,
maintained for 48 hr, did not augment the ability of the lactotroph of
estrogen-treated oophorectomized women to respond to TRH stimulation.
This finding agrees with data obtained in some previous studies in eugonadal

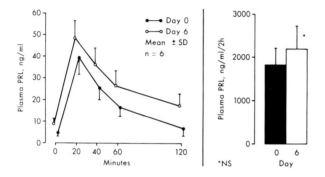

Fig. 1. Mean (±SD) plasma PRL levels during TRH tests on days 0 and 6 and
corresponding cumulative responses.

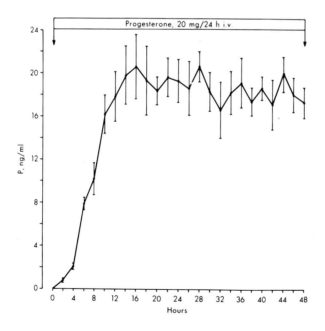

Fig. 2. Mean (±SD) plasma P levels during P-infusion.

women (Tyson and Friesen, 1973; McNeily and Hagan, 1974), thus indicating that PRL response to TRH did not vary throughout the menstrual cycle, i.e. that physiologically occurring changes in circulating E_2 and/or P do not enhance TRH-stimulated PRL levels. In a very recent study Sawin et al. (1978), who also measured E_2 and P levels, concluded that cyclic changes in these levels have indeed very little or no effect on the response. Others, however, have found enhanced PRL response to TRH during either the periovulatory (Lemarchand et al., 1977) or luteal phase (Boyd and Sanchez-Franco, 1977).

We confirmed that the PRL response to TRH is similar in post-menopausal and regularly menstruating women and that estrogen treatment did not induce a significantly greater TRH-stimulated PRL response, though basal PRL levels showed an exponential rise (Rutlin et al., 1977; Lachelin and Yen, 1978). Our data also indicate that the higher the basal PRL, the greater the $max_\triangle PRL$; nevertheless, these differences did not reach significant levels, at least within the present experimental design.

The role of P and other circulating steroids in the control of PRL secretion in humans should be investigated further. In ovariectomized rats large doses of P partially counteract the stimulatory effect of estrogen (Chen and Meites, 1970), and this has recently been confirmed in 'in vitro' experiments (Labrie, 1979) with pre-incubation of rat anterior pituitary cells with steroids, which showed that progestins and androgens could reverse the anti-dopamine effect of estrogens on PRL secretion at the pituitary level. Since, in the present experiment, the effect of P was studied in estrogen-pretreated women, and the P-infusion was of relatively short duration, it is unlikely that an inhibitory effect of P on PRL secretion and/or release would be detected. Therefore we have recently begun a series of experiments to investigate further the effects of P on the lactotroph in hypogonadal and post-menopausal women without estrogen pretreatment.

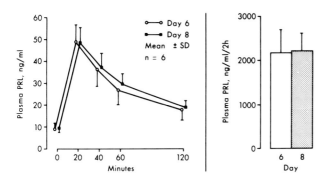

Fig. 3. Mean (±SD) plasma PRL levels during TRH tests on days 6 and 8 and corresponding cumulative responses.

References

Ajika, K., Krulich, L., Fawcett, C.P. and McCann, S.M. (1972): *Neuroendocrinology, 9,* 304.

Boyd, A.E., III and Sanchez-Franco, F. (1977): *J. Clin. Endocr., 44,* 985.

Chen, C.L. and Meites, J. (1970): *Endocrinology, 86,* 503.

Franchimont, P., Dourcy, C., Legros, J.J., Reuter, A., Vrindts-Gevaert, Y., v. Cauwenberge, J.R. and Gaspard, U. (1976): *Clin. Endocr., 5,* 643.

Friesen, H., Hwang, P., Guyda, H., Tolis, G., Tyson, J. and Myers, U. (1972): In: *Prolactin and Carcinogenesis,* p. 64. Editors: A.R. Boyns and K. Griffiths. Alpha Omega Alpha, Cardiff.

L'Hermite, M., Delvoye, P., Nokin, J., Vekemans, M. and Robyn, C. (1972): In: *Prolactin and Carcinogenesis,* p. 81. Editors: A.R. Boyns and K. Griffiths. Alpha Omega Alpha, Cardiff.

Labrie, F. (1979): In: *Abstracts of Lectures,* No. 9. IVth Intern. Symp. of the J. Steroid Biochem. "Recent Advances in Steroid Biochemistry", Paris.

Lachelin, G.C.L. and Yen, S.S.C. (1978): *J. Clin. Endocr., 46,* 369.

Lemarchand-Beraud, Th., Reymond, M. and Berthier, C. (1977): *Ann. Endocr. (Paris), 38,* 379.

McNeily, A.S. and Hagan, C. (1974): *Clin. Endocr., 3,* 427.

Meites, J. (1970): In: *Hypophysiotropic Hormones in the Hypothalamus,* p. 261. Williams and Wilkins, Baltimore.

Rutlin, E., Haug, E. and Torjesen, P.A. (1977): *Acta Endocr. (Kbh.), 84,* 23.

Sawin, C.T., Hershman, J.M., Boyd, A.E., III, Longcope, C. and Bacharach, P. (1978): *J. Clin. Endocr., 47,* 1296.

Tyson, J.E. and Friesen, H.G. (1973): *Amer. J. Obstet. Gynec., 116,* 337.

Effects of mid-cycle metoclopramide treatment on human menstrual cycle*

R. FLEMING[1], A. CRAIG[2], D.H. BARLOW[1] and J.R.T. COUTTS[1]

[1] *Department of Obstetrics and Gynaecology, Royal Maternity Hospital, Glasgow University, Rottenrow, Glasgow;* [2] *Clinpath Services Limited, High Wycombe, Bucks, U.K.*

Hyperprolactinaemia is a condition connected with both anovulatory (Bohnet et al., 1975) and ovulatory infertility (del Pozo et al., 1977) but the specific functions of prolactin (PRL) and its hypersecretion remain to be clarified. 'In vitro' evidence from McNatty et al. (1974) suggested that high concentrations of PRL caused inhibition of progesterone (P) biosynthesis by cultured human granulosa cells from a mature follicle. Hyperprolactinaemic anovulatory infertility, on the other hand, is usually associated with lowered gonadotrophin levels indicating a suppression of pituitary output of follicle stimulating hormone (FSH) and luteinising hormone (LH) in the presence of low concentrations of oestradiol (OE_2) (Bohnet et al., 1975). Strauck et al. (1977) produced data suggesting that hyperprolactinaemia in anovulatory women inhibited follicular development. There is considerable evidence, therefore, supporting pathological roles for hyperprolactinaemia at both ovarian and hypothalamo-pituitary levels. The involvement of hyperprolactinaemia in infertile women with normal menstrual rhythm is complicated and requires clarification. Although high PRL levels have been observed in a small group of patients with deficient luteal phases, hormonal measurement through complete menstrual cycles revealed a low incidence of long term hyperprolactinaemia (Coutts et al., 1978). However, in the latter study, a considerable proportion of the patients showed transient hyperprolactinaemia, with the highest frequency in the luteal phase. By dividing the cycle into the 4 compartments of follicular phase, mid-cycle, early luteal phase and late luteal phase, the correlations between mean PRL concentrations and 'total' OE_2 and P levels were assessed. The 'total' steroid levels were determined by summing all the respective OE_2 or P values within that phase. Linear regression analysis of these data showed no significant direct correlation between mean PRL levels and circulating steroid levels within any phase of the cycle (Table 1). However, indirect correlations were observed between mean mid-cycle PRL concentrations and reduced total late luteal levels of OE_2 and P (Fig. 1) indicating an association between mid-cycle hyperprolactinaemia and the short luteal phase. Patients with mid-cycle hyperprolactinaemia (mean concentration > 580 IU/l) had signi-

*This work was supported by a grant from Sandoz Laboratories (U.K.) Limited.

TABLE 1.

Correlations between mean prolactin concentrations and total levels of progesterone and 17β-oestradiol at different stages of the menstrual cycle**

		Total 17β-oestradiol				Total progesterone			
		F	M	EL	LL	F	M	EL	LL
Mean PRL	F	*	*	*	*	*	*	*	*
	M		*	*	−0.67		*	*	−0.44
	EL			*	*			*	*
	LL				*				*

*Correlation not significant.
**F = follicular phase (Days −12 to −3); M = mid-cycle (Days −2 to +2); EL = early luteal phase (Days +3 to +8 − PRL: Days +1 to +8 − steroids); LL = late luteal phase (Day +9 to end of cycle).

ficantly shorter luteal phases than those with normoprolactinaemia at mid-cycle (p < 0.01).

To investigate this association further, we have studied the effect of metoclopramide induced transient hyperprolactinaemia at mid-cycle in volunteers with normal menstrual history.

Material and methods

Blood samples

Each volunteer gave daily plasma samples for 2 consecutive menstrual cycles; the first was a control cycle and in the second metoclopramide (Maxolon®, Beecham Research Laboratories, 10 mg, 3 x daily) was administered for 6

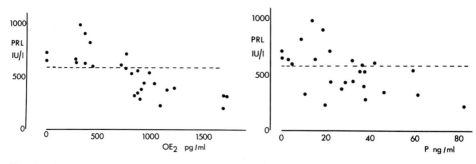

Fig. 1. Correlations between mean mid-cycle prolactin concentrations and late luteal phase steroid levels.

days over the estimated mid-cycle period. This treatment schedule was considered sufficient to maintain hyperprolactinaemia over 24 hr for the full 6-day period (Healy and Burger, 1977).

Hormone assays

Each sample was estimated for PRL, FSH, LH, OE_2 and P by specific radioimmunoassays. To avoid errors due to interassay variation all samples from each volunteer were analysed in the same assay for protein hormones and the samples from both luteal phases from one subject were assayed simultaneously for steroid hormones.

Results

Five subjects showed induced hyperprolactinaemia during the mid-cycle period; one subject from days −6 to −2, the last day of which was the first of the mid-cycle period, and the other 4 subjects over the whole mid-cycle

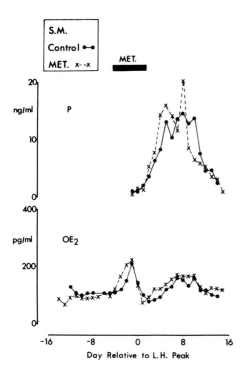

Fig. 2. Comparison between progesterone and oestradiol levels in control (−●——●−) and treatment (X−−X−−) cycles of a volunteer who took metoclopramide at mid-cycle.

TABLE 2.

Effects of mid-cycle metoclopramide on the positive feedback release of LH and FSH

Cycle	LH (IU/l)	FSH (IU/l)
Control*	137 ± 29 (S.D.)	45 ± 24 (S.D.)
Metoclopramide treatment*	120 ± 28 (S.D.)	40 ± 21 (S.D.)

*n = 5.

TABLE 3.

Effect of mid-cycle metoclopramide on total late luteal phase steroid levels

	Control cycle*	Metoclopramide treated cycle*
Total OE$_2$ (pg)	505 ± 156 (S.D.)	478 ± 188 (S.D.)
Total P (ng)	18 ± 9.4 (S.D.)	24 ± 5.9 (S.D.)

*n = 5.

TABLE 4.

Effect of mid-cycle metoclopramide on luteal phase length

Cycle	Luteal phase (days)
Control*	12.6 ± 1.5 (S.D.)
Metoclopramide treatment*	12.4 ± 1.9 (S.D.)

*n = 5.

period (days −2 to +2). The PRL concentrations induced by metoclopramide, estimated in the daily single samples, during treatment, ranged from 750 to 5,360 IU/l with a mean value of 2,495 ± 1,376 (S.D.) IU/l.

The effects of mid-cycle metoclopramide upon the positive feedback peaks of LH and FSH were studied by comparing the respective profiles before and during treatment in these 5 patients. The peaks were estimated by summing the respective gonadotrophin values for the mid-cycle period and there was no significant difference (Student's t test, unpaired data) between the control and treatment cycles (Table 2). The LH data analysed by Student's t test, paired data, were significantly lowered on metoclopramide (p < 0.01) but with these small sample numbers the physiological significance is debatable and in no case was the positive feedback eliminated.

The effects of mid-cycle metoclopramide on the steroid profiles of one typical subject are shown in Figure 2. There was no difference in either the peri-ovulatory or the late luteal steroid hormone profiles.

Late luteal steroid production was estimated by summing the daily concentrations of the respective hormones (OE_2 and P) observed from days +9 to the end of the luteal phase (the day when $P < 1.5$ ng/ml) inclusive. These data from control and metoclopramide treated cycles were compared (Table 3) and show no significant difference for either total late luteal OE_2 or P. Table 4 shows that metoclopramide treatment at mid-cycle had no effect upon luteal phase length.

Discussion

Delvoye et al. (1974) showed that sulpiride induced hyperprolactinaemia (over a prolonged period in normally menstruating women) climinated or reduced both the mid-cycle positive feedback peaks of LH and FSH and also luteal phase P levels. Luteal length was also shortened by sulpiride treatment which was initiated in the late follicular phase. In contrast, our results, using metoclopramide, failed to demonstrate a failure of positive feedback and neither follicular maturation, represented by pre-ovulatory OE_2 levels, nor luteal phase P profiles were affected. Glass et al. (1975) demonstrated a failure of positive feedback in hyperprolactinaemic anovulatory patients given oestrogen provocation tests. The present results suggest that this effect may not be due directly to the immediate PRL concentrations. The association between mid-cycle hyperprolactinaemia and short luteal phases (Coutts et al., 1978) is an indirect relationship which may reflect on the aetiology of the hyperprolactinaemia rather than as a consequence thereof.

References

Bohnet, H.G., Dahlen, H.G., Wuttke, W. and Schneider, H.P.G. (1975): *J. Clin. Endocr.*, *42*, 1114.

Coutts, J.R.T., Fleming, R., Carswell, W., Black, W.P., England, P., Craig, A. and Macnaughton, M.C. (1978): In: *Advances in Gynaecological Endocrinology*, p. 65. Editor: H.S. Jacobs. R.C.O.G., London.

Del Pozo, E., Wyss, H., Lancranjan, I., Obolensky, W. and Varga, L. (1977): In: *Ovulation in the Human*, p. 297. Editors: P.G. Crosignani and D.R. Mishell. Academic Press, London-New York.

Delvoye, P., Taubert, H.D., Jurgensen, O., L'Hermite, M., Delogne, J. and Robyn, C. (1974): *Acta Endocr. (Kbh.), Suppl., 184*, 110.

Glass, M.R., Shaw, R.W., Butt, W.R., Logan-Edwards, R., London, D.R. (1975): *Brit. Med. J., 3*, 274.

Healy, D.L. and Burger, H.G. (1977): *Clin. Endocr., 7*, 195.

McNatty, K.P., Sawers, R.S. and McNeilly, A. (1974): *Nature (Lond.), 250,* 653.
Strauch, G., Bonnefous, S., Paulian, B., Zaks, P., Pages, J.P. and Bricaire, H. (1977): In: *International Symposium on Prolactin, Nice,* p. 29. Editors: C. Robyn and H. Harter. Excerpta Medica, Amsterdam.

Relationship between hormonal status and clinical response in human fibrocystic disease

F. FRAIOLI[1], V. LA VECCHIA[1], F. VITA[1], F. SANTORO[3], C. ORZI[2] and L.R. MARCELLINO[2]

Istituto di V Clinica Medica, Università di Roma; [1] *Ospedale S. Camillo De Lellis, Ia Divisione Ostetrico Ginecologica, Roma;* [2] *Centro Tumori 'E. Medi' del Comune di Roma; and* [3] *RADIM, Laboratori di Ricerca, Pomezia (Roma), Italy*

The relationship between serum prolactin (PRL) and benign breast tumor mainly fibrocystic disease has not yet been fully elucidated and suitable treatment remains therefore to be established.

Some authors have found high or high-normal serum PRL levels (Cole et al., 1977) while according to others normal levels are present (Boyns et al., 1973; Gorins and Netter, 1974). It is generally accepted that PRL plays a specific role in the breast and this is also confirmed by the finding that breast tissue has specific receptors for PRL (Friesen et al., 1973). Fibrocystic disease of the breast can occur at any age. It is generally believed that this condition affects patients with endocrine disorders but a review of the literature in this field has failed to reveal any evidence of modifications in the hormonal pattern in the etiology of this disease.

The aim of the present investigation was to ascertain whether any correlation exists between the hormonal status, particularly PRL levels, and this condition. In addition various treatment schedules were employed in order to investigate etiology from a pharmacological point of view.

Material and methods

Studies were performed over the last 4 years on 987 females with fibrocystic disease who came spontaneously to the Prevention of Cancer Center, Rome, as part of a population cancer screening program.

Diagnosis of fibrocystic disease was based upon the clinical picture and xerography and/or mammography. Of these patients 890 were aged between 30 and 45 yrs, the remainder were younger. 92% had normal menses or slight oligomenorrhoea, 8% had amenorrhea (Table 1). Blood samples collected in all menstruating patients during the early, middle and late phase of the cycle (or every 7 days for 3 weeks in the non-menstruating patients) were assayed for serum PRL, 17β-estradiol (E_2), progesterone and gonadotropin, by specific, sensitive radioimmunoassay (RIA) techniques. Results were vali-

TABLE 1.

Patients with fibrocystic disease studied

Under 30 years	97
Between 30 and 45 years	890
Total	987
With normal menstrual cycle or slight oligomenorrhea	908
With amenorrhea	79
Given traditional treatment	909
Given CB 154	78

dated in terms of inter- and intra-assay variations not exceeding 8% and 11%, respectively, as coefficient of variation.

As far as concerns treatment schedules, patients receiving conventional therapy were also given vitamins A and E, progesterone and ∝-methyl-diol, according to the clinical schedules generally used. Seventy-eight patients received 2.5 mg 2-bromo/ergocriptine (CB 154, Parolodel®, Sandoz) continuously t.i.d. for a period of 3 months. Patients were randomly allotted to these drugs on the basis of the physical examination and at the discretion of the experienced consultant.

All patients returned to the clinic each month for 6 months for control examinations. Improvement or remission of disease was assessed on the basis of clinical examinations and xerography and/or mammography carried out at the end of the 6 months observation period.

Results

The results of hormonal assays are expressed as percentage of the values obtained in the various stages of the cycle (Table 2). It can be seen that most of the patients had a normal profile of the hormones considered, but in 46% progesterone failed to rise and the cycle was considered anovulatory. PRL levels are shown in Table 3. It is important to stress the incidence of hyperprolactinemia. It should not be overlooked that this hyperprolactinemia is of a slight proportion (25 ± 6 ng/ml SD) and that some patients were taking minor psychotropic drugs.

Table 4 gives the results of CB 154 treatment in 78 patients divided into 2 groups: one with high PRL values, the other with normal or low values. As already pointed out therapy was effective in a large percentage of cases, independent of PRL values. The other patients in our series received different therapeutic schedules: namely treatment with vitamins A and E, progesterone, hCG and alpha methyldiol. Patients were randomly allotted to those drugs since no change was observed in the hormone pattern.

TABLE 2.

Hormone levels in patients under study

Menstrual phase	Early			Middle			Late		
	High	Normal	Low	High	Normal	Low	High	Normal	Low
FSH	6	85	9	11	60	29	5	91	4
LH	8	88	8	13	45	42	6	91	3
17β-Estradiol									
(E$_2$)	4	85	11	2	58	40	4	69	27
Progesterone	1	80	20	1	85	14	0	54	46

Results are expressed as % of patients presenting high, normal or low values for each hormone in the various phases of the cycle. Patients presenting a mid-cycle peak of FSH, LH and E$_2$ were considered normal. Patients presenting elevations of progesterone > 2 ng/ml in the late phase were considered normal.

TABLE 3.

Serum prolactin values in the present series

	Early			Middle			Late		
	High	Normal	Low	High	Normal	Low	High	Normal	Low
Prolactin	66	29	5	27	72	1	60	35	5

Values referring to severe hyperprolactinemia (100 ng/ml) were discarded. Results are expressed as percentage of patients presenting high, normal, or low values of serum PRL. Normal values were based on the normal range obtained in the healthy female population (4-16 ng/ml).

TABLE 4.

Results of treatment with 2-bromoergocriptine in 70 patients

Patients with high values of serum prolactin (36):

No response	5%
Improvement	60%
Complete recovery	35%

Patients with normal or low values of serum prolactin (42):

No response	8%
Improvement	52%
Complete recovery	40%

The percent improvement and/or recovery was about 55%, being significantly less than that obtained in the CB 154 treatment (data not shown).

Comment

The exact course of fibrocystic disease, one of the most common breast lesions is not yet completely understood. Although no experimental evidence has been provided to show the PRL dependence of the disease, it appears reasonable to speculate on a possible role of PRL in this condition.

Despite the fact that a large percentage of the present patients display slight hyperprolactinemia, no conclusion can be drawn, however, from our data, on a possible etiologic relation between serum PRL and fibrocystic disease of the breast. This is also supported by the fact that the improvement obtained following bromocriptine treatment seems to be independent of PRL levels. For the other hormones studied it was not possible to find any alteration which could be attributed to an etiologic role.

Nevertheless, administration of CB 154 seems, in our experience, to be the most effective treatment. Other studies are needed in order to better understand the mechanisms responsible for this improvement.

References

Boyns, A.R., Cole, E.N., Griffiths, K., Roberts, M.M., Buchan, R., Wilson, R.G. and Forrest, A.P.M. (1973): *Europ. J. Cancer, 9,* 99.
Cole, E.N., Sellwood, R.A., England, P.C. and Griffiths, K. (1977): *Europ. J. Cancer, 13,* 597.
Friesen, H.G., Tolis, G. and Shiu, R. (1973): In: *Human Prostaglandin,* p. 11. Editors: J.L. Pasteels and C. Robyn. Excerpta Medica, Amsterdam.
Gorins, A. and Netter, A. (1974): *Nouv. Presse Méd., 3,* 73.

Endocrinological and therapeutic remarks about hyperprolactinaemic amenorrhoea

A. VOLPE, ANNA MARGHERITA SASSONE, CARLA BARBIERI, R. PELLATI, E. DALLA VECCHIA, ANNA GRASSO, G. MACCARRONE and V. MAZZA

Istituto di Ostetricia e Ginecologia, Università di Modena, Modena, Italy

An investigation has been carried out on the efficacy of some hormonal dynamic tests to discriminate between functional hyperprolactinaemia and pituitary adenoma. Moreover the efficacy of bromocriptine in the treatment of hyperprolactinaemic disorders of the menstrual cycle has been investigated.

Material and methods

Studies were performed on 105 amenorrhoeic hyperprolactinaemic patients coming to our department over the last 2 years, representing 22.4% of 468 amenorrhoeic patients who consulted us during that period. Only 19 out of the 105 patients in our series presented galactorrhoea in addition to hyperprolactinaemic amenorrhoea. Skull stratigraphy revealed pituitary adenoma in 14 patients.

Basal levels of gonadotropins FSH, LH, prolactin (PRL), triodothyronine (T_3) and thyroxine (T_4) were evaluated, and dynamic tests such as GnRH (100 μg i.v.) and TRH (200 μg i.v.) stimulation were performed in each case. Tests with sulpiride (100 mg i.m.) and bromocriptine (2.5 mg per os) were performed in all subjects with adenoma; the former was also performed in 36 cases of functional hyperprolactinaemia and the latter in 30 of these cases. PRL levels during sleep were measured hourly and the electroencephalogram was continuously recorded in 3 cases with adenoma and in 2 with functional hyperprolactinaemia. Skull stratigraphy was performed in anteroposterior and lateral projections. FSH, LH, PRL, T_3 and T_4 levels were measured by radioimmunoassay using commercially available kits.

Results and discussion

All patients showed normal FSH and LH levels. In patients with adenoma PRL levels exceeded 50 ng/ml in all cases; 2 of these patients had a poor gonadotropin response to GnRH. PRL response to TRH stimulus was normal

TABLE 1.

Dynamic tests in patients with pituitary adenoma and functional hyperprolactinaemia

	Pituitary adenoma			Functional hyperprolactinaemia		
	No. cases	Normal response	% Normal response	No. cases	Normal response	% Normal response
Bromocriptine test (2.5 mg per os)	14	10	71	30	28	93
Nomiphensine test (200 mg per os)	5	1	20	6	4	66
TRH test (200 μg i.v.)	14	2	12	91	52	58
Sulpiride test (100 mg i.m.)	14	2	12	36	18	50

TABLE 2.

Effects of post-operative bromocriptine therapy in 5 patients with prolactin secreting adenoma

Name	Age (yrs)	PRL (ng/ml) before surgery	PRL (ng/ml) after surgery	Post-operative bromocriptine (mg/day)	Results
V.R.	27	1,900	1,500	7.5	Normalization ovulatory cycles after 12 weeks
S.V.	24	1,420	660	10	Normalization ovulatory cycles after 12 weeks
P.A.	21	1,300	140	5	Normalization ovulatory cycles after 8 weeks
C.A.M.	36	482	132	5	Pregnancy after 10 weeks (miscarriage at 11 weeks)
idem	idem	idem	idem	5	Pregnancy at 12 weeks (twin delivery at term)
B.C.	31	615	252	7.5	Normalization ovulatory cycles after 10 weeks

TABLE 3.

Clinical results of bromocriptine therapy in 9 patients with pituitary adenoma

Name	Age (yrs)	PRL (ng/ml) before therapy	Bromocriptine (mg/day)	Results
C.M.	27	75	5	Pregnancy after 8 weeks (miscarriage at 20 weeks)
idem	idem	idem	5	Pregnancy after 14 weeks
G.T.	28	110	5	Pregnancy after 3 weeks
D.M.S.	35	80	5	Normalization ovulatory cycles after 12 weeks
S.F.	30	180	7.5	Pregnancy after 2 weeks
D.L.G.	31	80	5	Normalization ovulatory cycles after 6 weeks
C.M.	23	250	10	Normalization ovulatory cycles after 6 weeks
M.R.	26	190	5	Normalization ovulatory cycles after 6 weeks
I.D.	32	210	7.5	Normalization ovulatory cycles after 12 weeks
M.A.	28	180	7.5	Pregnancy after 6 weeks

in 12% of patients with adenoma and in 58% of patients with functional hyperprolactinaemia. Similarly, the PRL response to sulpiride was normal in 12% of adenomas and 50% of patients with functional hyperprolactinaemia. Bromocriptine caused a normal PRL inhibition in 71% of adenomas and in 93% of cases with functional hyperprolactinaemia. The nomiphensine test was normal in 20% of adenomas and 66% of patients with functional hyperprolactinaemias (Table 1).

Variations in PRL levels during sleep were found in only one subject, with microadenoma, but who was normoprolactinaemic as a result of treatment with bromocriptine given before the test was performed; no PRL fluctuations during sleep were found in the other patients who were still hyperprolactinaemic.

From the above data we may conclude that those hormonal tests which have been reported to be always negative in cases of prolactinoma and positive in cases of functional hyperprolactinaemia (Jaffe et al., 1973; Van Verder et al., 1974; Müller et al., 1978) did not give the same results in our hands. In our opinion it is not possible to discriminate between the 2 conditions on the basis of the available hormonal tests only. Five out of 14 adenomas have been operated; amenorrhoea was still present until bromocriptine therapy was instituted (5 to 10 mg/day). Such treatment restored

330   *A. Volpe et al.*

ovulatory cycles after a period ranging from 8 to 15 weeks; one of these patients became pregnant twice; the first pregnancy ended in miscarriage, the second ended in delivery at term of normal twins as shown in Table 2. Bromocriptine 7.5 mg/day (average dose) was given in all other cases of microadenoma, and normal ovulatory cycles were observed within a few weeks. Four of these patients, although informed of the risks (Peillon et al., 1970; Kaplan, 1971; Child et al., 1975; Thorner et al., 1975; Jewelewicz et al., 1977) became pregnant and gave birth to normal babies at term (Table 3).

Bromocriptine therapy was effective in all cases of functional hyperprolactinaemia; galactorrhoea, when present, was eliminated and normal ovulatory cycles were re-established as demonstrated by progesterone assays. Nine of these patients conceived after a few weeks treatment and delivered normal babies at term.

References

Child, D.F., Gordon, H., Mashiter, K. and Jophin, G.F. (1975): *Brit. Med. J., 4,* 87.
Jaffe, R.B., Yven, B.H., Kaye, W.R. and Midgley, A.R. (1973): *Amer. J. Obstet. Gynec., 117,* 757.
Jewelewicz, R., Zimmerman, E.A. and Carmel, P.W. (1977): *Fertil. and Steril., 28,* 35.
Kaplan, N.M. (1971): *J. Clin. Endocr., 21,* 1139.
Müller, E.E., Genazzani, A.R., Camanni, F., Cocchi, D., Massara, F., Picciolini, E., Locatelli, V. and Molinatti, G.M. (1978): In: *International Symposium on Pituitary Microadenomas. Milano, 1978. Serono Symposia,* p.56.
Peillon, F., Vila-Porcile, F., Oliver, L., Racadot, J.A. (1970): *Ann. Endocr., 31,* 259.
Thorner, M.O., Besser, G.M. and Jones, A.E. (1975): *Brit. Med. J., 4,* 694.
Van Verder, K., Pickordt, C.R., Glockner, B., Rjosk, H.K., Gottsman, M. and Serba, P.C. (1974): *Acta Endocr. (Kbh.), Suppl. 184,* 108 (Abstract).

20α-Hydroxy/17α-hydroxyprogesterone relationships with prolactin and androgens in normal, hyperprolactinemic and hirsute women*

G. MAGRINI, F. MÉAN and J.P. FELBER

Division de Biochimie Clinique, Département de Médecine, C.H.U.V., Lausanne, Switzerland

17β-Estradiol, progesterone and androgens are produced at different rates by granulosa and/or theca cells depending on the stage of the menstrual cycle.

Progesterone (P) and 17α-hydroxyprogesterone (17αOHP) were shown to be major products of human granulosa cells from preovulatory Graafian follicles in control short-term cultures with endogenous and exogenous substrates (Fowler et al., 1978). On the other hand, high activity of 20α-hydroxysteroid-dehydrogenase (20αOHSD), as observed in the secretory phase of the human menstrual cycle, may lead to a decrease in intracellular P (Pollow et al., 1975). The metabolism of P into 20α-hydroxyprogesterone (20αOHP) may thus be a local regulator of P intracellular concentration and action.

It has also been reported that prolactin (PRL) may influence steroidogenesis in women and has therefore been implicated in abnormal ovarian functions. A biphasic action of PRL on P secretion in cultured human adrenal cells, as well as an enhanced androgen production in cultured human adrenal cells was reported (McNatty et al., 1974; McKenna, 1978). It was hypothesized that the immediate decline in serum P observed after prostaglandin induced luteolysis of rat ovary probably triggers an increase in pituitary PRL. This increase in PRL, in turn, stimulates 20αOHP production (Torjesen et al., 1978). However, this hypothesis conflicted with the inhibitory effect of PRL observed on 20αOHSD activity 'in vivo' (Strauss and Stambaugh, 1974; Lamprecht and Poyser, 1976) and 'in vitro' (Lahav et al., 1977).

As conflicting data on the possible effects of PRL on P metabolism and androgen secretion have appeared in the literature, P, androgen and cortisol (F) levels were measured in various groups of women presenting hyperprolactinemia of different origin or hyperandrogenic hirsutism. The ratios between individual androgens and between 20αOHP and 17αOHP were analyzed.

The results were compared with those obtained at different stages of the menstrual cycle in normal controls.

*Presented in part at the IV International Symposium on Radioimmunology, Lyon, April 19-21, 1979.

Material and methods

Eighteen women with hyperprolactinemia of various origin were studied: 8 hyperprolactinemic women (H-PRL) before, and 10 during bromocriptine treatment (H-PRL + CB) at the dose of 2.5 mg twice a day for 3 months. Plasma samples were obtained in middle-late follicular and/or luteal phase.

Two groups of normoprolactinemic hirsute women were also studied, each patient presenting elevation of at least one plasma androgen: 13 of these patients had normal menstrual cycles (HNC) and 19 irregular or no cycles (HIC). Plasma samples were obtained in the morning (8 a.m.) in the follicular phase.

Finally 20 normally menstruating women were investigated at different stages of the cycle: early (E: days 1-5), middle-follicular (M: days 6-9), periovulatory (P: days 10-15) and luteal (L: days 19-26) phases.

Plasma 20αOHP, 17αOHP, P, testosterone (T), androstenedione ($\triangle$4), dehydroepiandrosterone sulfate (D-S), F, 17β-estradiol (E2) and PRL were measured by specific radioimmunoassays (Magrini et al., 1979).

Results

The steroid profiles in the 20 normally menstruating women at different stages of their cycles are shown in Figures 1 and 2. A sharp reduction of the 20α/17α ratio was observed at the periovulatory phase (p < 0.01 vs early follicular), which inversely correlates with an increase in $\triangle$4 levels (p < 0.05 vs early follicular). E2 and P showed the well known pattern, but no significant variations were observed for the other steroids in this group of women. F, however, showed a tendency to decrease from the early follicular to the periovulatory phase and inversely D-S.

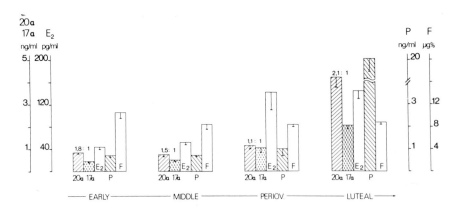

Fig. 1. Plasma 20α-hydroxy-progesterone (20α), 17α-hydroxy-progesterone (17α), estradiol (E$_2$), progesterone (P) and cortisol (F) in normally menstruating women during different stages of the cycle.

The results in the hyperprolactinemic patients are shown in Figure 3. The mean 20α/17α ratio decreased in the follicular phase from 1.9 (controls) to 0.9 in the H-PRL group (P = 0.025) but returned to 1.8 during bromocriptine treatment (H-PRL + CB; p < 0.025). In the luteal phase, the 20αOHP/17αOHP ratio changed respectively from 2.1 to 1.5 and 2.5, but not significantly.

In the follicular phase of the H-PRL group, the increase in mean levels of 17 OHP and △4 were highly significant compared with controls, being p < 0.001 and p < 0.05, respectively.

Alterations in steroid levels, although not statistically significant, appeared in the H-PRL group: the increase in △4 levels disappeared in the luteal phase; the slight mean increase in D-S levels in the follicular phase became pronounced during bromocriptine treatment but disappeared in the luteal phase of both groups.

The findings in the hirsute hyperandrogenic women are shown in Figure 4. The decrease in the 20αOHP/17αOHP ratio was not significant in the HNC group (from 1.9 in controls to 1.5). However, in the group HIC, the decrease became highly significant (from 1.9 to 1.1; p = 0.001). △4 and T were significantly elevated in both groups (p < 0.001) and especially in the HIC group. D-S was also significantly elevated (p < 0.02) but only in HIC.

Discussion

Significant variations in the 20αOHP/17αOHP ratio occur during the normal menstrual cycle: the sharp decrease in the periovulatory phase (1.1 vs 1.8 in the early follicular, p = 0.01) is mostly related to the 17αOHP increase at

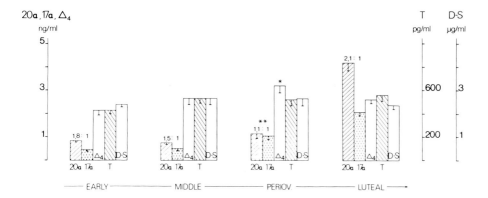

Fig. 2. Plasma 20α-hydroxy-progesterone (20α), 17α-hydroxy-progesterone (17α), androstenedione (△4), testosterone (T), and DHEA-sulfate (D-S) in normally menstruating women during different stages of the cycle. Statistical significance: *p < 0.05 vs early follicular; **p < 0.01 vs early follicular.

mid-cycle during the follicular development. A shift in the relative proportions of progestin formation seems then to occur in the periovulatory
phase, with a much higher increase in 17αOHP, compared to 20αOHP
production. The 20αOHP/17αOHP ratio returns to early follicular values
during the luteal phase (2.1) when the increase in 20αOHP production
appears to restore the balance. Mean values of the two hormones are in
agreement with those previously reported by other authors (Abraham et al.,
1977; Abraham, 1978). The decrease in the 20αOHP/17αOHP ratio
inversely correlates with the increase in △4 levels at mid-cycle. The pattern of
mean cortisol levels however does not seem to correlate with the adrenal
androgen D-S: the latter shows a slight increase at mid-cycle while, as
previously reported (Genazzani et al., 1977), the former tends to decrease.

Compared with controls, the mean 20αOHP/17αOHP ratio shows a sharp

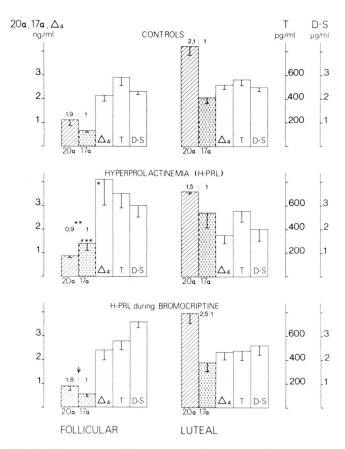

Fig. 3. Plasma steroid hormone levels in the follicular and luteal phase of the menstrual
cycle in hyperprolactinemic women before and during bromocriptine treatment (same
hormones measured as in Fig. 2). Statistical significance: *p $<$ 0.05 vs controls; **p =
0.025 vs controls; ***p $<$ 0.001 vs controls; Ψp $<$ 0.025 vs H/PRL.

decline in the hyperprolactinemic patients, which is statistically significant in the follicular phase. It returns close to control levels during bromocriptine treatment.

The decrease is mainly due to the highly significant rise in 17αOHP levels while the mean 20αOHP values show only minor changes.

This pattern is consistent with variations observed during the normal menstrual cycle where a marked reduction occurs in the 20αOHP/17αOHP ratio from the early to the periovulatory phase.

Moreover, △4 levels are significantly higher in the H-PRL group but return to control values after bromocriptine. The integrated values of △4, T and D-S show higher mean levels in the H-PRL group compared with controls and the H-PRL + CB group.

D-S is increased in the H-PRL patients in agreement with Bassi et al. (1977) and Vermeulen et al. (1977), but remains high during bromocriptine, probably on account of the relatively short period of observation. The increase in △4 and/or D-S levels in the follicular phase disappears in the luteal phase, apparently correlating with the parallel increase in the 20αOHP/ 17αOHP ratio, and particularly with the relatively greater increase in 20αOHP compared with 17αOHP formation. This change in the luteal phase appears to be accompanied by an overall decrease in the adrenal contribution to androgenic steroid production.

These findings, supporting possible modulating effects of hyperprolactinemia on the 20αOHP/17αOHP ratio and/or 17αOHP formation are in keeping with recent studies suggesting a possible role of PRL in regulating ovarian cell function and activity of 20αOHSD (McNatty et al., 1974; Lamprecht and Poyser, 1976; Torjesen et al., 1978).

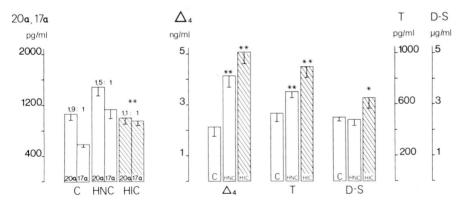

Fig. 4. Plasma steroid hormone levels in the follicular and luteal phase of the menstrual cycle in hirsute-hyperandrogenic women with normal (HNC) and irregular (HIC) cycles (same hormones measured as in Fig. 2). Statistical significance: *p < 0.02 vs controls; **p ⩽ 0.001 vs controls.

336   G. Magrini et al.

As far as concerns the H-PRL group, a similar behavior in the 20αOHP/17αOHP ratio and androgen levels is found in the hirsute patients, particularly in those with cycle disturbances. Comparing controls to HNC and HIC groups, in fact, a progressive decrease in the mean 20αOHP/17αOHP ratio ($1.9 - 1.47 - 1.09$; $p < 0.001$) is observed, accompanied by a rise in $\Delta 4$, T and D-S. Mean D-S in particular, is significantly increased only in the HIC group, in agreement with Abraham et al. (1975).

In conclusion, these findings suggest that in both conditions studied hypersecretion of PRL and/or androgens lead to a decrease in the 20αOHP/17αOHP ratio, and modulated ovarian and/or adrenal steroidogenesis, resulting in higher 17αOHP production.

Acknowledgements

The authors wish to thank G. Chiodoni, P. Bianchi, U. Reich and M.F. Planche for their excellent technical assistance, Dr. M. Gasperi for scientific assistance in editing the text and Miss M.C. Evraere for preparing the manuscript.

References

Abraham, G.E., Chakmakjian, Z.H., Buster, S.E. and Marshall, J.R. (1975): *Obstet. and Gynec., 46*, 2.
Abraham, G.E. (1978): In: *Endocrine Causes of Menstrual Disorders*, p. 15. Editor: J.R. Givens. Year Book Medical Publishers Inc., Chicago – London.
Abraham, G.E., Manlimos, F.J. and Garza, R. (1977): In: *Handbook of Radioimmunoassay*, p. 591. Editor: L.E. Abraham. Marcel Dekker Inc., New York – Basel.
Bassi, F., Giusti, G., Borsi, L., Cattaneo, S., Annotti, P., Forti, G., Pazzagli, M., Viginai, C. and Serio, M. (1977): *Clin. Endocr., 6*, 5.
Fowler, R.E., Fox, N.L., Edwards, R.G., Walter, D.E. and Steptoe, P.C. (1978): *J. Endocr., 77*, 171.
Genazzani, A.R., Magrini, G., Facchinetti, F., Romagnino, S., Pintor, C., Felber, J.P. and Fioretti, P. (1977): In: *Androgens and Antiandrogens*, p. 247. Editors: L. Martini and M. Motta. Raven Press, New York.
Lahav, M., Lamprecht, S.A., Amsterdam, A. and Lindner, H.R. (1977): *Molec. Cell. Endocr., 6*, 293.
Lamprecht, E.W. and Poyser, N.L. (1976): *Physiol. Rev., 56*, 595.
Magrini, G., Iselin, H., Ebiner, S.R. and Felber, J.P. (1979): *Arch. Androl., 2*, 141.
McKenna, T.J. (1978): In: *Endocrine Causes of Menstrual Disorders*. p. 371. Editor: J.R. Givens. Year Book Medical Publsihers Inc., Chicago – London.
McNatty, K.P., Sawers, R.S. and McNeilly, A.S. (1974): *Nature (Lond.), 250*, 653.
Pollow, K., Lubbert, H., Boqnoi, E. and Pollow, B. (1975): *J. Clin. Endocr., 41*, 729.
Strauss, J.R. and Stambaugh, R.L. (1974): *Prostaglandins, 5*, 73.
Torjesen, P.A., Dahlin, R., Hug, E. and Aakvaag, S. (1978): *Acta Endocr. (Kbh.), 87*, 625.
Vermeulen, A., Suy, E. and Rubens, R. (1977): *J. Clin. Endocr., 44*, 1222.

Androgen secretion and skin metabolism in hirsutism*

P. MAUVAIS-JARVIS, F. KUTTENN and I. MOWSZOWICZ

Department of Reproductive Endocrinology, Faculté de Médecine Necker-Enfants-Malades, Paris, France

Hirsutism in women may be defined as excessive hair growth in anatomical sites where such growth is considered to be a secondary male characteristic. This abnormality is related to increased activity of two androgen-dependent structures of human skin: the sebaceous gland and the hair follicle. From different studies it can be argued that hirsutism may arise from two causes: an increased secretion of active androgens by the adrenal glands or ovaries, and/or an increased utilization of androgens in the blood by the target cells of the skin. The first possibility has already been extensively reviewed by several authors (Bardin and Lipsett, 1967; Kirschner and Bardin, 1972). The raised metabolic clearance rate of testosterone reported by Bardin and Lipsett (1967) in hirsutism supports the second possibility. It results mainly from an increased metabolism of testosterone by extra-hepatic tissues as shown by the higher rate of conversion of testosterone to dihydro-testosterone (DHT) and 5α-androstane-3α,17β-diol (androstanediol, Adiol) in the blood of hirsute women than in that of normal women (Mahoudeau et al., 1971). This increased metabolic clearance rate of testosterone is facilitated by the low concentration of testosterone binding globulin in the plasma (TeBG) (Dray et al., 1968; Southren et al., 1969; Vermeulen et al., 1969) and a concentration of unbound testosterone in the plasma which is higher than normal (Rosenfield, 1972; Clark et al., 1975).

The pilosebaceous gland is a key androgen receptor, since all events involved in androgen activity in male accessory organs (prostate, seminal vesicles, etc.) have been described in this tissue. Indeed, the skin is capable of transforming free testosterone into DHT due to the 5α-reductase present in the microsomes (Voigt et al., 1970). A specific receptor for DHT has been isolated from human fibroblasts obtained in culture (Keenan et al., 1974). It is known further that human skin is capable of converting dehydro-epiandrosterone and especially androstenedione into testosterone and DHT (Gomez and Hsia, 1968). Skin thus appears to participate not only in the catabolism of androgens but also in the formation of active androgens from inactive precursors supplied through the blood (Fig. 1).

*This work was supported by grant No. 77.7.0969 from the Délégation Générale à la Recherche Scientifique et Technique.

Material and methods

The aim of our investigation was to examine the respective roles of overproduction of active androgens and excessive transformation of testosterone to 5α-reduced metabolites in the skin of women with hirsutism. Our study consisted of a hormonal investigation of 40 hirsute women compared with 20 normal women and 20 normal men of the same age. Among the 40 hirsute women were 12 patients with polycystic ovaries, 4 with adrenal virilism due to an acquired congenital hyperplasia and 24 women presenting with idiopathic hirsutism on the basis of purely clinical criteria (absence of menstrual abnormality, absence of signs of adrenal dysfunction).

In vivo, plasma testosterone, androstenedione and DHT were measured using radioimmunoassays (RIA) previously described (Kuttenn et al., 1977). Urinary androstanediol was determined by the RIA described by Wright et al. (1978).

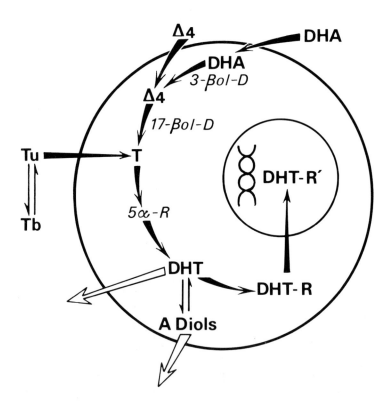

Fig. 1. Androgen metabolism in human skin. Tu = unbound testosterone (T); Tb = T bound to TeBG; △4 = androstenedione; Adiols = 3α- and 3β-androstanediols; R = cytosolic receptor; R_1 = nuclear receptor; 3β-ol-D = 3β-hydroxysteroid dehydrogenase; 17β-ol-D = 17β-hydroxysteroid dehydrogenase; 5α-R = 5α-reductase.

In vitro, 5α-reductase activity was measured in samples of 200 mg of pubic skin obtained under local anesthesia. The conversion of radioactive testosterone to DHT and androstanediols in skin homogenates was studied according to the method previously described (Kuttenn and Mauvais-Jarvis, 1975; Kuttenn et al., 1977).

Results

Polycystic ovary syndrome

The 12 patients studied had the clinical, anatomical, and hormonal features of polycystic ovary syndrome type I (Yen et al., 1970). Basal plasma LH level was 3 times higher than in normal women at the beginning of the follicular phase (Mauvais-Jarvis et al., 1978). After LHRH stimulation (100 μg i.v.) the peak LH level was excessively high (70.3 ± 10 mIU/ml) whereas FSH response was normal. As regards plasma androgens (Fig. 2) androstenedione was 3 times higher than in normal women (320 ± 20 ng/100 ml instead of 130 ± 20 ng/100 ml). Plasma testosterone and DHT were only slightly elevated. The urinary excretion of androstanediol was markedly increased (80 ± 25 μg/24 hr). Ovarian stimulation with 15,000 IU of hCG did not significantly elevate plasma T and DHT; however there was a slight but significant increase in plasma androstenedione and urinary androstanediol. In vitro, the calculated 5α-reductase activity in pubic skin homogenates (Fig. 3) was significantly higher than in normal women.

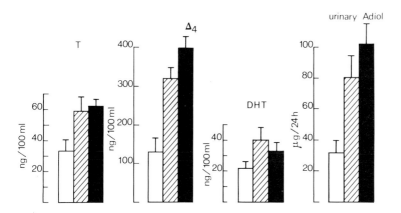

Fig. 2. Plasma testosterone (T), androstenedione (Δ4), DHT, and urinary androstanediol (Adiol) in 12 cases of polycystic ovarian syndrome (PCO). Normal women:⬜; PCO, base:▨ ; PCO, after hCG:⬛.

340   *P. Mauvais-Jarvis et al.*

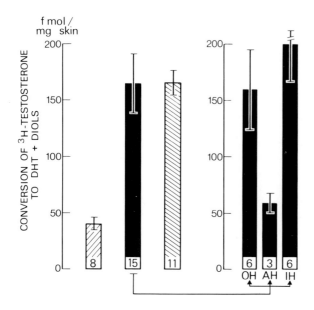

Fig. 3. Conversion rate of radioactive testosterone to 5α-reduced metabolites (DHT + androstanediols) in homogenates of pubic skin ▨: normal women; ◩: men; ▰:hirsute women; OH: hirsutism of ovarian origin (polycystic ovary syndrome); AH: hirsutism of adrenal origin (partial defect in 21-hydroxylase); IH: idiopathic hirsutism.

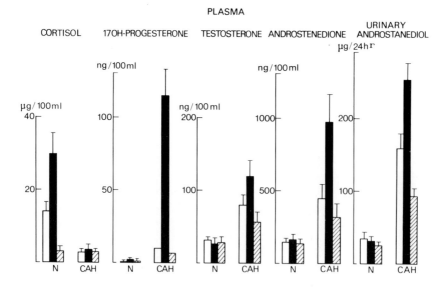

Fig. 4. Plasma steroids and urinary androstanediol in 4 patients with adrenal virilism due to a partial 21-hydroxylase deficiency (CAH) compared to 5 normal women (N). □ : baseline; ■ : after ACTH; ▨ : after dexamethasone.

Delayed onset congenital adrenal hyperplasia

Four cases of acquired virilism without abnormalities of the external genitalia and due to delayed onset congenital adrenal hyperplasia have been explored. The hormonal features observed in these patients aged 23-25 years were characteristic of partial 21-hydroxylase deficiency (Fig. 4). Indeed, 17-hydroxyprogesterone was only slightly elevated in basal conditions (9.0 ± 2.0 ng/ml), but increased dramatically after ACTH stimulation (125 ± 20 ng/ml). Plasma cortisol was low or normal but did not increase after ACTH. As regards circulating androgens, plasma testosterone was slightly elevated (80 ± 30 ng/100 ml) but increased after ACTH (120 ± 10 ng/100 ml). Plasma DHA and DHA sulfate were in the normal female range (Fig. 5). By contrast, plasma androstanedione was frankly elevated in basal conditions (420 ± 50 ng/100 ml) and increased significantly after ACTH stimulation (960 ± 60 ng/100 ml). Dexamethasone administration (2.5 mg daily for 5 days) completely suppressed the elevated plasma levels of 17-hydroxyprogesterone and androgens (Fig. 4).

In these patients the 5α-reductase activity calculated in vitro in pubic skin homogenates was not significantly increased when compared with results obtained in normal women (Fig. 3 and 5). However, the urinary excretion of androstanediol was very elevated in basal conditions (160 ± 50 μg/24 hr) and even more after ACTH stimulation (250 ± 50 μg/24 hr).

Idiopathic hirsutism

These 24 patients had abnormal hair growth of various degrees of density and extent. Their menstrual cycles were ovulatory; ovaries were normal at pelvic or culdoscopic examination. No abnormalities in the fractionated 17-ketosteroid excretion was noted after adrenal stimulation by ACTH or adrenal suppression by dexamethasone associated with ovarian stimulation by hCG. Plasma 17-hydroxyprogesterone was in the normal female range either in basal conditions or after ACTH stimulation. In these patients plasma testosterone was slightly higher than in normal women (51.1 ± 22 ng/100 ml). However this value was below that observed in patients with polycystic ovaries or adrenal virilism. By contrast plasma androstenedione was significantly elevated in all cases (203 ± 50 ng/100 ml). Here also, the observed values were lower than those in women with ovarian or adrenal hirsutism. On the other hand although the concentrations of DHT of the women with idiopathic hirsutism were higher than those of the normal women, they did not differ from the values of the women with ovarian or adrenal virilism. The urinary excretion of androstanediol (Fig. 6) was very significantly elevated in the women with idiopathic hirsutism compared with the normal women (137 ± 52 μg/24 hr instead of 44 ± 23 μg/24 hr). This value was, however, lower than that observed in the women with polycystic ovaries. Testosterone 5α-reductase activity measured in vitro (Figs. 3 and 6) was markedly elevated in the women with idiopathic hirsutism. The conversion of radioactive testosterone to DHT and androstanediols in these patients reached 200 fmol/mg skin. This figure is comparable to that observed in normal men. It differs significantly from that of the normal women. In addition it is clearly higher than that seen in adrenal virilism.

Discussion

In normal women about 70% of plasma testosterone is derived from prehormones, essentially dehydroepiandrosterone and androstenedione. Androstenedione is by far the most important prehormone, being the precursor of at least 50% of plasma testosterone (Horton and Tait, 1966). Thus the concurrent determination of plasma testosterone and androstene-

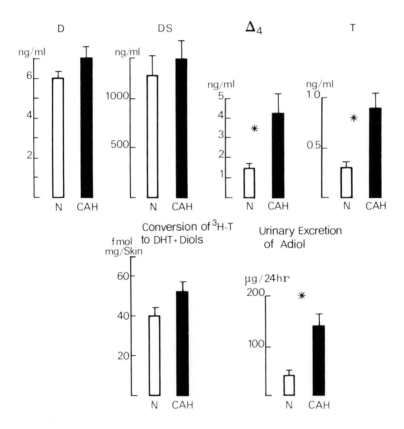

Fig. 5. Plasma dehydroepiandrosterone (D), dehydroepiandrosterone sulfate (DS), androstenedione (△4), testosterone (T), urinary androstanediol (Adiol) and conversion rate of radioactive testosterone 5α-reduced metabolites by pubic skin homogenates in 4 patients with partial 21-hydroxylase deficiency (CAH) compared to 5 normal women (N).

dione gives useful information about the production of active androgens in hirsute women.

Androstanediol and DHT are 2 potent androgens that do not seem to be secreted directly by the gonads or adrenal glands. In fact, DHT in the plasma is produced mainly by hepatic and extrahepatic 5α-reduction of testosterone and androstenedione (Ito and Horton, 1971; Mahoudeau et al., 1971) and the same assumption has been made regarding androstanediol in the urine (Mauvais-Jarvis et al., 1973; Wright et al., 1978). However, the various studies on the sources of plasma DHT, and plasma and urinary androstanediol, cannot distinguish between the synthesis of these androgens by liver or by target tissues. Therefore the evaluation of the capacity of sexual skin to metabolize testosterone into DHT and androstanediol in vitro seems the most reliable method for determining the actual rate of 'utilization' of androgens in the blood by target cells. The 5α-reductase enzyme of human skin uses unbound testosterone as substrate, which may originate either from testosterone in the blood or from the transformation of prehormone, notably androstenedione, within the target cells (Ito and Horton, 1971). In our study, the production of androgens seemed to be increased in all hirsute women, since the levels of testosterone and androstenedione were abnormally high in all the patients studied. As the major active androgen in the bloodstream is testosterone, it is interesting to note that the concentration of testosterone was especially high in the plasma of patients with either ovarian or adrenal dysfunction, whereas it was close to the normal range in patients with idiopathic hirsutism. In fact, the only androgen with a constantly and

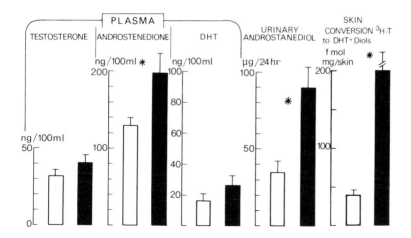

Fig. 6. Plasma testosterone, androstenedione, DHT, urinary androstanediol and conversion rate of radioactive testosterone to 5α-reduced metabolites by pubic skin homogenates in 24 patients with idiopathic hirsutism (▬) compared to 20 normal women (▭) p < 0.001.

significantly increased concentration in all cases of hirsutism is androstenedione. This is consistent with data reported elsewhere (Bardin and
Lipsett, 1967; André and James, 1974). It is interesting to note that plasma
androstenedione is particularly increased in women with delayed onset
congenital adrenal hyperplasia. In these, indeed, the elevated level of plasma
testosterone may be only due to the peripheral conversion of androstenedione secreted by the adrenals and there is no definitive proof of a direct
over-secretion of testosterone in this disease. The same assumption can be
made in the case of polycystic ovary disease. However, in this syndrome,
the origin of androstenedione seems to be exclusively the ovary (Yen et al.,
1970; Mauvais-Jarvis et al., 1978).

With regard to the parameters of peripheral androgen metabolism, it
appears clear that in hirsute patients, the rate of excretion of androstanediol
in the urine is a better discriminant of hirsutism than the level of DHT in the
plasma. This observation is probably best explained as follows. Since most of
the DHT synthesized in tissues is reduced in situ to 3α- and 3β
-androstanediols, only a small fraction of DHT enters the blood. By contrast,
almost all of the 3α- and 3β-androstanediols formed in tissues are excreted
into the urine. This conclusion is substantiated by the fact that the estimated
rate of production of 3α- and 3β-androstanediols in the blood (Bird et al.,
1974; Kinouchi and Horton, 1974) is similar to the daily excretion rate.
These observations support the assumption that 3α- and 3β-androstanediols
are end products of androgen metabolism. In so far as androstenedione
appears to be the major source of DHT in women (Ito and Horton, 1971),
the raised concentration of DHT in the plasma of hirsute patients could be
due to the peripheral conversion of this prehormone. The raised excretion
rate of androstanediol observed in hirsute patients reflects an increase in
both the amount of androstenedione produced and its peripheral conversion.
Indeed, the rate of production of androstenedione, which is around 3.0
mg/24 hr in normal women, may rise to 8.0 mg/24 hr in hirsute women. The
contribution of androstenedione to the androstanediol found in the urine
was calculated after i.v. injection of radioactive androstenedione (Baulieu
and Mauvais-Jarvis, 1964) and ranges from 0.5% in normal women to 1.0% in
hirsute patients (Mauvais-Jarvis, unpublished results). The variations in these
two parameters may account for the striking difference in androstanediol
excretion observed between normal and hirsute women (40-140 μg/24 hr)
and the wide range of variation within the group of hirsute women in the
present study. The same calculation of the contribution of testosterone in
the blood to the level of androstanediol in the urine of hirsute patients leads
to the conclusion that, at most, 20μg of the urinary androstanediol excreted
per 24 hr could arise from testosterone. The rate of excretion of androstanediol in the urine therefore gives a good estimate of the peripheral
metabolism of androstenedione. This is of particular importance, since
contrary to what was observed for testosterone, an increase in androstenedione metabolism by extrahepatic tissues is not reflected by an increase

in the metabolic clearance rate for androstenedione (MCR_A). There is, in fact, no difference between the MCR_A of normal and hirsute women (Bardin and Lipsett, 1967; Kirschner et al., 1976). The differences observed between normal and hirsute women in the contribution made by testosterone and androstenedione to the level of androstanediol in the urine 'in vivo' are directly related to the differences observed in the potential capacity of sexual skin to transform testosterone into DHT and 3α- and 3β-androstanediols 'in vitro' (Kuttenn and Mauvais-Jarvis, 1975). Since androstenedione may be converted into testosterone by human skin (Gomez and Hsia, 1968; Flamigni et al., 1971), the level of 5α-reductase activity present in this tissue is the major factor controlling the amount of androstenedione that is effectively metabolized into DHT and 3α- and 3β-androstanediols. In patients with idiopathic hirsutism, the increase in the concentration of androstenedione in the plasma reflects an excessive secretion of androstenedione by the ovaries as reported by Kirschner and Bardin (1972) and Kirschner et al. (1976), but it is reasonable to suggest that the abnormally high conversion of androstenedione into testosterone and DHT by sexual skin plays a major role in the production of hirsutism. In other words, the observation in patients with idiopathic hirsutism of a very high 5α-reductase activity, contrasting with only a moderate increase in the levels of testosterone and androstenedione in the plasma, supports the thesis that idiopathic hirsutism is caused by an increase in the sensitivity of the target organs to androgens. However, in ovarian and adrenal hirsutism, the increased production of androgens is the most important factor and in some cases can be responsible itself for the increase in the amount of androstanediol excreted.

In conclusion, the determination of both the level of androgens in the plasma and the capacity of skin to transform testosterone into 5α-reduced metabolites is necessary to elucidate the respective roles of abnormal androgen secretion and/or skin 'utilization' in the production of hirsutism.

References

André, C.M. and James, V.H.T. (1974): *Steroids, 24,* 295.

Bardin, C.W. and Lipsett, M.B. (1967): *J. Clin. Invest., 46,* 891.

Baulieu, E.E. and Mauvais-Jarvis, P. (1964): *J. Biol. Chem., 239,* 1578.

Bird, C.E., Choong, A., Knight, L. and Clark, A.F. (1974): *J. Clin. Endocr., 38,* 372.

Clark, A.F., Marcellus, S., De Lory, B. and Bird, C.E. (1975): *Fertil. Steril., 26,* 1001.

Dray, F., Sebaoun, J., Delzant, G., Ledru, M.J. and Mowszowicz, I. (1968): *Rev. Franç Etud. Clin. Biol., 13,* 622.

Flamigni, C., Collins, W.P., Koullapis, E.N., Craft, I., Dewhurst, C.J. and Sommerville, I.F. (1971): *J. Clin. Endocr., 32,* 737.

Gomez, E.C. and Hsia, S.L. (1968): *Biochemistry, 7,* 24.

Horton, R. and Tait, J.F. (1966): *J. Clin. Invest., 45,* 301.

Ito, T. and Horton, R. (1971): *J. Clin. Invest., 50,* 1621.

Keenan, B.S., Meyer, W.J., III, Hadjian, A.J., Jones, H.W. and Migeon, C.J. (1974): *J. Clin. Endocr., 38,* 1143.

Kinouchi, T. and Horton, R. (1974): *J. Clin. Invest., 54,* 646.

Kirschner, M.A. and Bardin, C.W. (1972): *Metabolism, 21,* 667.

Kirschner, M.A., Zucker, I.R. and Jespersen, D. (1976): *New Engl. J. Med., 294,* 637.

Kuttenn, F. and Mauvais-Jarvis, P. (1975): *Acta Endocr. (Kbh.), 79,* 164.

Kuttenn, F., Mowszowicz, I., Schaison, G. and Mauvais-Jarvis, P. (1977): *J. Endocr., 75,* 83.

Mahoudeau, J.A., Bardin, C.W. and Lipsett, M.B. (1971): *J. Clin. Invest., 50,* 1338.

Mauvais-Jarvis, P., Charransol, G. and Bobas-Masson, F. (1973): *J. Clin. Endocr., 36,* 452.

Mauvais-Jarvis, P., Lecomte, P., Kuttenn, F., Mowszowicz, I., Mandelbaum, J. and Wright, F. (1978): *Ann. Endocr. (Paris), 39,* 191.

Rosenfield, R.L. (1972): *J. Clin. Endocr., 32,* 717.

Southren, A.L., Gordon, G.G., Tochimoto, S., Olivo, J., Sherman, D.H. and Pinzon, G. (1969): *J. Clin. Endocr., 29,* 1356.

Vermeulen, A., Verdonck, L., Van der Straeten, M. and Orie, N. (1969): *J. Clin. Endocr., 29,* 1470.

Voigt, W., Fernandez, E.P. and Hsia, S.L. (1970): *J. Biol. Chem., 245,* 5594.

Wright, F., Mowszowicz, I. and Mauvais-Jarvis, P. (1978): *J. Clin. Endocr., 47,* 850.

Yen, S.S.C., Vela, P. and Rankin, J. (1970): *J. Clin. Endocr., 30,* 435.

Correlation between hirsutism, cycle disturbances, normal menstrual cycle stages and plasma androgen levels*

G. MAGRINI, F. MÉAN, P. BURCKHARDT, B. RUEDI and J.-P. FELBER

Division de Biochimie Clinique, Département de Médecine, C.H.U.V., Lausanne, Switzerland

The evaluation of peripheral levels of androgens in hirsute patients gives a first insight into their overall production. However, many authors have emphasized the multiglandular source of the excess androgens secreted in the majority of women with hirsutism: both the adrenal and the ovary may therefore contribute to the abnormal hormonal profile.

Although it is possible to find abnormalities such as raised plasma testosterone and/or androstenedione in most hirsute women, a significant proportion remains in whom these parameters are normal: in these cases an increased conversion of androgen precursors to more potent androgenic hormones at target organ levels might take place (Abraham et al., 1975; London and Shaw, 1978; McKenna, 1978).

The incidence of isolated and/or simultaneously elevated steroid levels in hirsutism is still a matter of controversy. This point is of great importance for screening purposes and in assessing the diagnostic value of single and/or combined hormonal evaluations.

The present report deals with the correlations and relative frequencies of elevated plasma androgen (or precursor) levels in hyperandrogenic hirsute patients, and the relation between elevated androgen levels and the menstrual histories.

Material and methods

Eighty hirsute normoprolactinemic women, 70 of whom had increased levels of at least one androgen were divided into 3 groups: 40 had normal cycles, 30 irregular cycles and 10 amenorrhea.

Plasma samples were obtained in the morning (8 a.m.), during the middle-late follicular phase.

A control group of 20 normally menstruating women was also studied in the early (day 1-5) and middle-late (days 6-9) follicular, periovulatory (days 10-15) and luteal (days 19-26) phases.

Plasma testosterone (T), androstenedione ($\triangle$4), 17α-hydroxyprogesterone (17αOHP), dehydroepiandrosterone sulfate (D-S), cortisol (F)

*Presented in part at the XII Acta Endocrinologica Congress Munich, June 26-30, 1979.

and progesterone (P) were measured by specific radioimmunoassays (Magrini et al., 1979a).

Results

The hormonal values in different phases of the menstrual cycle in the group of normal women are shown in Figures 1 and 2.

T, F and D-S do not vary consistently throughout the cycle, whereas 17$\propto$OHP and P show a sharp increase from the periovulatory to the luteal phases, as expected. In particular, the androgen precursor 17$\propto$OHP increases from the early follicular value of 471.0 ± 66.3 pg/ml (mean ± SEM) to reach 1062.5 ± 204.18) (p < 0.01) in the periovulatory and 2035.0 ± 155.59 pg/ml (mean ± SEM) in the luteal phases. However, F and D-S show

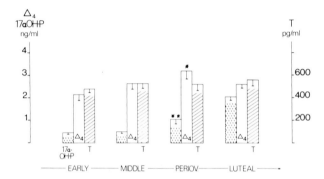

Fig. 1. Plasma testosterone (T), 17$\propto$-hydroxyprogesterone (17$\propto$OHP) and androstenedione ($\triangle$4) in normally menstruating women during different stages of the cycle. *p < 0.05 vs early follicular; **p < 0.01 vs early follicular.

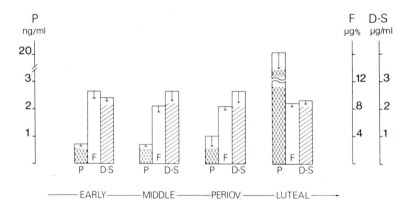

Fig. 2. Plasma progesterone (P), cortisol (F) and DHEA-sulfate (D-S) in normally menstruating women during different stages of the cycle.

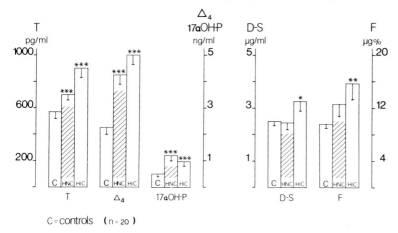

C = controls (n = 20)

Fig. 3. Hirsute hyperandrogenic women with normal (HNC) and irregular (HIC) cycles (same hormones measured as in Figs. 1 and 2). Statistical significance: *p < 0.02; **p < 0.005; ***p < 0.001.

decreasing and increasing trends, respectively, from the early follicular to the periovulatory phases, but neither variation is significant. The only androgen that shows a definite change in the periovulatory phase is $\triangle 4$ (p < 0.05), rising to 3187.5 ± 328.78 pg/ml from the early follicular value of 2189.5 ± 250.98 pg/ml (mean ± SEM, p < 0.05).

Results obtained in the hirsute hyperandrogenic women with normal (HNC) and irregular (HIC) cycles are given in Figure 3.

In the HNC and HIC groups, both mean T and $\triangle 4$ levels are increased, compared with the control group (p < 0.001). Although the mean values in the HIC group appear to be higher than in the HNC group, no statistically significant difference is detected between the two groups. The mean 17αOHP level in the pathological groups shows an increase compared with the controls (p < 0.001). Mean plasma D-S levels are slightly increased in the HIC group (p < 0.02) as well as mean F levels in both pathological groups (significantly in HIC: p < 0.005).

Finally Table 1 shows the frequency of individually and simultaneously elevated steroid levels and their (mean ± SEM) absolute values.

Discussion

No significant variations in plasma steroid levels occur in the present 20 normal menstrual cycles, except for the androgen precursor 17αOHP which showed a definite increase in the periovulatory phase (p < 0.05 vs early follicular) and for androstenedione (p < 0.05).

This observation is however in agreement with other authors (Judd and Yen, 1973; Abraham, 1974) who also found a rise in testosterone levels at

TABLE 1.

Frequency of elevated steroid levels (individually and simultaneously) and their absolute values (mean ± SEM)

	Hyperandrogenic hirsutism			
	N = 40 Hirsutism with normal cycles	N = 30 Hirsutism with irregular cycles	N = 10 Hirsutism with amenorrhea	N = 80 All hirsutism
Elevated levels of:				
Testosterone (T)	38%	72%	60%	53%
Androstenedione ($\triangle_4$)	73	93	100	83
17$\propto$OHProgest (17$\propto$OHP)	92	74	–	–
DHEA-Sulfate (D-S)	20	45	50	34
Cortisol (F)	43	31	43	38
Simultaneously elevated levels of:				
T + $\triangle_4$ + D-S	3.5%	20%	12.5%	14%
T + $\triangle_4$	44	69	58	47
T + $\triangle_4$ + 17$\propto$OHP	42	37	–	–
$\triangle_4$ + 17$\propto$OHP	75	68	–	–
$\triangle_4$ + D-S	7	15	25	12
D-S + F	14	13	12	5
Mean ± SEM				
T (pg/ml)	699 ± 36	907 ± 60.5	807 ± 118	
$\triangle_4$ (pg/ml)	4233 ± 315	5043 ± 374	5890 ± 557	
17$\propto$OHP (pg/ml)	1187 ± 115	976 ± 65	–	
D-S (pg/ml)	2.45 ± 0.24	3.23 ± 0.38	3.48 ± 0.38	
F (μg%)	12.3 ± 1.45	15.65 ± 1.6	13.3 ± 3.6	

mid-cycle, and with findings reported in a previous study (Genazzani et al., 1977).

The present investigation on hirsute hyperandrogenic women demonstrates a high incidence of elevated peripheral levels of both 17$\propto$OHP and $\triangle$4 and more seldom of testosterone.

T, $\triangle$4 and 17$\propto$OHP are significantly increased both in the HNC and HIC groups, confirming the tendency reported in our preliminary studies (Magrini et al., 1979b).

The mean rise in androgen levels is higher in the HIC group, especially for D-S. This adrenal steroid shows in fact a significant increase in the group with irregular cycles compared to controls and HNC patients, partly in agreement with the observations of Abraham et al. (1975) who reported that D-S was the only steroid showing a significant difference in mean levels between two similar groups of hirsute women. The increase in mean F levels in both groups (significant in HIC) (p < 0.005) confirms our previous observations (Magrini et al., 1979b) and reports of other authors (Abraham et al., 1975; McKenna, 1978). The data support the role of the adrenal in the altered steroidogenesis of hirsutism syndromes.

Comparative studies (Table 1) indicate that whereas more than two thirds of cases with hyperandrogenic hirsutism have elevated 17$\propto$OHP and/or $\triangle$4 levels, plasma T is increased in only half of them and D-S and F in one third. Moreover, $\triangle$4 alone is elevated in 93% of the HIC subjects and in 73% of the HNC patients, but percentages fall to 69 and 44 respectively, when T is simultaneously considered. When $\triangle$4 is paired with 17$\propto$OHP, percentages of 68 and 75 are obtained in the two groups, respectively which decrease to 37% and 42% when simultaneous elevations of the three hormones are considered.

These data also show that while simultaneously elevated levels of 3 or more androgens are not frequently found, the combined evaluation of T and $\triangle$4 gives elevated levels of at least one androgen in 96% of the HIC subjects and 73% in the HNC group: this combined evaluation therefore seems to be useful for clinical screening purposes.

Furthermore, determination of 17$\propto$OHP may provide additional information on the androgen profile and rule out the possibility of an adrenogenital syndrome.

Increased plasma levels of the most potent androgenic steroid, T, seem to be well correlated with the presence of cycle disturbances. In fact, the percentage of increased $\triangle$4 and 17$\propto$OHP levels in hirsutism with irregular cycles (90-95%; 70-80%) was not substantially greater than in the group with normal cycles (70-80%; 90-95%) whereas the percentage of increased T levels doubled (72% vs 38%; p < 0.005).

In the amenorrheic group androgen values were similar to those observed in the HIC group.

It is worth noting that F levels are significantly increased in a relatively small (31%) percentage of HIC subjects.

The present data show that in the groups of hirsute women studied, only 17$\propto$OHP and $\triangle$4 showed a very high frequency of clearly increased levels: however this pattern may be observed during the periovulatory phase of the normal menstrual cycle.

On the other hand, elevated plasma levels of the adrenal androgen D-S do not frequently correlate with the increase in the other steroids studied.

Finally, menstrual cycle disturbances associated with hirsutism are often accompanied by increased androgen plasma levels; moreover qualitative differences among the various androgens can be observed.

Acknowledgements

The authors wish to thank G. Chiodoni, P. Bianchi, A.M. Aeberhardt and D. Gander for their excellent technical assistance, Dr. M. Gasperi for scientific assistance in editing the text and Miss M.C. Evraere for preparing the manuscript.

This hormonal study was performed mainly on plasma samples from patients of Dr. P. Burckhardt or Prof. B. Ruedi to whom we are grateful.

References

Abraham, G.E. (1974): *Clin. Endocr., 39,* 340.
Abraham, G.E., Chakmakjian, Z.H., Buster, J.E. and Marshall, J.R. (1975): *Obstet. and Gynec., 46,* 169.
Genazzani, A.R., Magrini, G., Facchinetti, F., Romagnino, S., Pintor, C., Felber, J.P. and Fioretti, P. (1977): In: *Androgens and Antiandrogens.* p. 247. Editors: L. Martini and M. Motta. Raven Press, New York.
Judd, H.L. and Yen, S.S.C. (1973): *Clin. Endocr., 36,* 475.
London, D.R. and Shaw, R.W. (1978): In: *Recent Advances in Endocrinology and Metabolism.* p. 91. Editor: J.L.H. O'Riordan, Churchill-Livingstone, Edinburgh-London-New York.
Magrini, G., Iselin, H., Ebiner, J.R. and Felber, J.P. (1979a): *Arch. Androl., 2,* 141.
Magrini, G., Mean, F. and Felber, J.P. (1979b): In: *Radioimmunology.* p. 213. Editor: Ch.A. Bizollon. Elsevier/North Holland Biomedical Press, Amsterdam.
McKenna, T.J. (1978): In: *Endocrine Causes of Menstrual Disorders.* p. 371. Editor: J.R. Givens. Year Book Medical Publishers Inc., Chicago-London.

Spironolactone as an antiandrogen in the treatment of hirsutism

M. MESSINA, P. BIFFIGNANDI, C. MANIERI, E. GHIGO and
G.M. MOLINATTI

Cattedra di Endocrinologia, Università di Torino, Torino, Italy

Long-term therapy with spironolactone at doses exceeding 100 mg/day may cause side effects such as gynaecomastia, impotence, loss of libido, and seminal abnormalities in men, and menstrual irregularities and mammary tension in women (Greenblatt and Koch-Weser, 1973).

The competitive interaction of this drug with cytoplasmic and nuclear receptors has been demonstrated in several different animal and human target organs (Pita et al., 1975; Rifka et al., 1977). In addition, it has been shown that spironolactone causes a reduction in the concentration of cytochrome P-450 and of many related enzymatic activities (particularly 17α-hydroxylase and 17,20-desmolase) in testicular and adrenal tissues (Menard et al., 1974 a, b).

In view of these considerations the aim of this work was to determine the therapeutic effectiveness of spironolactone in the treatment of idiopathic hirsutism.

Material and methods

Eight women (17-26 yrs old) with severe idiopathic hirsutism were treated daily with 400 mg of spironolactone during the first 10 days and subsequently with 300-200 mg. The treatment with spironolactone was associated with oral contraceptives in 4 patients who showed menstrual irregularities (cases 3, 4, 6 and 7 on days 36, 96, 44 and 70 of therapy, respectively).

Clinical assessment of body hair growth (according to Ferrimann and Gallway, 1961) and hormonal estimations (plasma testosterone and plasma FSH and LH) were carried out every third day during the first 10 days and every 7th-15th day afterwards. Treatment was interrupted early in cases 2 and 5 (who are therefore included for hormonal results only). Our analysis of results was made with respect to 2 different periods of time (50-100 days and 100-150 days of therapy).

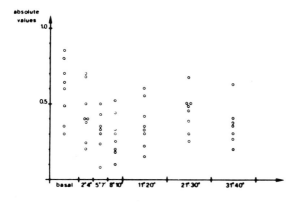

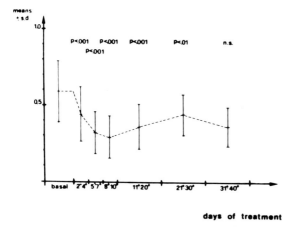

days of treatment

Fig. 1. Plasma testosterone in hirsute female subjects before and during administration of spironolactone; p values were obtained with the paired t-test.

Results

The clinical results are summarized in Table 1. In all patients, a significant decrease of plasma testosterone levels during administration of spirono-lactone was noted, especially in the first 20 days of treatment (Fig. 1); on the other hand, FSH and LH levels seemed to lose their cyclic pattern but did not increase above normal values (Fig. 2). Menstrual irregularities (polymenorrhoea or amenorrhoea) were seen in all cases. Except for menstrual alterations, spironolactone was well tolerated in all patients and, in particular, no abnormal changes in arterial pressure and in electrolyte pattern were observed.

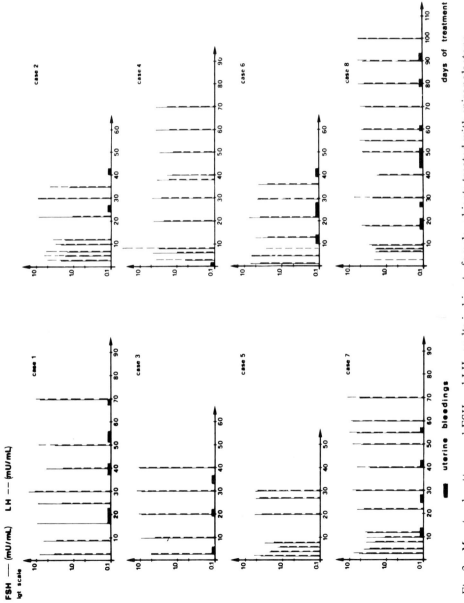

Fig. 2. Menstrual pattern and FSH and LH results in hirsute female subjects treated with spironolactone.

TABLE 1.

Clinical results. Clinical assessment refers to a comprehensive evaluation and principally according to the index of Ferrimann and Gallway (I.F.G.)

Cases (Age in yrs)	Days of treatment and clinical results		Ferrimann and Gallway's index changes
	Period A 50th → 100th	Period B 100th → 150th	
1 S.G. 26	Highly significant	–	33 → 20
3 B.G. 26	Significant	Highly significant	23 → 13
4 D.G. 21	Significant	Highly significant	22 → 13
6 C.C. 18	No result	Significant	19 → 11
7 D.P. 22	Highly significant	Highly significant	26 → 12
8 S.A. 22	No result	Significant	13 → 7

Discussion

The data show that the therapeutic effectiveness of spironolactone in female hirsutism is similar to that obtained with cyproterone acetate. We emphasize our work as one of the first clinical studies employing this drug for its antiandrogenic properties. In our opinion the combination with oral contraceptives does not modify the therapeutic findings that we ascribe to the interaction of spironolactone with the dihydrotestosterone binding proteins in target organs.

The decreased plasma testosterone levels noticed in the first period of treatment are difficult to explain since, at the regimen used (3-8 mg/kg body weight), the action of the drug on cytochrome P-450 is not remarkable. An increased metabolic clearance rate of testosterone, caused by spironolactone, has been demonstrated only in male subjects (Loriaux et al., 1976).

Acknowledgements

These studies were partly carried out in the Radioimmunology Laboratory of the Department of Endocrinology of the University of Turin. The laboratory equipment was supplied by 'Cassa di Risparmio di Torino'.

References

Ferrimann, D. and Gallway, J.D. (1961): *J. Clin. Endocr., 21,* 1440.
Greenblatt, D.J. and Koch-Weser, J. (1973): *J. Amer. Med. Ass., 225,* 40.
Loriaux, D.L., Menard, R., Taylor, A., Pita, J.C. and Santen, R. (1976): *Ann. Intern. Med., 85,* 630.
Menard, R., Stripp, B. and Gillette, J.R. (1974a): *Endocrinology, 94,* 1638.

Menard, R., Stripp, B., Loriaux, D.L., Bartner, F.C. and Gillette, J.E. (1974b): *56th Annual Meeting of the Endocrine Society.* Abstract 98, p. A-104.

Pita, J.C., Lippmann, M.E., Thompson, E.B. and Loriaux, D.L. (1975): *Endocrinology, 97,* 1521.

Rifka, S.M., Pita, J.C., Vigersky, R.A., Wilson, Y.A. and Loriaux, D.L. (1977): *J. Clin. Endocr., 46,* 338.

Chronic intermittent administration of LH-RH: a new approach to the treatment of infertility in hypothalamic amenorrhea

G. LEYENDECKER, T. STRUVE, W. NOCKE and M. HANSMANN

Department of Obstetrics and Gynecology, University of Bonn, F.R.G.

Hypothalamic amenorrhea constitutes more than two-thirds of all forms of amenorrhea diagnosed (Rjosk et al., 1979) indicating its clinical significance. Knowledge concerning the etiological factor(s), however, is still incomplete. There is indirect evidence that hypothalamic amenorrhea is associated with reduced and deficient hypothalamic LH-RH secretion (Leyendecker, 1979; Leyendecker et al., 1980). This view is strongly supported by the observation that presumably deficient endogenous LH-RH can be readily substituted by exogenous administration resulting in improved or normalized pituitary and ovarian function (vide infra) (Leyendecker et al., 1980).

Hypothalamic amenorrhea may occur as a primary or a secondary form. Although this distinction merely points to the stage of sexual development at which the menstrual disorder became clinically evident in an individual case, from a *heuristic* point of view it may be of interest to consider at least in some cases different etiological factors and mechanisms responsible for and involved in the occurrence of primary and secondary hypothalamic amenorrhea, respectively. (Olfacto-genital dysplasia is not included in these considerations). Functional tests usually demonstrate that primary hypo-thalamic amenorrhea is more serious than the secondary form. Moreover, the latter exhibits a great degree of spontaneous reversibility while primary hypothalamic amenorrhea is usually permanent.

Results from studies on chronic intermittent administration of LH-RH to prepubertal female rhesus monkeys (Wildt et al., 1980) suggest that the gradual start of ovarian function during puberty may largely depend upon a gradual onset of an adequate circhoral hypothalamic release of LH-RH. It is therefore tempting to speculate that in some cases of primary hypothalamic amenorrhea the 'maturation' of structures and mechanisms responsible for the circhoral release of LH-RH did not, or only insufficiently, occur. Further studies of the mechanisms involved in the onset of puberty in the experimental animal may provide a better understanding of the pathogenesis of primary hypothalamic amenorrhea.

Secondary hypothalamic amenorrhea is, by definition and indirect evidence, the result of a reduction of an initially more or less established hypothalamic LH-RH activity and thus, functionally, a relapse of the pituitary-ovarian axis into the prepubertal state. The central nervous system has long been recognized as a primary site of functional disturbances leading to ovarian failure. Thus, terms like psychogenic stress or situational amenorrhea have been introduced to characterize these conditions (Reifenstein, 1946; Tietze, 1948; Fries and Nillius, 1973; Frick, 1974). The more or less overt psychogenic background of some cases of secondary hypothalamic amenorrhea, the frequently observed spontaneous reversibility after environmental changes and/or improvement after psychotherapy caused Schneider and Leyendecker (1980) to conceive secondary hypothalamic amenorrhea not as a *disturbance* but rather as a phylogenetically inherited *potential* of the organism to react with reduced fertility towards endogenous and exogenous irritation. The potential benefit of this view of secondary hypothalamic amenorrhea is the possible availability of animal models for the study of this clinical condition. It is conceivable, of course, that psychogenic ovarian failure may also become manifest as a primary amenorrhea.

History and observation of patients suffering from secondary hypothalamic amenorrhea often reveal that corpus-luteum insufficiency, anovulatory cycles, oligomenorrhea are transitory stages during the development of or recovery from amenorrhea. Therefore, the concept had been developed (Leyendecker, 1979) that, in hypothalamic ovarian failure, these disturbances form a pathophysiological entity on the basis of a gradually reduced hypothalamic LH-RH release, of which the amenorrhea is only the most serious one.

Diagnosis of hypothalamic amenorrhea and the assessment of the residual hypothalamic function

Endogenous LH-RH cannot be measured reliably in peripheral blood and, thus, direct evaluation of the hypothalamic LH-RH function is presently not possible. Therefore, the diagnosis of hypothalamic amenorrhea is essentially based upon the exclusion of other causes which are known to lead to amenorrhea (Table 1). Once the diagnosis of hypothalamic amenorrhea has been established, the severity of the impairment of the hypothalamic-pituitary-ovarian axis may be readily assessed by clomiphene-, progestogen- and LH-RH tests, respectively. Pathophysiological studies in hypothalamic amenorrhea could demonstrate that the results of these functional tests are a precise reflection of the residual function of the hypothalamic-pituitary-ovarian axis in hypothalamic amenorrhea and therefore provide a subtle evaluation of the severity of the impairment of the hypothalamic LH-RH secretion (Leyendecker, 1979).

In hypothalamic amenorrhea, a positive clomiphene test indicates that there is little impairment of the hypothalamic function. Following the temporary elevation of serum FSH (and LH) during clomiphene administration the residual hypothalamic function is sufficient to further promote

TABLE 1.

Hypothalamic amenorrhea

Diagnosis	Tests for evaluation of residual hypothalamic function	Subclassification with respect to severity of impairment of hypothalamic function	Therapeutic principles

Exclusion of other forms of amenorrhea on the basis of clinical and laboratory findings, i.e. primary ovarian failure, primary pituitary failure, hyperprolactinemia, androgen excess, internal and endocrine diseases, anatomical abnormalities	Clomiphene
	
	Progestogen
	
	LH-RH
		1. Clomiphene positive with bleeding following
		  − a normal luteal phase
		  − an insufficient luteal phase
		  − an anovulatory cycle
		
		2. Clomiphene negative progestogen positive
		
		3. Progestogen negative
		  − LH-RH positive
		  − LH-RH negative
			Mobilization of endogenous gonadotropins with antiestrogenic compounds
			
			Exogenous gonadotropins (hMG/hCG)
			
			Exogenous LH-RH (chronic intermittent)

follicular maturation and eventually cause ovulation. Thus the positive test may be subclassified according to the occurrence of a normal luteal phase, an insufficient luteal phase or an anovulatory bleeding following the administration of the test dose of clomiphene, reflecting different degrees of the hypothalamic impairment within the clomiphene positive group (Table 1).

Patients who are clomiphene positive usually exhibit withdrawal bleeding following the administration of a progestogen. Some patients, who are progestogen positive do not bleed following the administration of clomiphene. Patients displaying these results are suffering from an intermediate form of hypothalamic amenorrhea on account of the severity of the hypothalamic impairment (Leyendecker, 1979).

In severe hypothalamic LH-RH deficiency there is little or no stimulation of the pituitary gonadotropes and thus little follicular stimulation. Due to the low serum estradiol levels in these patients the endometrium is not sufficiently proliferated to allow a secretory transformation following administration of a progestogen: The progestogen test is negative. Since the progestogen negative group is comprised of LH-RH responsive as well as unresponsive patients (Figs. 1-3), the LH-RH test allows a subclassification of the progestogen negative group. On the basis of a negative LH-RH test no conclusion can be drawn as to the primary site (pituitary vs suprapituitary) of the lesion, since neither a primarily deficient nor a long-term unstimulated

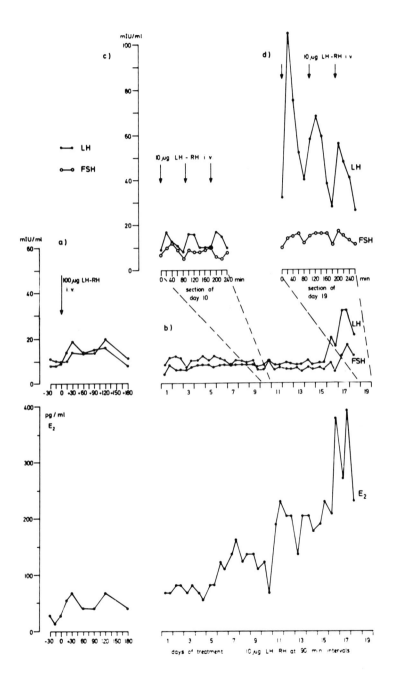

Fig. 1. FSH, LH and estradiol serum levels in a 22-year-old woman with progestogen negative primary amenorrhea during chronic intermittent treatment with 10 μg of LH-RH per bolus.

pituitary — as in the most severe form of hypothalamic amenorrhea — would respond to a single LH-RH stimulus. Only long term stimulation of the pituitary with LH-RH would allow differentiation in this respect.

LH-RH substitution in hypothalamic amenorrhea

Presently, in clinical practice, the treatment of infertility in hypothalamic amenorrhea consists either in the mobilization of endogenous gonadotropins by the administration of antiestrogenic compounds which may be supported by the properly timed additional administration of hCG, LH-RH and/or estrogen, or by gonadotropin substitution, the latter being usually restricted to the more serious forms of hypothalamic amenorrhea (Table 1).

It was predictable that synthetic LH-RH would be used therapeutically as soon as it was available in larger amounts. However, previous attempts to induce follicular maturation and ovulation in severe hypothalamic amenorrhea or anorexia nervosa were not successful (Breckwoldt et al., 1974; Gual and Lichtenberg, 1976) or required high doses and multiple injections per day (Nillius et al., 1975).

Recent experimental data on the endocrine regulation of the hypothalamic-pituitary unit resulted in a better understanding of the regulatory principles and provided a basis for a more physiological approach to LH-RH therapy in hypothalamic amenorrhea. It is now well established that hypothalamic LH-RH secretion is pulsatile in character with a rather circhoral frequency of pulses during the proliferative and periovulatory phases of the cycle (Dierschke et al., 1970; Yen et al., 1972; Carmel et al., 1976). In the rhesus monkey it could be established that pulsatility in the LH-RH stimulation of the pituitary gonadotropes is a prerequisite of normal pituitary gonadotropic function (Belchetz et al., 1978). Furthermore, it was demonstrated that, in the primate, hypothalamic LH-RH function is 'permissive' in character (Nakai et al., 1978; Leyendecker, 1979; Leyendecker et al., 1980) in that the cyclicity of the endocrine events during the menstrual cycle is solely regulated at the pituitary and ovarian level. The clinical application of this new understanding of the hypothalamic-pituitary function would be a pulsatile substitution of deficient endogenous LH-RH as a mode of treatment of infertility in hypothalamic amenorrhea.

Patients suffering from progestogen negative primary and secondary hypothalamic amenorrhea were treated with LH-RH. The treatment consisted of the i.v. administration of 10-15 μg of LH-RH every 90 min over a period of 9-19 days. The dose of 10-15 μg per bolus was chosen because it resulted in a pulsatile pattern of serum LH similar to that of the normal proliferative phase of the cycle (Yen et al., 1972). Furthermore, this dose of LH-RH resulted in venous and thus pituitary blood levels of LH-RH similar to those found in the pituitary stalk effluent of the rhesus monkey (Carmel et al., 1976).

This treatment regimen was applied (Fig. 1) in a 22-year-old woman with progestogen negative primary hypothalamic amenorrhea. Following a test dose of 100 μg of LH-RH a slight pituitary response was observed. During chronic intermittent treatment with 10 μg of LH-RH per bolus started on the next day estradiol levels in serum steadily increased indicating an improvement in pituitary-ovarian function. When preovulatory serum estradiol levels were reached an abrupt pituitary release of LH and to a lesser extent of FSH occurred similar to the respective peaks of a normal cycle. On day 19 the induced pulsatile pattern of serum LH corresponded to the typical pattern during the descending limb of a normal midcycle peak.

In a 20-year-old woman (Fig. 2) with progestogen negative secondary

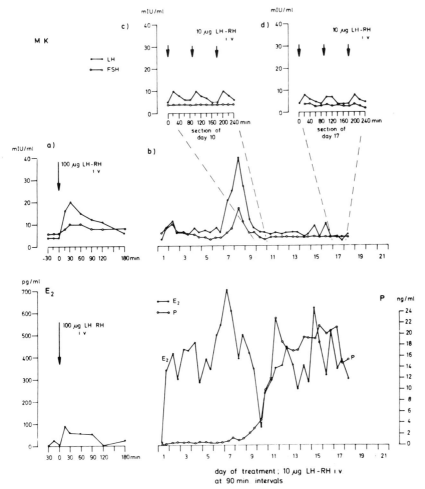

Fig. 2. FSH, LH, estradiol and progesterone serum levels in a 20-year-old woman with progestogen-negative secondary amenorrhea during chronic intermittent treatment with 10 μg of LH-RH per bolus.

hypothalamic amenorrhea the pituitary response to 100 μg of LH-RH revealed that the function of the hypothalamic-pituitary axis was impaired to a lesser extent compared to the patient in Figure 1. Within 9 hrs of the beginning of the chronic intermittent administration of LH-RH with 10 μg per bolus, estradiol levels in serum rose abruptly. This rise was followed by a further increase in serum estradiol and on days 6 and 7 LH and FSH peaks in serum occurred. The progesterone levels reached normal midluteal phase values subsequently indicating ovulation and subsequent corpus luteum formation.

As indicated by the results obtained in these 2 women the residual hypothalamic function as reflected by the LH-RH test results seems to be very important with respect to the duration of treatment and probably also dose of LH-RH required for the induction of ovulation. This is demonstrated in Figure 3 which is a composite picture of findings in 6 patients showing on the left the results in 3 patients with the most severe form of hypothalamic amenorrhea as reflected by the poor or absent pituitary response towards a 100 μg LH-RH test dose (upper left). All these patients were suffering from progestogen negative *primary* hypothalamic amenorrhea. The duration of treatment until a LH peak or ovulation occurred was 14-16 days in this group of patients. One patient exhibited only a moderate elevation of serum estradiol during treatment. The patient with an ovulatory response was treated with 15 μg of LH-RH per bolus and ovulation occurred 14 days after the start of treatment.

The patients, however, who exhibited a significant response to the 100 μg test dose of LH-RH (Fig. 3; upper right) were all suffering from progestogen negative *secondary* hypothalamic amenorrhea. All patients ovulated with a dose of 10-15 μg of LH-RH per bolus, and the duration of chronic intermittent treatment required for the induction of ovulation was only 5-7 days. Also in contrast to the other patients, serum LH and FSH levels fell well into the normal range. Estradiol levels, however, rapidly rose above the normal range. This finding is interpreted that, in the women with a less impaired hypothalamic function, a follicle or a set of follicles had already gained a certain degree of maturation prior to the start of therapy which allowed immediate secretion of estradiol as soon as the gonadotropin levels had normalized.

The requirement of a circhoral administration of LH-RH certainly impedes the clinical application of chronic intermittent administration of LH-RH as a regimen for the treatment of infertility in hypothalamic amenorrhea, unless a portable device is used which administers the required dose of LH-RH automatically. The construction of such a portable computerized minipump is facilitated by the fact that LH-RH function is only permissive. Thus, in substitution therapy, no readjustments in the dose of LH-RH during follicular maturation and ovulation are required once the appropriate substitution dose has been established. For the purpose of treatment of patients with clomiphene negative hypothalamic amenorrhea

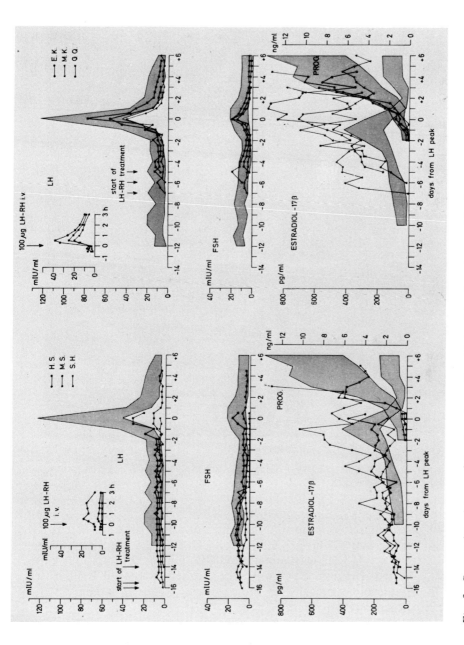

Fig. 3. Composite picture of treatment results obtained in 6 patients with chronic intermittent administration of LH-RH. Left: results in patients with primary hypothalamic amenorrhea. Right: results in patients with secondary hypothalamic amenorrhea. All patients were progestogen negative. Shaded areas: normal mean value ± SEM.

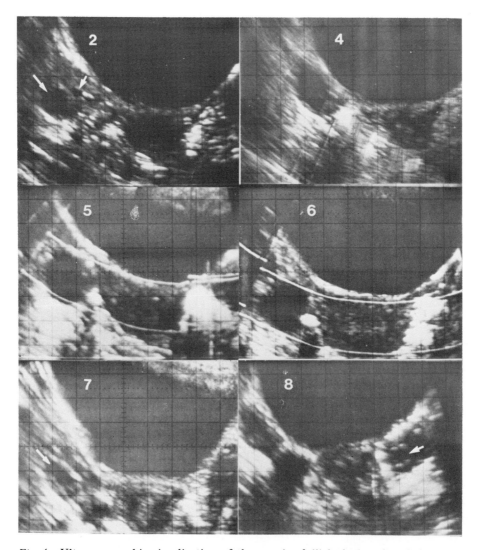

Fig. 4. Ultrasonographic visualization of the growing follicle during chronic intermittent administration of LH-RH in a 29-year-old woman with progestogen negative secondary hypothalamic amenorrhea (E.K.).

on an outpatient basis with chronic intermittent administration of LH-RH, a portable minipump (Ferring GmbH, Kiel, F.R.G.) was constructed which delivers a LH-RH containing solution via a chronic indwelling antecubital i.v. catheter every 90 min. The pump was applied for the first time to a 29-year-old woman with progestogen negative secondary hypothalamic amenorrhea (Figs. 4 and 5).

The LH-RH test (Fig. 5, upper left) revealed a significant response of the

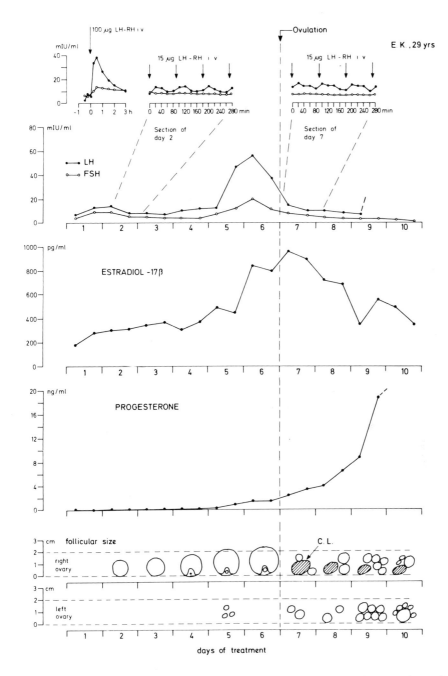

Fig. 5. Composite picture of endocrinological and ultrasonic findings in patient E.K. during chronic intermittent administration of LH-RH by means of a portable computerized minipump.

pituitary towards the 100 μg bolus. On the basis of this result and previous experience with chronic intermittent administration of LH-RH (Fig. 3) it was predicted that the patient would ovulate approximately one week after the beginning of treatment. The treatment was monitored by the measurements of LH, FSH, estradiol and progesterone in the serum as well as by ultrasonographic visualization of the growing follicle (Figs. 4 and 5). Ultrasonography was performed daily starting on the second day of treatment (Fig. 4), when a follicular diameter of already 14 mm was determined. The follicle grew steadily during therapy and had reached a diameter of 24 mm on day 6 of treatment. On day 7 the follicle could no longer be visualized and structures were found which correspond to a corpus luteum of the normal menstrual cycle (Hackelöer et al., 1979).

The levels of estradiol in serum increased from below 200 pg/ml to values in the range of 400 pg/ml prior to the LH surge and corresponded well to the maturation of only one follicle (Fig. 5). In contrast to the normal cycle, however, there was no rapid decline of serum estradiol during and following the LH peak but a further rise to levels in the range of 900 pg/ml after ovulation. Presumably, the gonadotropin surges on days 5 and 6 had induced the growth of accompanying follicles of the right and left ovary, which could be visualized by ultrasonography and which were probably the sources of the additional estradiol. However, none of these follicles ovulated as judged from ultrasonography. The pump was removed on day 9 of treatment and on days 9, 11 and 13, respectively, single i.m. doses of 2500 IU of hCG were administered for further support of corpus luteum function. Starting on day 18 of treatment a steady rise of hCG in serum was observed which was not attributable to the exogenous hCG, indicating that implantation had occurred. Further endocrinological and ultrasonographic follow-up revealed normal development of a singleton pregnancy.

Conclusions

Hypothalamic amenorrhea constitutes merely the most severe form of a whole spectrum of disturbances of the pituitary-ovarian axis of which the common denominator is a more or less expressed reduction of the hypothalamic LH-RH secretion. Depending upon the degree of hypothalamic LH-RH deficiency hypothalamic ovarian failure may present as corpus-luteum insufficiency, anovulatory cycle, oligomenorrhea and amenorrhea. Clinical and experimental data hint at the possibility that at least in some cases primary and secondary hypothalamic amenorrhea constitute different disturbances of which, however, the etiologies remain to be defined.

Administration of gonadotropins has been the treatment of choice of infertility in clomiphene negative hypothalamic amenorrhea. The data presented indicate that chronic intermittent administration of LH-RH by means of a portable computerized minipump, however, may be an attractive alternative. The inconvenience of this treatment mode caused by the inevitability of wearing the pump is outbalanced by some apparent advantages: (1) The substitution of a lacking hormone with a defined dose of this hormone in a mode which simulates the physiological secretory pattern of this hormone. (2) During chronic intermittent administration of LH-RH the regulatory mechanisms which govern pituitary-ovarian interaction are operating. Thus, the incidence of overstimulation could be minimized. (3) The pituitary-ovarian response during treatment seems to correlate with the severity of the hypothalamic dysfunction. Typical response patterns, however, facilitate the prediction of the time of ovulation. (4) On the basis of the present result it seems legitimate to foresee that chronic intermittent administration of LH-RH by means of a pump, once fully established, might be monitored only by the measurement of the basal body temperature. Then treatment of infertility would become available for patients who are presently excluded from adequate treatment because they cannot, for various external reasons, follow the strict regimen of frequent gynecological controls mandatory in gonadotropin substitution therapy.

References

Belchetz, P.E., Plant, T.M., Nakai, Y., Keogh, E.J. and Knobil, E. (1978): *Science, 202,* 631.

Breckwoldt, M., Czygan, P.J., Lehmann, F. and Bettendorf, G. (1974): *Acta Endocr., (Kbh.), 75,* 209.

Carmel, P.W., Araki, S. and Ferin, M. (1976): *Endocrinology, 99,* 243.

Dierschke, D.J., Battacharya, A.N., Atkinson, L.E. and Knobil, E. (1970): *Endocrinology, 87,* 850.

Frick, V. (1974): In: *The Family:* 4th Int. Congr. Psychosomatic Obstetrics and Gynecology, p. 246. Editor: H. Hirsch. Karger, Basel.

Fries, H. and Nillius, S.J. (1973): *Acta Psychiatr. Scand., 49,* 653.

Gual, C. and Lichtenberg, R. (1976): In: *Ovulation in the Human,* p. 243. Editors: P.G. Crosignani and D.R. Mishell. Academic Press, London.

Hackelöer, B.J., Fleming, R., Robinson, H.P., Adam, A.H. and Coutts, J.R.T. (1979): *Am. J. Obstet. Gynec., 135,* 122.

Leyendecker, G. (1979): *Europ. J. Obstet. Gynec. Reprod. Biol., 9,* 175.

Leyendecker, G., Struve, T. and Plotz, E.J. (1980): *Arch. Gynec.,* in press.

Nakai, Y., Plant, T.M., Hess, D.L., Keogh, E.J. and Knobil, E. (1978): *Endocrinology, 102,* 1008.

Nillius, S.J., Fries, H. and Wide, L. (1975): *Amer. J. Obstet. Gynec., 122,* 921.

Reifenstein, E.C. (1946): *Med. Clin. N. Amer., 30,* 1103.

Rjosk, H.K., Fahlbusch, R. and von Werder, K. (1979): *Arch. Gynec., 228,* 518.

Schneider, H.P.G. and Leyendecker, G. (1980): In: *Advances in Steroid Biochemistry and Pharmacology,* Vol. 7, p. 24. Editors: M.H. Briggs and A. Corbin. Academic Press, London.

Tietze, K. (1948): *Zbl. Gynäk., 70,* 377.

Wildt, L., Marshall, G. and Knobil, E. (1980): *Science, 207,* 1373.

Yen, S.S.C., Tsai, C.C., Naftolin, F., Van den Berg, G. and Ajabar, L. (1972): *J. Clin. Endocrinol. Metab., 34,* 671.

Infertility with normal menstrual rhythm: hormone profiles in response to HMG (Pergonal) treatment

W.P. BLACK[1], R. FLEMING[1], M.C. MACNAUGHTON[1], A. CRAIG[2], P. ENGLAND[3] and J.R.T. COUTTS[1]

[1] Department of Obstetrics and Gynaecology, Royal Maternity Hospital, University of Glasgow, Rottenrow, Glasgow; [2] Clinpath Services Limited, High Wycombe, Bucks; [3] Department of Pathological Biochemistry, Glasgow Royal Infirmary, Glasgow, U.K.

Investigation of hormone profiles in infertile women with normal menstrual rhythm has revealed a number of abnormalities of both the follicular and luteal phases. It is probable that many abnormal luteal profiles are derived from an abnormal follicle and it has been suggested that poor follicular maturation occurs in some patients with long standing infertility (Dodson et al., 1975; Cooke et al., 1977). Dodson et al. (1975) investigated a series of such patients and, by means of daily plasma sampling and hormone assessment, discerned a group with poor preovulatory oestradiol (OE_2). This poor follicular maturation appeared to be related to a low profile of follicle stimulating hormone (FSH) during the peri-menstrual period. For this reason, a protocol was instituted to study the effect of supplementation of gonadotrophin levels on days 1, 3 and 5 of the cycle.

Material and methods

The patients for this trial were extensively investigated to exclude other causes of their infertility which was of greater than 3 yrs duration. Laparoscopic examination revealed no abdominal abnormality and patent fallopian tubes were confirmed. Their husbands had normal sperm assessment. Each patient gave serial daily blood samples throughout 2 complete menstrual cycles; the first was an investigation cycle and in the second she received human menopausal gonadotrophin (HMG, Pergonal, Serono Ltd. (UK) 225 IU, FSH) on days 1, 3 and 5. Day 1 was the first day of menses. Blood samples were taken at the same time each day where possible. The plasma from each blood sample was assayed for OE_2, progesterone (P), FSH, luteinizing hormone (LH) and prolactin (PRL), using specific radio-immunoassays (RIA) and the hormone profiles were examined by reference to our laboratory normal data arranged relative to the mid-cycle LH peak-day 0.

Results

Results are presented from the investigation cycles of 27 infertile patients and 29 of their treatment cycles. The hormonal abnormalities observed during the investigation cycles were: (1) Poor follicular maturation (n = 7), diagnosed when the pre-ovulatory OE_2 rise above the normal early follicular phase range failed to occur before day −3. (2) Poor P surge (n = 13), diagnosed when P concentration fell below the normal range on at least 3 occasions between days +1 and +5 inclusive. This was often associated with luteal insufficiency but not always. (3) Short luteal phases (n = 2), diagnosed when the P concentration fell below 1.5 ng/ml prior to day +12. (4) Elevated LH levels (n = 8), diagnosed when > 50% of the LH concentrations in the follicular phase prior to day −2 lay above the 97.5% confidence limits.

In addition, 13 of these patients showed transient hyperprolactinaemia of variable extent and duration (Coutts et al., 1978).

The effects of the treatment were assessed under the categories of firstly, immediate hormonal responses, and secondly, the ensuing luteal phase hormonal profiles. The immediate hormonal responses were effectively HMG provocation tests and reflected the ability of the follicles to respond to gonadotrophin stimulation. These responses were very variable and have been divided into 3 types. A type I response was characterised by an absence of a significant rise of OE_2 above the normal early follicular phase range during the period of administration. This was associated with longer follicular phases (n = 7) or follicular phases of similar length (n = 3) to the

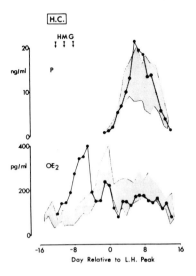

Fig. 1. Examples of a type II response of OE_2 to HMG therapy on days 1, 3 and 5 (↓) compared with normal ranges (hatched background).

patients' own investigation cycle. In these patients, the FSH levels fluctuated markedly during days 1-6 in the absence of increased OE_2 secretion and the LH levels were lower during days 1-6 than in the patients' own investigation cycle.

An example of a type II response can be seen in Figure 1. A significant OE_2 rise above the normal follicular phase range was observed, beginning during the treatment period and preceding a preovulatory OE_2 peak. The OE_2 rise in response to HMG was often of a similar order of magnitude to a normal pre-ovulatory peak but it failed to elicit a positive feedback response of gonadotrophins.

A type III response to HMG (n = 7) was characterised by an immediate and excessive rise in OE_2 to levels often well above the normal range (> 0.4 ng/ml). No ovulation followed, menstruation occurred on decline of the OE_2 and the 'cycles' were short. Significant rises in P were observed during such treatment cycles in 4 of the 7 patients and although coincident LH elevations were seen the concentrations of P never attained normal mid-luteal phase levels.

The ensuing luteal phase hormone profiles were assessed by reference to the patient's own investigation cycle on a qualitative basis. Where a diagnosed abnormality was absent after HMG treatment this was considered an improved luteal phase. When an abnormality was observed following HMG treatment, which was not diagnosed in the investigation cycle, this was considered adversely affected. Figure 2 shows the results of analyses of the treatment cycle luteal phases over the whole group of infertile patients irrespective of the observed immediate responses to HMG. A wide range of luteal phase responses was observed with only a moderate pregnancy rate. Two of the pregnancies reported were approaching the end of their treatment protocol and were given hCG empirically. The remaining 3 pregnancies were observed during the first or second treatment cycles; one showed improved luteal profiles and no immediate OE_2 response (type I),

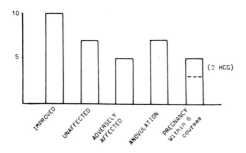

Fig. 2. Assessment of the effects of HMG on days 1, 3, 5 therapy on the production of steroid hormones during the luteal phase. For each individual patient the luteal phase steroid hormone production during a cycle on therapy was compared and contrasted with that in the luteal phase of her own investigational cycle.

whilst in 2 who showed significant OE_2 response to HMG (type II) the luteal phases were unaffected.

The abnormality observed in a patient's cycle was a poor indicator of the response to HMG. One exception to this rule was the group with elevated LH levels who responded as type I (4 of 8) or as type II with minimal OE_2 rises (4 of 8). None of this group responded with excessive OE_2 output (type III). The group with poor follicular maturation showed all types of immediate response (I, n = 3; II, n = 3; III, n = 1) and their following luteal phases were improved in only 2 cases. The group with a poor P surge also had various immediate responses (I, n = 4; II, n = 7; III, n = 2) and their luteal phases were improved in 4 cases only.

Discussion

The treatment scheme of HMG on days 1, 3 and 5 showed a disappointing pregnancy rate amongst this group of infertile women. Equally, the effects upon observed investigational abnormalities were, on the whole, disappointing. The immediate OE_2 responses to therapy indicated that amongst these women follicles in the peri-menstrual period ranged from unresponsive to hypersensitive. The endogenous LH and FSH levels during the treatment period showed marked fluctuations based on single daily sampling and this may indicate that the administration regime was instrumental in disturbing pituitary/hypothalamic function. The case for peri-menstrual ovarian stimulation in some of these patients probably still exists but an alternative regime must be found.

References

Cooke, I.D., Lenton, E.A., Adams, M., Pearce, M.A., Fahmy, D. and Evans, C.R. (1977): *J. Reprod. Fertil., 51,* 203.

Coutts, J.R.T., Fleming, R., Carswell, W., Black, W.P., England, P., Craig, A. and Macnaughton, M.C. (1978): In: *Advances in Gynaecological Endocrinology,* p.65. Editor: H.S. Jacobs. R.C.O.G., London.

Dodson, K.S., Coutts, J.R.T. and Macnaughton, M.C. (1975): *Brit. J. Obstet. Gynaec., 82,* 602.

Monitoring of ovarian activity by the radioimmunological determination of estrogen glucuronides, estrone and 17β-estradiol in urine

T. LEHTINEN, A.-L. KAIRENTO and H. ADLERCREUTZ

Department of Clinical Chemistry, University of Helsinki, Helsinki, Finland

Monitoring of ovarian function is important for the determination of the fertile period with the aim to achieve conception or for contraceptive purposes, and for evaluation of some pathological conditions. Methods for plasma and urinary hormones are available for that purpose. During the 20 years since 1955, when Brown (1955) introduced his chemical method for the assay of the 3 classical estrogens in urine, mainly urinary assays were used in routine clinical work. Recently radioimmunological (RIA) methods for the determination of estrogens in plasma have replaced the old chemical urinary assays because of their greater practicability. However, even more simple RIA-methods for direct assay of estrogen conjugates in diluted urine are now available (Kellie et al., 1972; Samarajewa and Kellie, 1975; Adlercreutz et al., 1976; Lehtinen and Adlercreutz, 1977; Baker et al., 1978; Collins et al., 1979).

The present investigation deals with the study of the excretion of several estrogen conjugates measured with these simple techniques in a large number of menstrual cycles in order to find the most suitable method for clinical use. For comparison a RIA method for estrone and estradiol in urine was developed and assays were carried out in 15 cycles.

Material and methods

Twenty one young healthy women collected urine during the menstrual cycle. The clinical data of these women are shown in Table 1. Nine cycles were studied starting immediately after the end of the menstrual period and ending about 5 days after the assumed ovulation time. Twenty complete cycles were studied. Seven of the subjects collected urine during 2 cycles with an interval of about one year. All collections were made separately during day and night time. The day-collection included the urine excreted during the day including the last void before going to bed. The night-collection included the urine excreted during the night and the first morning sample. 24-hr urine was obtained by combining specimens from these 2 collections. All samples were pooled daily and frozen immediately after the

TABLE 1.

Clinical data of the 21 women studied

Subject	Age (yrs)	No. of children	IUD*	Length of cycle (days)	Day of LH peak
1a	32	—		27	14
1b	33	—		28	14
2a	32	1	+	26	14
2b	33	1	+	27	17
3	32	—		29	18
4a	30	2	+	28	16
4b	31	2	+	28	14
5a	28	—		27	12
5b	29	—		27	11
6	40	2		26	18
7	32	1	+	28	19
8a	34	2	+	27	16
8b	35	2	+	25	14
9a	36	3		24	13
9b	36	3		25	15
10a	27	2	+	28	17
10b	28	2	+	31	20
11	26	—	+	28	19
12	26	—		28	15
13a	25	—		30	16
13b	27	—		23	10
14	34	—		25	11
15	32	—		32	17
16	20	—		37	23
17	21	—		26	14
18	28	1	+	29	16
19	28	—		28	15
20	28	—	+	29	18
21	32	—		28	10
Mean	30			28	15
Range	20 – 40			23 – 37	10 – 23

*IUD = intrauterine device.

addition of 0.01% NaN_3. Blood samples were taken for 3 days around ovulation time. One blood sample was also taken during the luteal phase for progesterone determination. All cycles were ovulatory as judged from plasma and urinary luteinizing hormone (LH), urinary pregnandiol-3-glucuronide (P-3G) and plasma progesterone assays. The day of peak LH excretion in urine followed by an increase in P-3G was designated day 0 and the day before and after were designated day −1 and +1 etc.

Estriol-16α-glucuronide (E_3-16G) in urine was assayed by a solid-phase

376 T. Lehtinen et al.

TABLE 2.

Mean day of peak excretion, estrogen mean values of days −10 and −6 in day, night and 24-hr collections and between individual variation of mean basal values from days −8 to −6 in 24-hr collections

		Mean day of peak excretion	Mean values (nmol) of days −10 and −6	Between individual CV % (days −8 to −6)
Estriol-16∝-glucuronide	Day	0	10.5 − 13.7	
	Night	−1 − (0)	5.6 − 5.7	
	24-hr	(−1)−0	16.7 − 18.9	60
Estriol-3-glucuronide	Day	+1	22.8 − 29.8	
	Night	0	10.9 − 13.4	
	24-hr	0	38.2 − 48.4	30
Estrone-3-glucuronide	Day	0	25.4 − 33.5	
	Night	−1	13.5 − 15.9	
	24-hr	0	39.3 − 55.4	36
Estrone		−1	20.7 − 29.4	60
Estradiol		−1	9.5 − 11.9	30

radioimmunoassay as described by Lehtinen and Adlercreutz (1977). Estriol-3-glucuronide (E_3-3G) was assayed by an identical method (unpublished). Estrone-3-glucuronide (E_1-3G) and P-3G were assayed as described by Collins et al. (1977). The antisera to E_3-3G, E_1-3G and P-3G were kindly donated by Drs. Kellie and Samarajewa. Progesterone in plasma was assayed by RIA after extraction with petroleum ether as described by Haukkamaa (1974). LH in plasma and urine was determined by a double antibody solid-phase technique (DASP) as modified by Karonen et al. (1978). Urinary total estrone (E_1) and 17β-estradiol (E_2) were determined by RIA after acid hydrolysis of the conjugates, ether extraction and chromatographic separation of E_1 and E_2 on Sephadex LH-20 (to be published).

Results

The statistical analysis of the results indicated that the mean excretion of all estrogen metabolites assayed was fairly constant over days −10 to −6. The mean values of days −10 and −6 are shown in Table 2, together with the day of peak excretion of each metabolite in day-, night- and 24-hr urine. The between-individual coefficient of variation for the mean basal value over days −8 to −6 for each metabolite in the 24-hr urine specimen is also shown

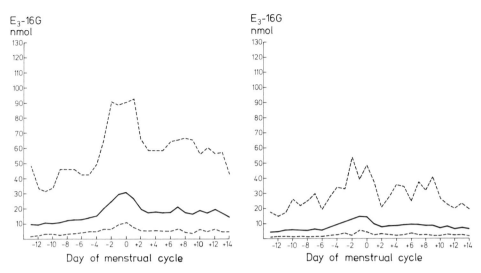

Fig. 1. Day excretion of estriol-16α-glucuronide (E_3-16G) in urine of 29 subjects. Mean with 95% confidence limits.

Fig. 2. Night excretion of estriol-16α-glucuronide (E_3-16G) in urine of 29 subjects. Mean with 95% confidence limits.

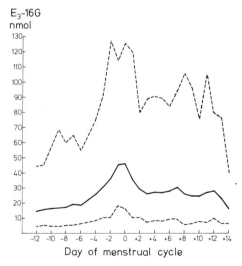

Fig. 3. 24-hr excretion of estriol-16α-glucuronide (E_3-16G) in urine of 29 subjects. Mean with 95% confidence limits.

in Table 2. As 8 subjects collected urine during 2 cycles, within-individual variation could be calculated for the mean basal values for E_3-16G. This was only 21% in 24-hr urine samples. Figures 1, 2 and 3 show mean (with 95% confidence limits) excretion of E_3-16G during day, night and 24-hr, respec-

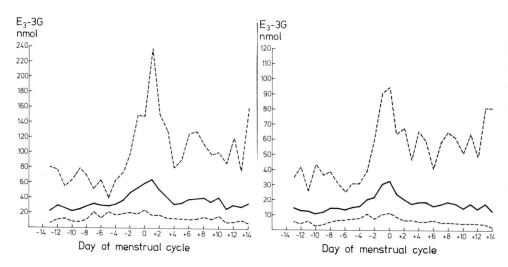

Fig. 4. Day excretion of estriol-3-glucuronide (E₃-3G) in urine of 10 subjects. Mean with 95% confidence limits.

Fig. 5. Night excretion of estriol-3-glucuronide (E₃-3G) in urine of 10 subjects. Mean with 95% confidence limits.

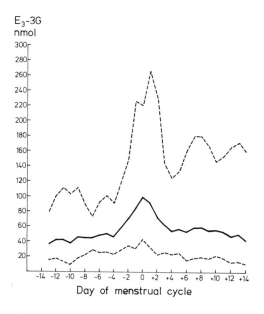

Fig. 6. 24-hr excretion of estriol-3-glucuronide (E₃-3G) in urine of 10 subjects. Mean with 95% confidence limits.

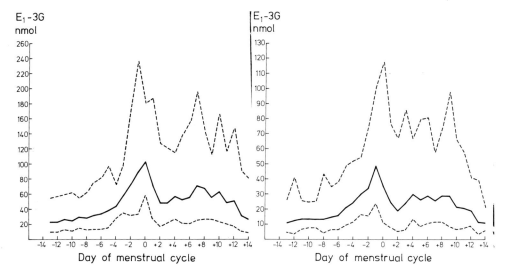

Fig. 7. Day excretion of estrone-3-glucuronide (E$_1$-3G) in urine of 20 subjects. Mean with 95% confidence limits.

Fig. 8. Night excretion of estrone-3-glucuronide (E$_1$-3G) in urine of 20 subjects. Mean with 95% confidence limits.

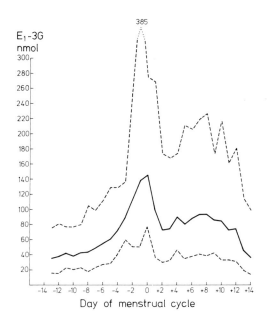

Fig. 9. 24-hr excretion of estrone-3-glucuronide (E$_1$-3G) in urine of 20 subjects. Mean with 95% confidence limits.

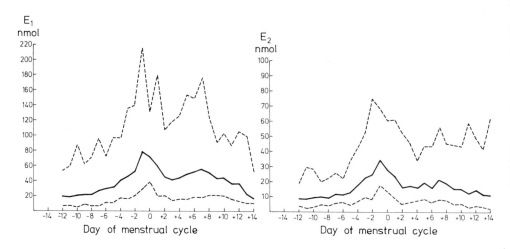

Fig. 10. 24-hr excretion of estrone (E_1) in urine of 15 subjects. Mean with 95% confidence limits.

Fig. 11. 24-hr excretion of estradiol (E_2) in urine of 15 subjects. Mean with 95% confidence limits.

tively. The same is shown for E_3-3G in Figures 4, 5 and 6, and for E_1-3G in Figures 7, 8 and 9. The excretion of E_1 and E_2 in 24-hr urine is shown in Figures 10 and 11, respectively. It is seen from the figures that E_1-3G is excreted in highest concentration of all conjugates, followed by E_3-3G and E_3-16G. The cusum plots for the rise of concentration before ovulation indicated that the mean output of the estrogen metabolites in urine increased significantly from a basal level by day −5 with the exception of E_3-3G. The mean value of the latter first started to rise on day −3.

Discussion

The present study shows that by measuring directly unhydrolyzed conjugates of estrogens, as good a picture of ovarian activity can be obtained as by measuring total estrone or estradiol. The basal excretion of all conjugates during the follicular phase is fairly constant before the rise prior to ovulation which, however, is not as pronounced for the estriol conjugates as in the case of E_1-3G. This conjugate starts to rise significantly earlier than all the conjugates especially if 24-hr collections are used and reaches peak excretion immediately before the time of the LH-peak and hence could also be of value in the prediction of ovulation (Adlercreutz et al., 1980). Baker et al. (1978) came to a similar conclusion. The use of the ratio of E_1-3G to P-3G excretion to detect the fertile period has also recently been suggested (Baker et al., 1978; Collins et al., 1979). The present study was performed on a very large amount of material, and various statistical methods have been used to establish the most suitable assay for clinical purposes. Some of these results have been presented elsewhere (Adlercreutz et al., 1980). These analyses are still in progress. Creatinine was assayed in all 3 urine collections in all cycles and the ratio of E_3-16G to creatinine was calculated. However, this approach did not improve the results by decreasing day to day variability in this material, possibly because the subjects had collected the urine specimen very carefully. The results given in Figures 8 and 9 and those in our previous study (Adlercreutz et al., 1980) suggest that for clinical purposes, the data from E_1-3G assays in night collections of urine will be almost as useful as that from measurements of this conjugate in 24-hr urine collections. This would be a very useful clinical approach. The large amount of data from normal subjects presented here provides comprehensive reference material which is useful for future clinical studies.

Acknowledgements

The skillful technical assistance of Ms Inga Wiik and Mrs Rauni Lehtola is gratefully acknowledged. This work was supported by the World Health Organization and Ford Foundation. We also thank NIAMDD (Bethesda, U.S.A.) for gifts of LH and its antiserum.

References

Adlercreutz, H., Lehtinen, T. and Kairento, A.-L. (1980): *J. Steroid Biochem.*, *12*, 395.
Adlercreutz, H., Lehtinen, T. and Tikkanen, M.J. (1976): *J. Steroid Biochem.*, *7*, 105.
Baker, T., Jennison, K.M. and Kellie, A. (1979): *Biochem. J.*, *177*, 729.
Brown, J.B. (1955): *Biochem. J.*, *60*, 185.
Collins, W.P., Collins, P.O., Kilpatrick, M.J., Manning, P.A., Pike, J.M. and Tyler, P.P.P. (1979): *Acta Endocr. (Kbh.)*, *90*, 336.
Haukkamaa, M. (1974): *J. Steroid Biochem.*, *5*, 631.
Karonen, S.-L., Lähteenmäki, P., Hohenthal, U. and Adlercreutz, H. (1978): *Scand. J. Clin. Lab. Invest.*, *38*, 97.
Kellie, A.E., Samuel, V.K., Riley, W.J. and Robertson, P.M. (1972): *J. Steroid Biochem.*, *3*, 275.
Lehtinen, T. and Adlercreutz, H. (1977): *J. Steroid Biochem.*, *8*, 99.
Samarajewa, P. and Kellie, A. (1975): *Biochem. J.*, *151*, 369.

Anatomic-functional evaluation of the ovaries*

. N. GARCEA, A. CARUSO, S. CAMPO, P. SICCARDI and V. PANETTA

Istituto di Clinica Ostetrica e Ginecologica, Università Cattolica del Sacro Cuore, Rome, Italy

Recent studies on menstrual disorders due to chronic anovulation (Yen and Jaffe, 1978) have led to a better understanding of the physiopathology of the hypothalamic-hypophyseal-ovarian axis, but various aspects of the pathogenesis and mechanism responsible for the condition remain to be elucidated.

The aim of the present investigation was to demonstrate the usefulness of celioscopic examinations in establishing the functional status of the ovary.

Material and methods

A retrospective study was made of 553 celioscopies carried out in patients with chronic anovulation. Basal plasma levels of FSH, LH, prolactin (PRL), 17β-estradiol (E_2) and progesterone were measured by radioimmunoassay.

Results

Patients were divided into 6 groups according to celioscopic findings: Patients with (1) normal ovaries, (2) mild, moderate or severe hypoplasia of the ovaries, or streak-like gonads, (3) ovaries of normal volume and smooth surface, (4) polycystic ovaries, (5) Stein Leventhal ovaries (smooth translucent surface with superficial vascular network and firm consistency), (6) ovarium gyratum (aged ovaries, similar to those of menopausal females) (Garcea et al., 1976 a, b).

Correlating celioscopic findings and menstrual disorders (Fig. 1) a peculiar distribution of results in the different groups of patients is observed. Hypoplastic ovaries are seen to prevail in primary amenorrhea, and hypoplastic and polycystic ovaries in secondary amenorrhea or oligomenorrhea. A relationship between ovarian morphology and basal values of LH, FSH and PRL is evident in only a few cases (Fig. 2), e.g. high FSH levels in the presence of streak-like or extremely hypoplastic ovaries typical of primary

*This work was supported in part by a grant from the 'Ministero di Pubblica Istruzione', Rome, 1979.

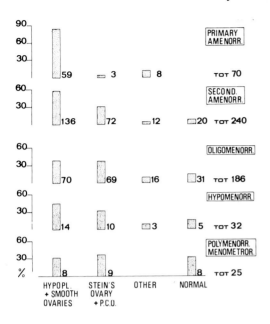

Fig. 1. Celioscopic findings in different types of menstrual disorders.

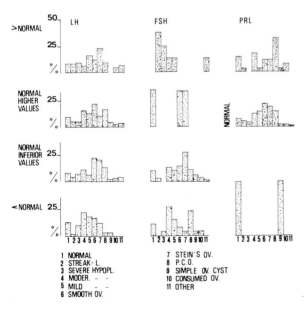

Fig. 2. Results of hormone assays compared to celioscopic findings.

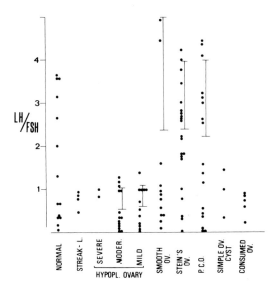

Fig. 3.   Relationship between LH-FSH ratio and ovarian findings.

ovarian failure. High LH values were found in the majority of patients with polycystic or Stein Leventhal's ovaries, but several cases of polycystic ovaries presented LH values in the low or normal range. In 30% of the cases with hyperprolactinemia the celioscopic findings revealed polycystic or Stein Leventhal's ovaries. However various ovarian diseases and presumably different disturbances of the hypothalamic-hypophyseal-ovarian axis may be associated with hyperprolactinemia. In fact some patients with hyperprolactinemia present normal, hypoplastic or smooth ovaries. In our series of patients the LH-FSH ratio (Fig. 3) in ovarian hypoplasia did not exceed 1.5 (mean 0.5). On the contrary smooth, polycystic and Stein Leventhal's ovaries showed a wide range of LH-FSH ratios, average values lying between 2 and 2.3.

Discussion and conclusions

Menstrual disorders due to anovulation depend in most cases on hypothalamic-pituitary hypofunction, which may be 'tonic' or cyclic'.

Data emerging from the present study appear to indicate that 'tonic' hypothalamic-pituitary hypofunction, a characteristic of primary amenorrhea, causes trophic damage of varying degree to the gonads, resulting in hypoplastic ovaries. In cases of oligomenorrhea and secondary amenorrhea, on the other hand, in which cyclic gonadotropin secretion is frequently altered, ovaries are often of the polycystic type with all its variants. Thus about 30% of subjects with these menstrual disorders present ovaries of this type. It is evident nevertheless that different types of ovaries and therefore presumably different forms of dysfunction of the hypothalamic-pituitary axis can cause the same type of menstrual disorder. In fact only in 3 situations do basal hormone levels provide satisfactory information for diagnostic purposes, i.e. in patients with: (1) high FSH values and primary or secondary amenorrhea indicating ovarian failure, (2) high LH and an LH-FSH ratio exceeding 2-3 indicating polycystic ovary, and (3) high PRL levels which demonstrate a peculiar organic or functional impairment of the pituitary. It is worthwhile pointing out that in cases presenting high FSH values celioscopy associated with ovarian biopsy may be useful to distinguish the resistant ovary syndrome from premature ovarian failure. In almost all other cases, basal hormone values fail to provide specific diagnostic information or indications regarding choice of therapy. Celioscopy, on the contrary, reveals the anatomic and functional status of the ovaries in all these patients and simultaneously defines the stage of the disorder.

In our opinion celioscopy may be usefully employed not only for diagnostic purposes but also, and in particular, in establishing appropriate treatment of the disease.

References

Garcea, N., Caruso, A., Micchia, T. and Morace, E. (1976a): *Minerva Ginecol., 28,* 124.
Garcea, N., Caruso, A., Montemurro, A. and Bompiani, A. (1976b): *Acta Europ. Fertil., 7,* 63.
Yen, S.S.C. and Jaffe, R.B. (1978): *Reproductive Endocrinology.* W.B. Saunders Co., Philadelphia, London, Toronto.

Influence of SHBG on activity of 17β-hydroxysteroid oxido-reductase in human erythrocyte

M. EGLOFF, N. SAVOURE, J. TARDIVEL-LACOMBE, C. MASSART, M. NICOL and H. DEGRELLE

U.E.R. Biomédicale des Saints Pères (Laboratoire Associé au CNRS No 87), Paris CEDEX 06; U.E.R. Médicales de Rennes, Villejean, Rennes, France

The impact point of sex hormone binding globulin (SHBG) on peripheral conversion of androstenedione to testosterone has been studied 'in vitro' with a simple experimental model. The human erythrocytes have been shown to contain a 17β-hydroxysteroid dehydrogenase interconverting androstenedione and testosterone and it has been assumed that this conversion in the blood itself might be considered as an important source of testosterone, especially in women (Blaquier et al., 1967; Van der Molen and Groen, 1968).

In blood circulation, SHBG strongly binds testosterone, which is the product of the reaction, but not androstenedione. Thus, it was of interest to investigate the possible role of this plasma protein, comparatively to serum albumin, in the intra-cellular conversion of androstenedione to testosterone.

Material and methods

A highly purified preparation of SHBG was obtained from pregnant human serum, in 4 steps at 4°C: ammonium sulphate precipitation (30-50% saturation), affinity chromatography on blue Sepharose Cl-6B (Pharmacia; Uppsala), gel filtration on Ultrogel ACA-44 (Pharmindustrie) and preparative electrofocusing. The SHBG peak was detected by the ^{3}H-dihydrotestosterone bound radioactivity and the purification steps were checked by polyacrylamide gel electrophoresis. The binding capacity of the purified protein was determined by the method described by Corvol et al. (1971).

The enzymic conversion rate of ^{3}H-androstenedione to ^{3}H-testosterone was evaluated in human erythrocytes as followed: 4×10^9 washed cells were suspended in a final volume of 4 ml of Krebs-Ringer solution containing glucose (1 g/l) and 140 pmoles of ^{3}H-androstenedione. Following incubation at 37°C for 2 hr in a shaking bath, the steroids were extracted twice with 4 ml benzene and chromatographed on silica gel thin layer plate using continuous flow development with a benzene-acetone mixture (6: 1 v/v) together with unlabelled steroids (30 μg) used as carriers.

The testosterone and androstenedione areas were scraped off and the

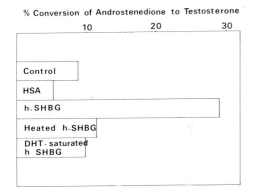

Fig. 1. Effect of SHBG on the percent conversion of androstenedione and testosterone in erythrocytes.

radioactivity was measured by liquid scintillation. All experiments were done in duplicate. The results were expressed as the percentage of conversion of androstenedione to testosterone.

Results and discussion

As shown in Figure 1, the purified SHBG increases more than 3 times the conversion rate of androstenedione to testosterone in erythrocytes. In order to test if the binding sites of the protein were involved in this effect, the same experiment was carried out with heated SHBG (60°C) and dihydro-testosterone-saturated SHBG: in both cases, the conversion rate fell dramatically. In comparison, it was found that human serum albumin (HSA) slightly decreases the enzymic conversion.

Since SHBG, as well as serum albumin, probably do not penetrate the erythrocytes, it is likely that these proteins have an effect upon the equilibrium of the flow rates of both steroids across the membrane. Within the cells, the glucose concentration available is sufficient to produce NADPH for the one-way reductive conversion (Fig. 2). Thus, it may be assumed that SHBG facilitates the diffusion of testosterone, which is the product of the reaction, out of the cell and therefore displaces the chemical equilibrium of the reaction within the cell. In contrast, serum albumin, which binds androstenedione as well as testosterone with a low affinity and a high capacity, would prevent the membrane transfer of the substrate.

The biological role of SHBG has been investigated mostly on the testosterone uptake and on metabolism by target organs or the liver (Mowszowicz et al., 1970; Mercier-Bodard et al., 1976; Vermeulen and Ando, 1979). It is generally accepted that the specifically bound hormone

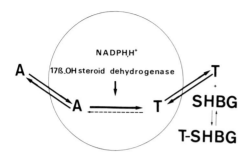

Fig. 2. Schematic representation of the role of NADPH in the one-way reductive conversion of androstenedione.

fraction is not biologically active. From this work, it may be concluded that SHBG could play an important physiological and pathological role in the extra-glandular production of testosterone.

References

Blaquier, J., Forchielli, E. and Dorfman, R.I. (1967): *Acta Endocr. (Kbh.), 55,* 697.
Corvol, P., Chrambach, A., Rodbard, D. and Bardin, C.W. (1971): *J. Biol. Chem., 246,* 3435.
Mercier-Bodard, C., Marchut, M., Perrot, M., Picard, M.T., Baulieu, E.E. and Robel, P. (1976): *J. Clin. Endocr., 43,* 374.
Mowszowicz, I., Kamm, D. and Dray, F. (1970): *J. Clin. Endocr., 31,* 584.
Van der Molen, H.J. and Groen, D. (1968): *Acta Endocr. (Kbh.), 58,* 419.
Vermeulen, A. and Ando, S. (1979): *J. Clin. Endocr., 48,* 320.

Sterility in Wobbler mice. A defect in cellular 17β-estradiol binding activity?

A. MOLTENI, E. FORS and J. LEESTMA

Department of Pathology, Northwestern University School of Medicine, Chicago, IL, U.S.A.

The Wobbler mouse is an important model for human motor neuron disease bearing considerable resemblance to Werdnig-Hoffman disease (Leestma, 1980). The condition is transmitted by an autosomal recessive gene which arose as a spontaneous mutation in a C57Bl/Fa mouse (Falconer, 1956). The pathology of the disease is that of a vacuolating degeneration of motor neurons in the spinal cord and brain stem (Duchen and Strich, 1968; Andrews and Andrews, 1976) which causes a typical neurogenic muscular atrophy in affected muscle groups. The muscular atrophy and paralysis become evident by about 3 weeks of age and may progress over many months leading to forelimb paralysis and contracture, atrophy of neck and masticatory muscles, and some weakness in the lower extremities. Heterozygous animals show no evidence of neurological disease and can only be identified when they produce a Wobbler in their litters (Andrews and Andrews, 1976). Wobblers of either sex have never been known to produce litters with each other, with heterozygous, or normal animals as mates. The male Wobbler is probably sterile because of immobile sperm which show altered axonemal geometry (Leestma and Sepsenwol, 1980).

Female Wobblers appear to be incapable of estrus cycles as monitored by vaginal cytology though they possess histologically normal appearing uteri and ovaries. An explanation for female Wobbler sterility may be anestrus due to impaired ability of target organs to respond to hormonal stimulation. It is this hypothesis that was examined in this study.

Material and methods

All animals were generated in a small colony maintained in our Department for the past 3 years. Male and female Wobblers (wr/wr), heterozygotes (wr/+), and controls (+/+) were killed using ether anesthesia and exsanguination. The inferior vena cava was injected with 0.05 ml of heparin solution and was then transected after a few seconds for blood collection by small pipette. Blood was pooled (generally 3 animals per tube) for each group, refrigerated, and centrifuged for later analysis for estradiol concentration. A radioimmunoassay procedure and kit (Micromedic Systems, Inc.,

Horsham, Pennsylvania) for estradiol was used. After bleeding, the liver, ovaries with uteri, and the brains were removed, snap-frozen in liquid nitrogen and stored individually in sealed vials at $-80°C$ until analysis for 17β-estradiol (E_2) receptors was made using the methods of Jensen et al. (1971) and Jensen and De Sombre (1977).

Liver has been selected as tissue for the study of E_2 binding activity since this property was reported by Aten et al. (1978). The tissue is available in amounts which allow measurement in single animals. Changes in E_2 binding ability in liver cells might reflect an abnormality of all tissues with respect to E_2 binding. Additionally the problem of analysis of uteri was that the organs of many animals (more than were available due to small colony size) had to be pooled to provide enough tissue for analysis. Furthermore, in order to provide adequate controls for the Wobbler, which does not show estrus, many controls in different stages of estrus would have been needed.

The data obtained were analyzed using SPSS, a statistical package (t-test) run on the CDC 8600 computer at the Vogelback Computing Center, Northwestern University (Nie et al., 1975).

Results

E_2 binding activity in 12 male Wobblers, 8 female Wobblers, 7 male heterozygotes, 9 female heterozygotes, 4 male controls, and 8 female controls is depicted in Figure 1. The combined Wobblers (males and females)

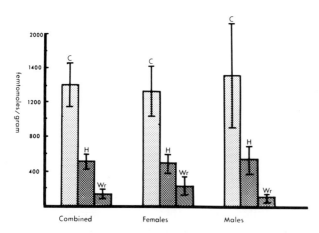

Fig. 1. Histogram illustrating the comparative levels of 17β-estradiol (E_2) binding in liver between combined male and female Wobbler mice, separated male and female Wobblers, and control animals negative for the *wr* gene. Vertical bars above the columns: Standard Errors of the Mean (SEM), C = control, H = heterozygote (wr/+), and Wr = Wobbler (wr/wr).

showed mean E$_2$ binding in liver of 135 fmol/g (S.E.M. = 46); heterozygotes showed 500 fmol/g (S.E.M. = 73); and controls showed 1392 fmol/g (S.E.M. = 260). Each group was significantly different from the other (p < 0.001) using a two-tailed t-test (Nie et al., 1975). A total of 48 animals were analyzed.

Male Wobblers showed E$_2$ binding in liver of 82 fmol/g (S.E.M. = 28), male heterozygotes, 528 fmol/g (S.E.M. = 133), and controls, 1508 fmol/g (S.E.M. = 590). Wobbler male E$_2$ binding was significantly different from that of heterozygotes (p < 0.001) and from controls (p < 0.001) but heterozygotes were not significantly different from controls.

Female Wobblers showed E$_2$ binding in liver of 215 fmol/g (S.E.M. = 105), heterozygotes, 477 fmol/g (S.E.M. = 85), and controls, 1334 fmol/g (S.E.M. = 813). Wobbler females E$_2$ binding was significantly different from controls (p < 0.005), as it was for the heterozygotes from control (p < 0.01), but heterozygotes were not significantly different from Wobblers. For purposes of this report the 8s and 4s E$_2$ binding were combined to yield total E$_2$ binding.

E$_2$ binding levels for uteri of Wobblers appeared to be lower than in heterozygotes or controls, though the number of analyses were small compared with those of liver and thus statistical analysis was not possible.

Serum estradiol levels in female Wobblers (pooled) was 420 pg/ml, female heterozygotes, 150 pg/ml, and in male heterozygotes, 250 pg/ml. A control group of Swiss white mice showed serum estradiol levels of 85 ± 15 pg/ml. These results appear significant though more determinations would be necessary to allow statistical analysis.

Discussion

The observation of E$_2$ binding ability of many tissues other than the female genital organs is well established having been shown to occur in liver (Aten et al., 1978), pancreas (Sandberg and Rosenthal, 1974; Molteni et al., 1979), salivary glands and kidney (Concolino et al., 1978; Molteni et al., 1979). These observations are not surprising when one considers the multiple roles that estrogens play in all systemic cells. It is logical to suppose then that if a defect in estrogen binding in one organ were found, it might also be seen in other organs. Such inability would logically also be accompanied by elevated serum levels of estrogen. This appears to be the case in the Wobbler.

The inability of the Wobbler to reproduce may be explained on the basis of at least two defects: in the male, sperm immobility and disordered axonemal geometry; in both male and female, tissue unresponsiveness to estrogen and correspondingly high serum levels of E$_2$. This inability to bind estrogen seems to affect several cells of the animal besides the reproductive tract. An intermediate pattern between Wobblers and controls may be seen in heterozygous animals who display less marked defects in estrogen binding and elevation of serum E_2 levels. The results support the hypothesis that female Wobbler sterility results from target organ unresponsiveness to estrogen on the basis of an unknown defect in the animal whose relationship to the neurological disease and other pathology is obscure. This defect, present in both males and females, may provide a model for the study of altered tissue responsiveness to estrogen in addition to a complex reproductive abnormality in the mouse.

Acknowledgements

The authors are grateful to Dr. D. Albertson and Ms. Rita M. Kaurs for the serum estradiol determinations.

References

Andrews, J.M. and Andrews, R.L. (1976): In: *Amyotrophic Lateral Sclerosis. Recent Research Trends*, p. 191. Editors: J.M. Andrews, R.T. Johnson and M.A.B. Brazier. Academic Press, New York.

Aten, R.F., Weinberg, M.J. and Eisenfeld, A.J. (1978): *Endocrinology, 102*, 435.

Concolino, G., Marrochi, A., Conti, C., Tenaglia, R., Di Silverio, F. and Bracci, U. (1978): *Cancer Res., 38*, 4340.

Duchen, L.W. and Strich, S.J. (1968): *J. Neurol. Neurosurg. Psychiat., 31*, 535.

Falconer, D.S. (1956): *Mouse News Letter, 15*, 23.

Jensen, E.V., Block, G.E., Smith, S., Kyser, K. and De Sombre, E. (1971): *Nat. Cancer Inst. Monogr., 34*, 55.

Jensen, E.V. and De Sombre, E. (1977): *Advanc. Clin. Chem., 19*, 57.

Leestma, J.E. (1980): *Amer. J. Path.*, submitted for publication.

Leestma, J.E. and Sepsenwol, S. (1980): *J. Reprod. Fertil.*, in press.

Molteni, A., Bahu, R., Battifora, H.A., Fors, E.M., Reddy, J.K., Rao, M.S. and Scarpelli, D.S. (1979): *Ann. Clin. Lab. Sci., 9*, 103.

Nie, N.H., Hull, C.H., Jenkins, J.G., Steinbrenner, K. and Bent, D.H. (1975): p. 203. *Statistical Package for the Social Sciences, 2nd Ed.* McGraw-Hill, New York.

Sandberg, A.A. and Rosenthal, M.E. (1974): *J. Steroid Biochem., 5*, 969.

Author index

Subject index

Prepared by E.A. van der Veen, Amsterdam